DECISION-MAKING IN
Adult Neurology

DECISION-MAKING IN
Adult Neurology

BRETT L. CUCCHIARA, MD
Associate Professor of Neurology
University of Pennsylvania
Philadelphia, Pennsylvania

RAYMOND S. PRICE, MD
Associate Professor of Neurology
Director, Neurology Residency
University of Pennsylvania
Philadelphia, Pennsylvania

ELSEVIER

3251 Riverport Lane
St. Louis, Missouri 63043

DECISION-MAKING IN ADULT NEUROLOGY   ISBN: 978-0-323-63583-7

Library of Congress Control Number: 2020936656

Content Strategist: Melanie Tucker
Senior Content Development Specialist: Anne Snyder
Publishing Services Manager: Shereen Jameel
Senior Project Manager: Umarani Natarajan
Design Direction: Renee Duenow

Printed in the United States of America

Last digit is the print number: 9 8 7 6 5 4 3

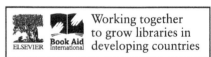

This book would not have been possible without the many teachers, colleagues, students, and patients from whom I have learned over the years. In particular, I owe a great debt to Dr. Leon Weisberg, who taught me neurology as a medical student and who 30 years ago created a book upon which this current one was modeled. My father, Dr. Roy Cucchiara, proofread the entirety of the early drafts of this book several times over; his keen insights and careful eye were a godsend. Most of all, though, I credit the persistent encouragement, love, and support of my wife Maia and my daughters Amelia and Eliza for whatever success this book achieves. This book is dedicated to them.

Brett L. Cucchiara

I have been fortunate to work with innumerable outstanding colleagues, co-residents, and trainees who motivated me to become a better physician and person. Dr. Steven Galetta, my residency director, inspired me to become a neurologist, and I still hear his voice every time I approach a challenging case. I also owe an infinite amount of gratitude to Dr. Amy Pruitt for her mentorship throughout my career. Finally, none of this would have been possible without the unwavering support and guidance of my mother, Joanne, and the endless love and patience of my wife, Anne Marie, and my daughters, Presley and Paige. I am eternally grateful to them.

Raymond S. Price

Section Editors

ANDRES DEIK, MD
Assistant Professor of Clinical Neurology
University of Pennsylvania
Philadelphia, Pennsylvania

CHRISTOPHER G. FAVILLA, MD
Assistant Professor of Neurology
University of Pennsylvania
Philadelphia, Pennsylvania

MICHAEL GELFAND, MD, PHD
Assistant Professor of Clinical Neurology
University of Pennsylvania
Philadelphia, Pennsylvania

JOSHUA P. KLEIN, MD
Associate Professor of Neurology and Radiology
Harvard Medical School
Vice Chair, Clinical Affairs, Department of Neurology
Chief, Division of Hospital Neurology
Brigham and Women's Hospital
Boston, Massachusetts

JOSHUA M. LEVINE, MD
Associate Professor of Neurology
Chief, Division of Neurocritical Care
University of Pennsylvania
Philadelphia, Pennsylvania

COLIN QUINN, MD, MSPT
Assistant Professor of Clinical Neurology
Department of Neurology
University of Pennsylvania
Philadelphia, Pennsylvania

ANA RECOBER, MD
Director, Headache Program
Main Line Health
Lankenau Medical Center
Wynnewood, Pennsylvania

DAVID RAIZEN, MD, PHD
Associate Professor of Neurology
University of Pennsylvania
Philadelphia, Pennsylvania

DANIELLE SANDSMARK, MD, PHD
Assistant Professor
Department of Neurology
University of Pennsylvania
Philadelphia, Pennsylvania

Contributors

WHITLEY AAMODT, MD
Movement Disorders Fellow
Department of Neurology
University of Pennsylvania
Philadelphia, Pennsylvania
Chapter 69: Intracranial Hypotension

STEPHEN ARADI, MD
Assistant Professor of Neurology
University of South Florida
Tampa, Florida
Chapter 24: Dysarthria

CHARLES J. BAE, MD
Associate Professor of Clinical Medicine and Neurology
University of Pennsylvania
Philadelphia, Pennsylvania
Chapter 77: Hypersomnia
Chapter 80: Parasomnias

RAMANI BALU, MD, PHD
Assistant Professor
Department of Neurology
Division of Neurocritical Care
University of Pennsylvania
Philadelphia, Pennsylvania
Chapter 105: Encephalitis
Chapter 106: Acute Meningitis

HAMID BASSIRI, MD, PHD
Assistant Professor of Pediatrics
The Children's Hospital of Philadelphia
Philadelphia, Pennsylvania
Chapter 108: Tuberculosis Affecting the Nervous System

JOHN BEST, MD
Department of Neurology
University of California–San Francisco
San Francisco, California
*Chapter 110: Lyme Disease Involving the Nervous System
(Neuroborreliosis)*

ALICE CAI, MD
Department of Neurology
University of Pennsylvania
Philadelphia, Pennsylvania
Chapter 80: Parasomnias

CHARLES CANTOR, MD
Professor of Clinical Neurology and Medicine
University of Pennsylvania
Philadelphia, Pennsylvania
Chapter 79: Restless Legs Syndrome

MEGHAN M. CAYLOR, PHARMD, BCPS, BCCCP
Clinical Pharmacy Specialist
Neurocritical Care
Hospital of the University of Pennsylvania
Philadelphia, Pennsylvania
Chapter 61: Paroxysmal Sympathetic Hyperactivity

NEENA CHERAYIL, MD
Assistant Professor of Neurology
Northwestern University
Chicago, Illinois
Chapter 22: Hearing Loss

MOLLY CINCOTTA, MD
Department of Neurology
University of Pennsylvania
Philadelphia, Pennsylvania
Chapter 37: Difficulty Walking

ERIN CONRAD, MD
Clinical Instructor
Department of Neurology
University of Pennsylvania
Philadelphia, Pennsylvania
Chapter 39: Transient Loss of Consciousness

H. BRANCH COSLETT, MD
William N Kelley Professor of Neurology
University of Pennsylvania
Philadelphia, Pennsylvania
Chapter 5: Aphasia
Chapter 9: Rapidly Progressive Dementia

DAVID COUGHLIN, MD, MTR
Assistant Professor
Department of Neurosciences
University of California San Diego
La Jolla, California
Chapter 36: Ataxia
Chapter 81: Abnormal Involuntary Movements
Chapter 82: Chorea
Chapter 83: Tremor
Chapter 84: Treatment of Essential Tremor
Chapter 85: Parkinson Disease: Treatment
Chapter 86: Treatment of Dystonia
Chapter 87: Treatment of the Patient With Tics

DANIEL CRISTANCHO, MD
Department of Neurology
University of Pennsylvania
Philadelphia, Pennsylvania
Chapter 4: Low Back Pain

BRETT L. CUCCHIARA, MD
Associate Professor of Neurology
University of Pennsylvania
Philadelphia, Pennsylvania
Chapter 9: Rapidly Progressive Dementia
Chapter 10: Delirium
Chapter 21: Recurrent Episodic Dizziness
Chapter 22 Hearing Loss
Chapter 23: Pulsatile Tinnitus
Chapter 24: Dysarthria
Chapter 34: Hyperreflexia and Hyporeflexia
Chapter 40: Transient Ischemic Attack
Chapter 43: Large Cerebellar Infarction
Chapter 107: Subacute and Chronic Meningitis
Chapter 108: Tuberculosis Affecting the Nervous System
Chapter 109: Neurosyphilis
Chapter 110: Lyme Disease Involving the Nervous System
    (Neuroborreliosis)
Chapter 114: Neurosarcoidosis
Chapter 116: White Matter Lesions on Magnetic Resonance Imaging

ANDRES DEIK, MD
Assistant Professor of Clinical Neurology
Parkinson's Disease and Movement Disorders Center
University of Pennsylvania
Philadelphia, Pennsylvania
Chapter 36: Ataxia
Chapter 81: Abnormal Involuntary Movements
Chapter 82: Chorea
Chapter 83: Tremor
Chapter 84: Treatment of Essential Tremor
Chapter 85: Parkinson Disease: Treatment
Chapter 86: Treatment of Dystonia
Chapter 87: Treatment of the Patient With Tics

ANNE G. DOUGLAS, MD
Department of Neurology
University of Pennsylvania
Philadelphia, Pennsylvania
Chapter 38: Bladder Dysfunction

CHRISTYN EDMUNDSON, MD
Assistant Professor of Neurology
University of Pennsylvania
Philadelphia, Pennsylvania
Chapter 90: Demyelinating Neuropathies
Chapter 95: Lumbosacral Plexus Syndromes
Chapter 97: Myasthenia Gravis: Diagnosis
Chapter 98: Myasthenia Gravis: Treatment

CHARLES ESENWA, MD
Assistant professor of Neurology
Albert Einstein College of Medicine
Bronx, New York
Chapter 56: Vascular Malformations

CHRISTOPHER G. FAVILLA, MD
Assistant Professor of Neurology
University of Pennsylvania
Philadelphia, Pennsylvania
Chapter 40: Transient Ischemic Attack
Chapter 41: Patient With Acute Ischemic Stroke
Chapter 44: Prevention of Recurrent Ischemic Stroke
Chapter 45: Ischemic Stroke in the Young
Chapter 46: Patent Foramen Ovale and Ischemic Stroke
Chapter 50: Acute Spontaneous Intracerebral Hemorrhage
Chapter 51: Intracerebral Hemorrhage in the Young

Chapter 52: Intracerebral Hemorrhage Due to Anticoagulant Therapy
Chapter 53: Restarting Antithrombotic Therapy After Intracerebral
    Hemorrhage
Chapter 54: Subarachnoid Hemorrhage
Chapter 57: Cerebral Venous Sinus Thrombosis

ANDREA FUENTES, MD
Neurology Resident
University of Pennsylvania
Philadelphia, Pennsylvania
Chapter 102: Glioma
Chapter 103: Meningioma

MICHAEL GELFAND, MD, PHD
Assistant Professor of Clinical Neurology
University of Pennsylvania
Philadelphia, Pennsylvania
Chapter 39: Transient Loss of Consciousness
Chapter 70: Adult with First Seizure
Chapter 71: Initial Treatment of Epilepsy
Chapter 72: Drug-Resistant Epilepsy
Chapter 73: Antiepileptic Drugs
Chapter 74: Status Epilepticus
Chapter 75: Comorbidities in Patients with Epilepsy
Chapter 76: EEG Interpretation

DONNA GEORGE, MD
Assistant Professor of Neurology
University of Pennsylvania
Philadelphia, Pennsylvania
Chapter 53: Restarting Antithrombotic Therapy After Intracerebral
    Hemorrhage

PHILIP GEHRMAN, PHD
Associate Professor of Psychology
Department of Psychiatry
University of Pennsylvania
Philadelphia, Pennsylvania
Chapter 78: Insomnia

ALEXANDER J. GILL, MD, PHD
Neurology Resident
University of Pennsylvania
Philadelphia, Pennsylvania
Chapter 104: Paraneoplastic Syndromes

FRANCISCO GOMEZ, MD
Neurocritical Care Fellow
University of Pennsylvania
Philadelphia, Pennsylvania
Chapter 105: Encephalitis
Chapter 106: Acute Meningitis

MURRAY GROSSMAN, MD
Professor of Neurology
University of Pennsylvania
Philadelphia, Pennsylvania
Chapter 6: Chronic Cognitive Decline

ALI G. HAMEDANI, MD, MHS
Instructor
Division of Neuro-ophthalmology
Department of Neurology
University of Pennsylvania
Philadelphia, Pennsylvania
Chapter 12: Transient Visual Loss
Chapter 13: Visual Field Loss

Chapter 14: Visual Hallucinations
Chapter 15: Ptosis
Chapter 16: Pupillary Asymmetry (Anisocoria)
Chapter 17: Diplopia
Chapter 18: Nystagmus
Chapter 111: Optic Neuritis

KATHERINE HAMILTON, MD
Assistant Professor of Clinical Neurology
University of Pennsylvania
Philadelphia, Pennsylvania
Chapter 1: Initial Headache

KELLEY A. HUMBERT, MD
Clinical Assistant Professor
Department of Neurology
NYU Langone Health
New York, New York
Chapter 57: Cerebral Venous Sinus Thrombosis

KOTO ISHIDA, MD
Associate Professor of Neurology
NYU Langone Health
New York, New York
Chapter 116: White Matter Lesions on Magnetic Resonance Imaging

JONATHAN JI, MD
Neurocritical Care Fellow
University of Pennsylvania
Philadelphia, Pennsylvania
Chapter 11: Coma

ERIC KAISER, MD, PHD
Instructor
Department of Neurology
University of Pennsylvania
Philadelphia, Pennsylvania
Chapter 2: Chronic Headache

ATUL KALANURIA, MD
Director, Penn Neurocritical Care Fellowship Program
Assistant Professor of Neurology
University of Pennsylvania
Philadelphia, Pennsylvania
Chapter 11: Coma

POUYA KHANKHANIAN, MD
University of Pennsylvania
Philadelphia, Pennsylvania
Chapter 73: Antiepileptic Drugs

JOSHUA P. KLEIN, MD
Associate Professor of Neurology and Radiology
Harvard Medical School
Vice Chair, Clinical Affairs, Department of Neurology
Chief, Division of Hospital Neurology
Brigham and Women's Hospital
Boston, Massachusetts
Chapter 117: Ring-Enhancing Lesions on Magnetic Resonance Imaging
Chapter 118: Sellar Lesions on Magnetic Resonance Imaging
Chapter 119: Cerebellopontine Angle Mass Lesions on Magnetic Resonance Imaging

DENNIS L. KOLSON, MD, PHD
Professor of Neurology
Vice Chair for Academic Affairs/Faculty Development
University of Pennsylvania
Philadelphia, Pennsylvania
Chapter 113: Transverse Myelitis

GLENN KONSKY, DO
Vascular Neurologist
St. Luke's University Health Network
Bethlehem, Pennsylvania
Chapter 48: Patient With Asymptomatic Carotid Stenosis

MICHAEL E. KRITIKOS, MD
University of Iowa Hospitals and Clinics
Iowa City, Iowa
Chapter 55: Unruptured Intracranial Aneurysm

MONISHA A. KUMAR, MD
Associate Professor of Neurology
University of Pennsylvania
Philadelphia, Pennsylvania
Chapter 59: Management of Increased Intracranial Pressure

DAVID KUNG, MD
Assistant Professor
Department of Neurosurgery and Radiology
University of Pennsylvania
Philadelphia, Pennsylvania
Chapter 54: Subarachnoid Hemorrhage
Chapter 55: Unruptured Intracranial Aneurysm

ERIC LANCASTER, MD
Assistant Professor of Neurology
University of Pennsylvania
Philadelphia, Pennsylvania
Chapter 115: Autoimmune Encephalitis

ANGELICA MARIA LEE, DO, MS
Assistant Professor of Neurology
Associate Clerkship Director of Neurology
Uniformed Services University of the Health Sciences–School of Medicine
Bethesda, Maryland
Chapter 74: Status Epilepticus

JOSHUA M. LEVINE, MD
Associate Professor of Neurology
Chief, Division of Neurocritical Care
University of Pennsylvania
Philadelphia, Pennsylvania
Chapter 11: Coma
Chapter 42: Malignant Middle Cerebral Artery Infarction
Chapter 58: Brain Death

NOAH LEVINSON, MD
Assistant Professor of Neurology
Temple University
Philadelphia, Pennsylvania
Chapter 90: Demyelinating Neuropathies
Chapter 92: Mononeuropathy Multiplex
Chapter 95: Lumbosacral Plexus Syndromes

AVA LIBERMAN, MD
Assistant Professor of Neurology
Albert Einstein College of Medicine
Montefiore Medical Center
Bronx, New York
Chapter 51: Intracerebral Hemorrhage in the Young

HANNAH MACHEMEHL, MD
Department of Neurology
University of Pennsylvania
Philadelphia, Pennsylvania
Chapter 25: Proximal Weakness

ELIZABETH MAHANNA-GABRIELLI, MD
Assistant Professor of Anesthesiology, Perioperative Medicine,
and Pain Management
University of Miami Miller School of Medicine
Miami, Florida
Chapter 60: Management of Neuromuscular Respiratory Failure

MICHAEL MCGARVEY, MD
Associate Professor of Neurology
University of Pennsylvania
Philadelphia, Pennsylvania
Chapter 47: Spinal Cord Infarction

ADYS MENDIZABAL, MD
Department of Neurology
Hospital of the University of Pennsylvania
Philadelphia, Pennsylvania
Chapter 67: Trigeminal Autonomic Cephalalgias: Treatment
Chapter 68: Trigeminal Neuralgia

STEVEN R. MESSÉ, MD
Associate Professor of Neurology
University of Pennsylvania
Philadelphia, Pennsylvania
Chapter 45: Ischemic Stroke in the Young
Chapter 46: Patent Foramen Ovale and Ischemic Stroke

SAAD MIR, MD
Stroke Director, Lower Manhattan Hospital
Weill Cornell Site Director, NYP Mobile Stroke Treatment Unit
Assistant Professor of Clinical Neurology
Weill Cornell Medical College
New York, New York
Chapter 44: Prevention of Recurrent Ischemic Stroke

MEGAN T. MOYER, MSN, ACNP-BC, CNRN
Nurse Practitioner
Clinical Traumatic Brain Injury Research Team
Department of Neurology
Penn Presbyterian Medical Center
Philadelphia, Pennsylvania
Chapter 64: Postconcussive Syndrome

MICHAEL MULLEN, MD
Assistant Professor of Neurology
University of Pennsylvania
Philadelphia, Pennsylvania
Chapter 48: Patient with Asymptomatic Carotid Stenosis
Chapter 49: Preoperative Neurovascular (Carotid) Clearance

CODY NATHAN, MD
Neurology Resident
University of Pennsylvania
Philadelphia, Pennsylvania
Chapter 109: Neurosyphilis

PAUL J. NOVELLO, MD
Assistant Professor of Neurology
University of Pennsylvania
Philadelphia, Pennsylvania
*Chapter 52: Intracerebral Hemorrhage Due to
Anticoagulant Therapy*

JESSICA OEHLKE, MD
White River Junction Veterans Affairs
Medical Center
Department of Medicine
White River Junction, Vermont
Chapter 78: Insomnia

SUSANNA O'KULA, MD
Epilepsy Fellow
Department of Neurology
NYU Langone Health
New York, New York
Chapter 72: Drug-Resistant Epilepsy

CARLYN PATTERSON-GENTILE, MD, PHD
Department of Neurology
Children's Hospital of Philadelphia
Philadelphia, Pennsylvania
Chapter 65: Migraine Headache: Acute Treatment
Chapter 66: Migraine Headache: Prophylactic Treatment

CHRISTOPHER PERRONE, MD
Assistant Professor of Clinical Neurology
University of Pennsylvania
Philadelphia, Pennsylvania
Chapter 107: Subacute and Chronic Meningitis
Chapter 108: Tuberculosis Affecting the Nervous System
Chapter 114: Neurosarcoidosis

RAYMOND S. PRICE, MD
Associate Professor of Neurology
Director, Neurology Residency
University of Pennsylvania
Philadelphia, Pennsylvania
Chapter 3: Neck Pain
Chapter 4: Low Back Pain
Chapter 18: Nystagmus
Chapter 19: Facial Weakness
Chapter 20: Acute Vertigo
Chapter 21: Recurrent Episodic Dizziness
Chapter 26: Wrist Drop
Chapter 27: Unilateral Hand Weakness
Chapter 28: Unilateral Hand Numbness
Chapter 29: Knee Extension Weakness
Chapter 30: Unilateral Foot Drop
Chapter 31: Fasciculations
Chapter 32: Sensory Disturbance: Pain and Temperature
Chapter 33: Sensory Disturbance: Vibration and Proprioception
Chapter 34: Hyperreflexia and Hyporeflexia
Chapter 35: Multiple Cranial Neuropathies
Chapter 37: Difficulty Walking
Chapter 38: Bladder Dysfunction
Chapter 69: Intracranial Hypotension
Chapter 88: Electromyography and Nerve Conduction Studies
Chapter 89: Distal Symmetric Polyneuropathy
Chapter 91: Paraprotein-Associated Neuropathies
Chapter 92: Mononeuropathy Multiplex
Chapter 93: Carpal Tunnel Syndrome
Chapter 94: Brachial Plexus Syndromes
Chapter 96: Motor Neuron Disease
Chapter 99: Myopathy

BRYAN PUKENAS, MD
Assistant Professor of Radiology
University of Pennsylvania
Philadelphia, Pennsylvania

COLIN QUINN, MD, MSPT
Assistant Professor of Clinical Neurology
University of Pennsylvania
Philadelphia, Pennsylvania

LINDSAY RAAB, MD
Neurocritical Care Fellow
University of Pennsylvania
Philadelphia, Pennsylvania

DAVID RAIZEN, MD, PHD
Associate Professor of Neurology
University of Pennsylvania
Philadelphia, Pennsylvania

PREETHI RAMCHAND, MD
Assistant Professor of Neurology,
Radiology, Neurosurgery, and Anesthesiology
University of Pennsylvania
Philadelphia, Pennsylvania

IZAD-YAR D. RASHEED, MD
Department of Neurology
University of Pennsylvania
Philadelphia, Pennsylvania

ANA RECOBER, MD
Director, Headache Program
Main Line Health
Lankenau Medical Center
Wynnewood, Pennsylvania

CHRISTOPHER RENNER, MD
WellSpan Neurology
York, Pennsylvania

ILENE M. ROSEN, MD
Associate Professor of Medicine
Vice Chair for Education
Department of Medicine
Assistant Dean for Graduate Medical Education
University of Pennsylvania
Philadelphia, Pennsylvania

JON ROSENBERG, MD
Department of Neurology
Columbia University College of Physicians and Surgeons

DANIELLE K. SANDSMARK, MD, PHD
Assistant Professor
Department of Neurology
University of Pennsylvania
Philadelphia, Pennsylvania

ARUN K. SHERMA, MD
Director, Neurological Intensive Care Unit
Sinai-Grace Hospital
Detroit Medical Center
Detroit, Michigan

LAURA A. STEIN, MD
Assistant Professor of Neurology
University of Pennsylvania
Philadelphia, Pennsylvania

ETSEGENET F. TIZAZU, MD, MS
Epilepsy Fellow
Department of Neurology
University of Pennsylvania
Philadelphia, Pennsylvania

JOSE TORRES, MD
Assistant Professor of Neurology
NYU Langone Medical Center
New York, New York

JESSY WALIA, MD
Neurocritical Care Fellow
University of Pennsylvania
Philadelphia, Pennsylvania

ERIC WILLIAMSON, MD
Associate Professor of Clinical Neurology
University of California Los Angeles
Director, Multiple Sclerosis Center of Excellence
West Los Angeles Veterans Administration Hospital
Los Angeles, California
Chapter 112: Treatment of Multiple Sclerosis

DAVID WOLK, MD
Associate Professor of Neurology
University of Pennsylvania
Philadelphia, Pennsylvania
Chapter 7: Acute Memory Loss
Chapter 8: Chronic Memory Loss

Contents

CONTENTS

Introduction

This is a book of flowcharts. Loved by many, viewed with suspicion by some, flowcharts can be seen as vital aids to decision making and powerful teaching tools—or they can be dismissed pejoratively as "cookbook medicine." As the authors of this book, we clearly see value in these charts, but we also think it useful to reflect on how they might be used, what they bring to the student and practitioner, and where their limits lie.

Clinical decision making is fraught with error and bias. As medical practitioners, we sometimes fail to ask the right questions, perform the right diagnostic testing, or, even worse, fail to consider a specific diagnosis entirely. Flowcharts help combat bias, frame and organize thinking, and provide a useful visual structure to aid in learning and remembering important clinical information. To illustrate this, consider a few clinical scenarios. A doctor sees a young woman who reports a new, severe retro-orbital headache; there is a strong family history of migraine. He jumps to the conclusion that this is migraine. That "jumping to conclusions" is *anchoring bias*—the doctor fails to consider a range of possible explanations for a symptom complex because he has fixated on the obvious fact that headache in a young woman is most often due to migraine, and this is supported by her family history. But has he developed a differential diagnosis and considered other possibilities? Has he asked the right questions to investigate the likelihood of these other possibilities? And importantly, what if he is wrong? Has he considered the most dangerous potential outcomes? Briefly reviewing a flowchart on headache will remind him to consider other possibilities—and to look for signs and symptoms that might support or refute these possibilities. Sure enough, he had forgotten to look carefully for a Horner syndrome. And with the lights dimmed, the pupillary asymmetry is obvious. The patient has a carotid dissection.

Alas, he is now primed to fall victim to a very different form of bias—*availability bias*. With his recollection of this near miss so vivid, he finds himself thinking maybe *every* patient with a headache has a carotid dissection. This may lead to ordering unnecessary tests and creating worry for both him and his patients, but also perhaps to failing to consider other unusual but similarly important diagnoses. Again, the flowchart can help—by reviewing the logical flow of a diagnostic pathway, and seeing the universe of potential diseases associated with a particular symptom, he can regain perspective.

There are numerous other types of bias, but consider one more in particular. A man presents with difficulty walking. The doctor examines him and the initial neurologic examination is normal; she has him walk, and his gait appears bizarre, with an unusual twisting of both his legs as he walks. She suspects a functional disorder, gently inquires about recent stressors and psychiatric disease, and discovers that he has a history of untreated anxiety and recently lost his job. He notes that his symptoms have been present for many months prior to this recent stressor. Focusing on his job loss and anxiety, she dismisses this last piece of information and refers him for psychiatric evaluation. A moment spent glancing

at a flowchart and she might have realized she had become a victim of *confirmation bias*, or "seeing what you want to see, and hearing what you want to hear." In fact, the patient has dystonia, and had she more carefully examined his gait, she might have noted the stereotyped quality of the twisting leg movements that remitted when walking backward. Capturing all the relevant data requires one to consider all the relevant possibilities—seeing and hearing even what you don't mean to see and hear. It is our contention that a flowchart can help with this.

Flowcharts, of course, also have limitations. Not all diagnostic assessment proceeds in a linear fashion. The ability to dynamically maneuver through reams of incoming data—probing, advancing, and retreating in response to new information as it is discovered—is the hallmark of the superb clinician. In this respect, the charts in this book should be seen as a supplement to and not a substitute for clinical training. By necessity, we have streamlined and condensed the decision-making pathways in this book to make them fit on the page. This means some potentially useful but less essential clinical features and diagnostic or treatment strategies may have been omitted, as have references to some very uncommon diseases. Much in medicine is based more on expert opinion than rigorous scientific data. We present here our approach to common diagnostic and therapeutic neurologic problems; however, there may be other alternative but also reasonable approaches to these same problems. Finally, while we have made our best effort to ensure the recommendations herein are timely and accurate at the time of publication, as with all medical textbooks we cannot anticipate how new scientific advances will alter practice in the coming years.

In the practice of medicine, one can go wrong in many ways. There are diagnostic errors. There are therapeutic errors. There are errors of omission and errors of commission. There is attribution bias, authority bias, premature closure, diagnostic momentum, search satisfaction, overconfidence. The list goes on and on. We propose that a good start at avoiding these pitfalls is actually to stop for a moment. Defy the demands of the electronic medical record and hospital administrators, and give yourself permission to take a minute to slow down, step away from the bedside, and think things over. We hope the flowcharts contained within this book facilitate this critical process.

Brett L. Cucchiara, MD
Raymond S. Price, MD

AUTHORS' NOTE:

We welcome comments and suggestions from our readers. If you disagree with something in this book, or identify something you think is in error, please contact us at decisionmakinginadultneurology@gmail.com. Include as much detail as possible. While it may not be possible for us to respond individually, be assured we will take your feedback seriously.

PART I
Symptoms and Signs

Initial Headache

Katherine Hamilton and Ana Recober

New headache is a common complaint in the outpatient or emergency room setting. Distinguishing between headaches due to a potentially dangerous cause and those that are benign is paramount. Speed of onset of the headache, associated medical conditions, and neurologic examination findings are important factors to consider.

A. Headaches commonly follow concussion. Decisions about imaging in this scenario are reviewed in Chapter 63. Cervical arterial dissection of the internal carotid or vertebral arteries may also be associated with headache following trauma; often there is a delay between injury and development of pain. There may be associated neck pain, and the headache is often notably focal over just one region (such as retro-orbital). When suspicion for dissection is present, computed tomography angiogram (CTA) or magnetic resonance angiogram (MRA) of the neck are indicated.

B. A sudden-onset ("thunderclap") headache is one that reaches maximum intensity within 1 minute. The intensity is not as significant as the rapidity of onset. This type of headache warrants emergent evaluation, starting with noncontrast head CT to evaluate for subarachnoid hemorrhage (SAH).

C. In addition to SAH, head CT may identify other causes of thunderclap headache, such as intracerebral or intraventricular hemorrhage, pituitary apoplexy, or third ventricular colloid cyst. Presence of ischemic changes on CT should raise concern for arterial dissection, reversible cerebral vasoconstriction syndrome (RCVS), or cerebral venous thrombosis (CVT). A hyperdense artery sign suggests ischemic stroke, and hyperdense venous sinuses suggest CVT.

D. With modern-generation scanners and expert neuroradiology interpretation, the sensitivity of head CT for SAH approaches 99% when done within 6 hours of headache onset. However, sensitivity diminishes with time from headache onset and with less skilled CT readers. Given this and the catastrophic results of failing to identify SAH (i.e., aneurysmal rebleeding), if CT is negative, lumbar puncture should be performed. Xanthochromia, a yellow tinge to cerebrospinal fluid (CSF) caused by red blood cell (RBC) degradation, or elevated RBCs that do not decrease in successive tubes of CSF samples suggest the presence of SAH. Xanthochromia is reliably present 12 hours after occurrence of SAH and may persist for 2 weeks.

E. Headaches developing slowly over hours to days are common and most often benign. Certain features suggest an increased likelihood of a dangerous cause. As most primary headaches (e.g., migraine) present in the second to third decade of life, older patients (>50 years) presenting with new headache should undergo brain magnetic resonance imaging (MRI). Similarly, imaging is indicated in the immunocompromised and those with recent dental, head or neck, or neurosurgical procedures (concern for infection), in those with known malignancy (concern for metastasis), and in women who are pregnant or postpartum (concern for preeclampsia, RCVS, CVT). Additional testing, such as sedimentation rate to evaluate for giant cell arteritis or lumbar puncture to evaluate for a chronic meningeal process, may be needed depending on the clinical context. Postural headache that consistently worsens with lying down or headache precipitated by Valsalva maneuvers (e.g., coughing) suggest increased intracranial pressure and warrants brain imaging.

F. Lumbar puncture should include measurement of opening pressure, protein, glucose, and cell counts. While infectious and inflammatory processes rarely present with thunderclap headache, marked inflammation in the CSF should raise concern. RCVS and CVT can be associated with mild elevations in white blood cells (<15 per mm³) and/or protein (<100 mg/dL). Opening pressure is often elevated in patients with CVT.

G. Characteristic clinical features suggest a specific underlying cause of thunderclap headache; however, even in the absence of these, a high suspicion for secondary cause of headache should be maintained. Multiple recurrent thunderclap headaches strongly suggest RCVS; this is a common feature of this condition. While very rare, pheochromocytoma may present similarly. Catheter angiography is typically necessary to diagnose RCVS, given involvement of smaller-caliber vessels that are unreliably imaged with CT or MR angiography. CVT can present with thunderclap headache. There are often additional neurologic findings on examination; superimposed slowly progressive headache is typical. Diagnosis is with MR or CT venography. Pituitary apoplexy is due to either hemorrhage into or infarction of the pituitary gland. The former is visible on head CT, while the latter typically requires brain MRI with contrast to identify. Ocular movement abnormalities due to cranial neuropathies and visual loss due to compression of the optic nerves, chiasm, or tracts point to this diagnosis. Arterial dissection should be suspected in the setting of coexistent neck pain, recent trauma, or when focal neurologic deficits are present. Horner syndrome may be present with carotid dissection. Diagnosis is with neck MRA or CTA. Spontaneous intracranial hypotension is characterized by postural headache with improvement when lying flat. The presence of subdural fluid collections, meningeal enhancement, venous engorgement, pituitary hyperemia, or brain sagging on contrast MRI suggests the diagnosis. More involved testing to identify a spinal CSF leak may be needed.

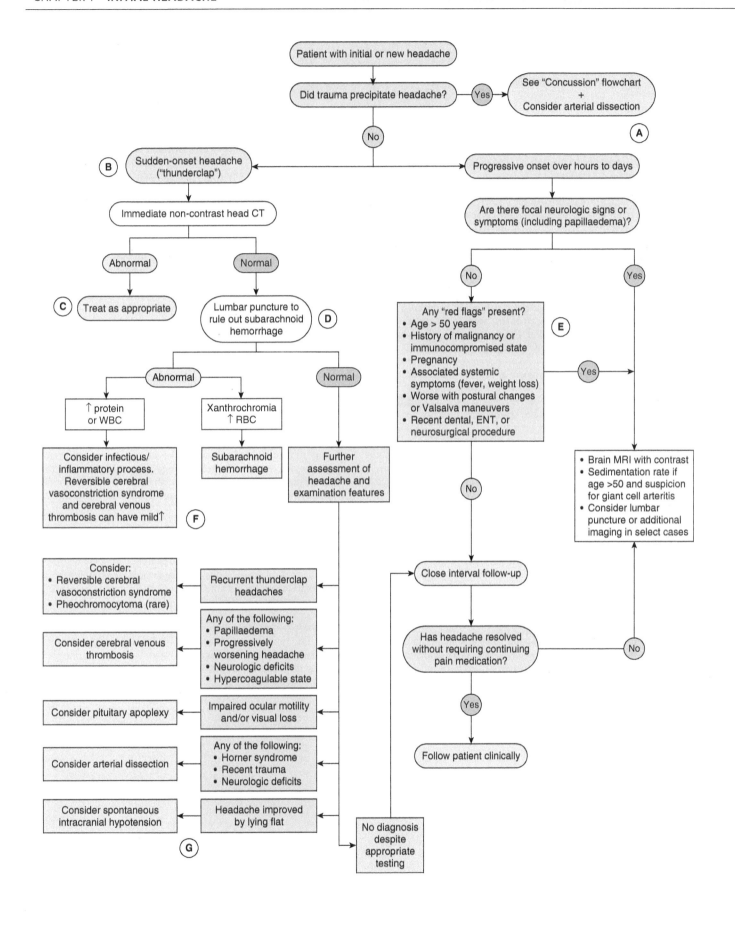

2 | Chronic Headache

Eric Kaiser and Ana Recober

Chronic headache is one of the most common neurologic symptoms. The main focus of the initial evaluation of a patient with chronic headache is to (1) determine if the headache is secondary to some underlying disease or is a primary headache disorder, and (2) classify the headache type to choose optimal treatment.

A. So-called "red flags" are features in the history that suggest headache may be due to an underlying disease. Most primary headache disorders present in adolescence or early adulthood, so headaches developing after age 50 should raise concern for a secondary cause and prompt brain imaging. Similarly, brain imaging is generally indicated for headaches following recent head trauma; that waken a patient from sleep, worsen with changes in body position or are triggered by Valsalva maneuvers including cough, exercise, or sexual activity; that occur in patients who are pregnant, immunocompromised, or have autoimmune disease or cancer; or that are associated with signs or symptoms of subacute infection. For patients with a known primary headache disorder, consider imaging if headaches develop new characteristics or patterns, or become progressively more severe or frequent. An abnormal neurologic examination should always prompt concern for a secondary cause and consideration of brain imaging. Be certain to evaluate for papilledema, which can indicate elevated intracranial pressure due to malignancy, infection, or idiopathic intracranial hypertension.

B. Migraine is a common primary headache disorder. Approximately 20%–40% of people with migraine experience an aura with at least some of their migraine attacks. Auras are unilateral, fully reversible neurologic symptoms that develop gradually over 5 minutes lasting up to 60 minutes and are typically followed by a headache with migrainous features. Aura symptoms are most often visual and binocular (scotomas with or without positive phenomena such as fortification spectra and/or scintillations), but can be monocular. They may also affect sensation (numbness or dysesthesias), language (aphasia), or motor function. Brainstem aura (dysarthria, vertigo, tinnitus, diplopia, ataxia, and/or decreased level of consciousness) is rare and additional work up should be considered. Typical migraine aura can also occur without headache.

C. For migraine without aura, an individual needs to have had at least five attacks of headache with migrainous features (see chart) that last between 4 and 72 hours when untreated or unsuccessfully treated. The associated symptoms help distinguish migraine from other headache disorders. Unless there are concerning features on history or examination, additional testing is not needed.

D. Trigeminal autonomic cephalalgias (TACs) are a group of primary headache disorders characterized by severe unilateral periorbital or temporal pain associated with ipsilateral cranial autonomic symptoms and a sense of restlessness or agitation. Duration and frequency of attacks are different for each disorder, as well as treatment response. Initial diagnostic evaluation for TACs should include magnetic resonance imaging (MRI) of the brain with contrast with special attention to the pituitary gland and cavernous sinus.

E. Ophthalmologic evaluation should be considered for orbital or periorbital pain, which may also occur with photophobia. Examples of primary ophthalmologic causes of pain include conjunctivitis, uveitis, keratitis, scleritis, corneal abrasions, dry eye syndrome, acute angle-closure glaucoma, orbital cellulitis, and optic neuritis.

F. Trigeminal neuralgia consists of attacks of very brief, lancinating pain in the distribution of the trigeminal nerve. The ophthalmic division of the trigeminal nerve is typically spared. Pain is often triggered by innocuous stimuli such as brushing teeth, cold air, talking, chewing, or touching the face. Rarely, trigeminal neuralgia is due to demyelination or neoplasm affecting the trigeminal nerve; more commonly it is idiopathic or associated with a compressive vascular loop. It is best evaluated with brain MRI with contrast and thin cuts through the trigeminal nerve and posterior fossa.

G. Temporomandibular disorders may also show abnormal movements of the mandible and/or decreased range of motion in addition to tenderness on examination. Patient education, dental referral for occlusional splints, and physical therapy may be helpful. The usefulness of imaging is controversial.

H. With occipital neuralgia, paroxysms of pain are brief and associated with dysesthesia and/or allodynia. Occipital nerve block is both diagnostic and therapeutic. Occipital neuralgia is often overdiagnosed in the setting of migraine, as occipital tenderness is commonly found on examination and occipital nerve blocks often provide pain relief, but they are distinct disorders.

I. Tension-type headache is the most common primary headache disorder, but most patients do not seek medical advice. Note that it does not have migrainous features such as aggravation by routine physical activity or nausea/vomiting, but may have photophobia or phonophobia. Unless there are concerning features on history or examination, additional testing is not needed.

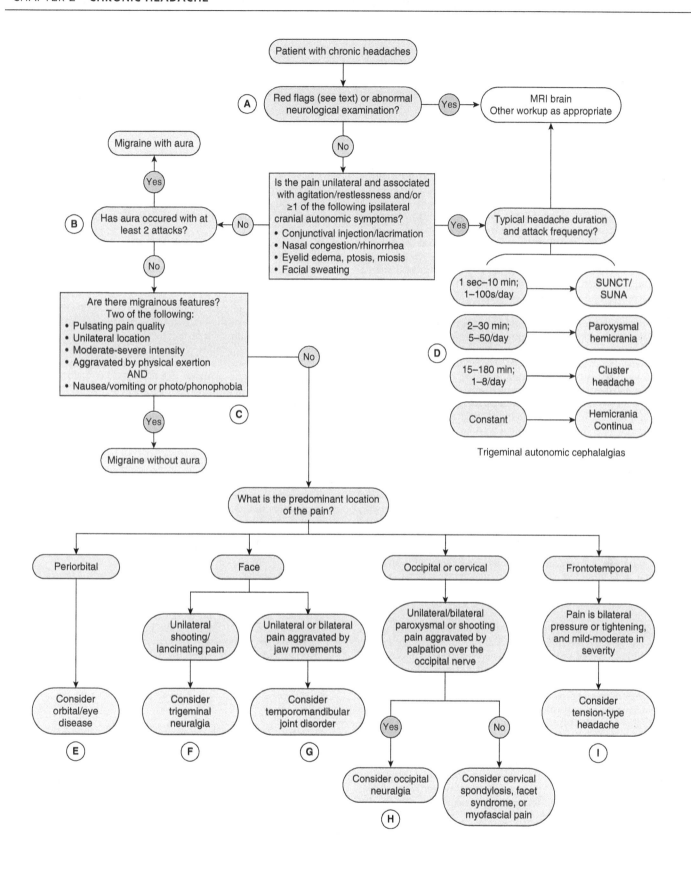

Trigeminal autonomic cephalalgias

3 | Neck Pain

Colin Quinn and Raymond S. Price

A. Neck pain resulting from trauma should be managed with particular caution to avoid causing or exacerbating damage to the cervical spine. When injury to the spinal column is suspected, immediate cervical immobilization is critical. Neurologic examination should be performed immediately to determine if there are neurologic deficits referable to a spinal level or vascular injury. Computed tomography (CT) of the cervical region is the imaging study of choice to examine the bony structure of spinal column. Magnetic resonance imaging (MRI) can provide more information regarding the spinal cord and the surrounding soft tissues and is recommended for patients with altered consciousness who cannot participate fully in the neurologic examination. Vascular imaging either with CT or MRI should be performed if there is suspicion for a vascular injury (see section B).

B. Dissection of the carotid or vertebral arteries should be considered in any patient with neck pain and symptoms or signs suggesting cerebral ischemia. While trauma is a significant risk factor for dissection, ~50% of dissections occur spontaneously without obvious antecedent trauma. Fibromuscular dysplasia, Marfan or Ehlers-Danlos syndrome, and a variety of other rare disorders of connective tissue predispose to dissection. An important diagnostic clue to carotid dissection is the presence of an ipsilateral Horner syndrome (anisocoria with an ipsilateral small pupil and ptosis) due to injury to the third-order sympathetic neurons ascending with the carotid artery.

C. If a patient has neck pain with difficulty walking or leg weakness, suspect cervical myelopathy. This requires emergent neuroimaging if acute and urgent neuroimaging if subacute or chronic to evaluate for the need for surgical decompression. If an intrinsic spinal cord lesion not related to compression is identified in a patient with acute or subacute onset of symptoms, refer to the evaluation of transverse myelitis in Chapter 113.

D. Pain radiating into and down the arm (radicular pain) suggests cervical radiculopathy. However, radicular pain is not always present and cervical radiculopathy must still be considered if there is arm weakness.

E. The absence of arm weakness in the setting of radicular pain suggests a mild or sensory-predominant cervical radiculopathy, although a pure musculoskeletal process without nerve compression cannot be entirely excluded. In either case, patients are treated with conservative symptomatic management with nonsteroidal antiinflammatory drugs (NSAIDs) and physical therapy. If pain is severe or persistent, medications for neuropathic pain (tricyclic antidepressants) may be used. Time-limited trials of opioids or benzodiazepines can be considered for severe, disabling pain but, given the potential for abuse and addiction should not be used as initial treatment for mild–moderate pain. Although frequently used, gabapentin, systemic steroids, or epidural steroid injections have not demonstrated clear long-term benefit. Failure to respond to conservative treatment should prompt reevaluation for progressive neurologic deficits.

F. Weakness of shoulder abduction along with neck pain radiating into the shoulder is most consistent with a C5 radiculopathy. Weakness of external rotation may also be present due to involvement of the muscles of rotator cuff.

G. Weakness of elbow flexion or a reduced biceps and brachioradialis reflex along with neck pain radiating into the anterior arm or lateral forearm is most consistent with a C6 radiculopathy.

H. Weakness of elbow and wrist extension or a reduced triceps reflex along with neck pain radiating into the posterior arm or forearm is most consistent with a C7 radiculopathy. For further localization of wrist drop, see Chapter 26.

I. Weakness of finger extension and abduction along with neck pain radiating into the posterior arm or forearm is most consistent with a C8/T1 radiculopathy. For further localization of hand weakness, see Chapter 27.

J. The presence of arm weakness in a presumed cervical radiculopathy indicates the loss of motor axons with the potential for further axonal loss if the underlying cause is not addressed. MRI of the cervical spine (with contrast if there is clinical suspicion for infection or malignancy) should be performed to evaluate for the need for surgical decompression. Be aware that degenerative cervical spine changes, such as disc herniation or osteophytes, are very common in older patients and may represent an incidental finding unrelated to symptoms. If there is clinical uncertainty regarding whether the degenerative changes seen on MRI are causing the patient's symptoms, nerve conduction studies/electromyography (NCS/EMG) should be performed. NCS/EMG can confirm the localization of the lesion in the peripheral nervous system, assess the severity of motor axon loss, and provide information on the acuity of the injury.

K. The absence of arm weakness or radicular pain suggests a musculoskeletal source of pain. In the acute phase, these patients may benefit from NSAIDs. With more chronic pain, an interdisciplinary approach including physical therapy, massage, yoga, and cognitive-behavioral therapy may be helpful. Patients should be instructed to resume normal activities and limit themselves to 1–2 hours of rest daily when the pain is most severe.

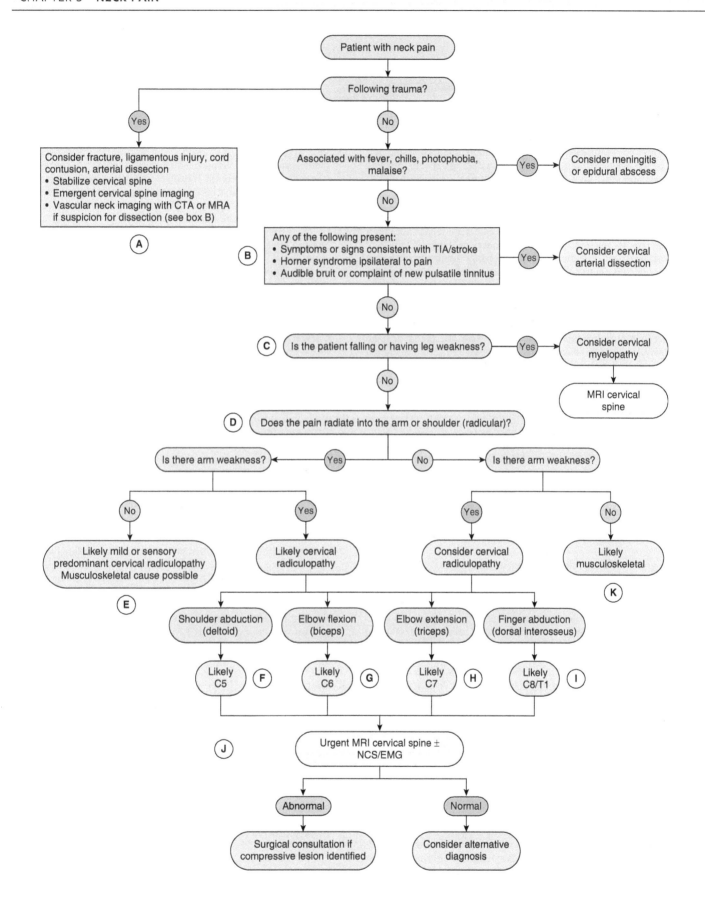

4 Low Back Pain

Daniel Cristancho and Raymond S. Price

Acute low back pain spontaneously resolves within 2–4 weeks in the majority of cases. Therefore, in the absence of trauma, fever, known malignancy, or focal neurologic signs or symptoms (such as incontinence or leg weakness), acute low back pain does not require imaging or intervention other than conservative symptomatic management.

A. Patients with new low back pain following trauma require emergent imaging of the lumbar spine, usually with computed tomography (CT), to identify conus medullaris or lumbosacral nerve root injury secondary to fracture, ligamentous injury, or compression from hematoma. Left untreated, such injuries may result in permanent neurologic disability. Other specific clinical features may suggest a cause for pain for which imaging is indicated. The most frequent presenting symptoms of epidural abscess are back pain (~50%) and fever or chills (~33%). Delayed diagnosis is common and a high index of suspicion is necessary. Recent systemic infection or spinal procedure, including lumbar puncture, epidural anesthesia, or spine surgery, should raise concern for this diagnosis. Spinal cord infarction and Guillain-Barré syndrome, while rare, often feature prominent low back pain. In neither condition, however, is pain the only symptom; associated leg weakness and reflex abnormalities, along with the temporal course of symptoms, suggests these diagnoses.

B. Nontraumatic low back pain involving new bowel or bladder incontinence, regardless of the presence of other symptoms, requires emergent imaging of the lumbar spine. Magnetic resonance imaging (MRI) provides better visualization of the conus medullaris, nerve roots, and intervertebral disc pathology compared to CT and is therefore preferred if available. Asymmetric weakness, pain radiating into the legs (radicular pain), or absent knee reflexes suggests cauda equina pathology. In contrast, symmetric leg weakness with absent Achilles and preserved patellar reflexes suggests a conus medullaris lesion.

C. The presence of radicular pain suggests lumbosacral radiculopathy. Nonradicular low back pain associated with unilateral leg weakness should also prompt consideration of lumbosacral radiculopathy. A forward flexed stance when standing or walking to reduce low back pain suggests the lumbosacral radiculopathy is due to spinal canal stenosis. This posture provides symptomatic relief by widening the spinal canal.

D. The absence of leg weakness or radicular low back pain is most suggestive of a musculoskeletal source of pain. In the acute phase, these patients may benefit from nonsteroidal antiinflammatory drugs (NSAIDs). With more chronic pain, an interdisciplinary approach including physical therapy, massage, yoga, and cognitive-behavioral therapy may be helpful. Patients should be instructed to resume normal activities and limit themselves to 1–2 hours of rest daily when the pain is most severe.

E. Radicular pain without leg weakness suggests a mild or sensory-predominant lumbosacral radiculopathy, though a musculoskeletal source of pain cannot be excluded. Acute symptomatic treatment may include NSAIDS and physical therapy. Additionally, treatment for neuropathic pain with gabapentin may be beneficial. Time-limited trials of opioids or benzodiazepines can be considered for severe, disabling pain but, given their potential for abuse and addiction, should not be used as first-line treatment. Although frequently used, systemic steroids or epidural steroid injections have not clearly demonstrated a long-term benefit. Failure to respond to conservative treatment should prompt reevaluation for progressive neurologic deficits. For chronic low back pain, additional approaches such as tricyclic antidepressants and radiofrequency ablation are frequently used in addition to the treatments above.

F. Isolated unilateral weakness of hip flexion suggests an L2 radiculopathy, which is quite uncommon. Weakness of unilateral hip flexion, hip adduction, and knee extension with a reduced or absent patellar reflex suggests an L3 radiculopathy. These findings can also be seen with a lumbar plexopathy (see Chapter 95).

G. The evaluation of unilateral knee extension weakness is discussed in Chapter 29.

H. Unilateral foot drop is commonly caused by L5 radiculopathy and peroneal neuropathies. The evaluation of foot drop from ankle dorsiflexion weakness is discussed in Chapter 30.

I. Unilateral ankle plantarflexion weakness and a reduced or absent Achilles reflex suggests an S1 radiculopathy or tibial neuropathy.

J. The presence of leg weakness in a presumed lumbosacral radiculopathy indicates the loss of motor axons with the potential for further axonal loss if the underlying cause is not addressed. MRI of the lumbar spine (with contrast if there is clinical suspicion for infection or malignancy) should be performed to evaluate for the need for surgical decompression. Be aware that degenerative lumbar spine changes, such as disc herniation or osteophytes, are very common in older patients and may represent an incidental finding unrelated to symptoms. If there is clinical uncertainty regarding whether the degenerative changes seen on MRI are causing the patient's symptoms, nerve conduction studies/electromyography (NCS/EMG) should be performed. NCS/EMG can confirm the localization of the lesion in the peripheral nervous system, assess the severity of motor axon loss, and provide information on the acuity of the injury. Symptomatic treatment of these patients consists of the conservative treatment approach discussed in section E.

K. If lumbar spine MRI is normal in patients with leg weakness or bowel or bladder incontinence, consider imaging of the thoracic and cervical spine to evaluate for myelopathy.

REFERENCES

1. Chou R, Qaseem A, Snow V, et al. Diagnosis and treatment of low back pain: a joint clinical practice guideline from the American College of Physicians and the American Pain Society. *Ann Intern Med.* 2007;147:478.
2. Hartvigsen J, Hancock MJ, Kongsted A, et al. What low back pain is and why we need to pay attention. *Lancet.* 2018;391:2356–2367.
3. Tavee JO, Levin KH. Low back pain. *Continuum (Minneap Minn).* 2017;23:467–486.

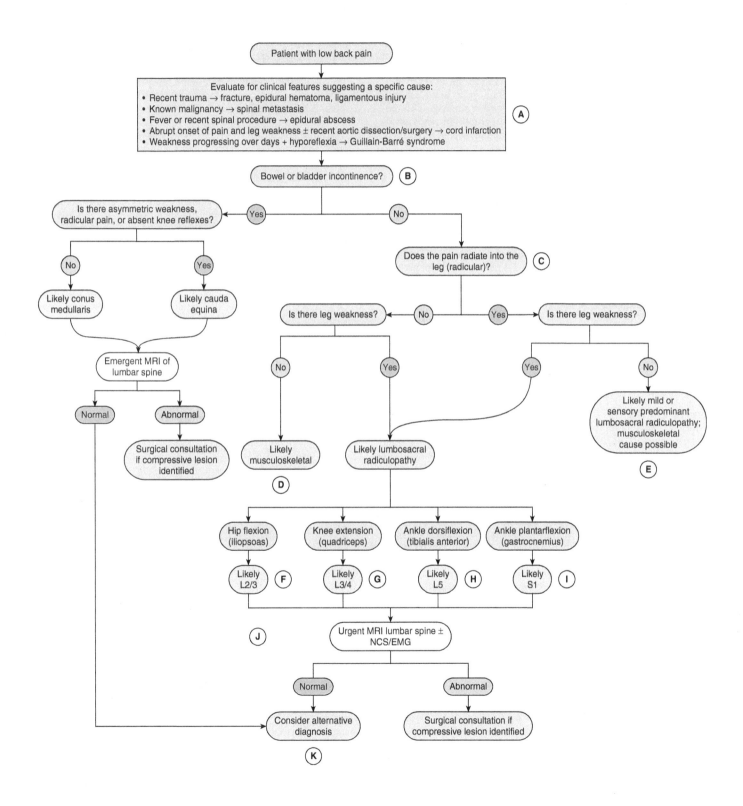

Patient with low back pain

Evaluate for clinical features suggesting a specific cause:
- Recent trauma → fracture, epidural hematoma, ligamentous injury
- Known malignancy → spinal metastasis
- Fever or recent spinal procedure → epidural abscess
- Abrupt onset of pain and leg weakness ± recent aortic dissection/surgery → cord infarction
- Weakness progressing over days + hyporeflexia → Guillain-Barré syndrome

(A)

Bowel or bladder incontinence?   (B)

Yes   No

Is there asymmetric weakness, radicular pain, or absent knee reflexes?

No   Yes

Likely conus medullaris   Likely cauda equina

Does the pain radiate into the leg (radicular)?   (C)

Emergent MRI of lumbar spine

Normal   Abnormal

Surgical consultation if compressive lesion identified

Is there leg weakness?   No   Yes   Is there leg weakness?

No   Yes   Yes   No

Likely musculoskeletal   (D)   Likely lumbosacral radiculopathy   Likely mild or sensory predominant lumbosacral radiculopathy; musculoskeletal cause possible   (E)

Hip flexion (iliopsoas)   Knee extension (quadriceps)   Ankle dorsiflexion (tibialis anterior)   Ankle plantarflexion (gastrocnemius)

Likely L2/3   (F)   Likely L3/4   (G)   Likely L5   (H)   Likely S1   (I)

(J)

Urgent MRI lumbar spine ± NCS/EMG

Normal   Abnormal

Consider alternative diagnosis   Surgical consultation if compressive lesion identified

(K)

5 Aphasia

H. Branch Coslett

Aphasia is an acquired disorder of language that is frequently observed in patients with lesions in the left hemisphere. Stroke is one of the most common causes of aphasia; slowly progressive aphasia may be seen with mass lesions, or with neurodegenerative diseases such as primary progressive aphasia. Symptoms of aphasia, which may be observed individually or in different combinations, include poor word retrieval (anomia), difficulty accessing meaning from spoken language (comprehension deficits), and inability to repeat words, phrases or sentences or to apply the grammatical and syntactic rules to understand or generate language.

When evaluating a patient with suspected aphasia, the following parameters should be assessed. First, *naming* should be tested by asking subjects to name objects that differ in frequency from high to low (e.g., thumb vs. eyebrow) and length (e.g., bat vs. propeller). The nature of the errors should be noted. Patients will frequently be unable to generate a response or produce a sound-based error; less commonly, patients may substitute a word that is similar in meaning. *Fluency* should be assessed by noting the rate and ease with which language is produced. Non-fluent patients may generate only a few words at a time whereas fluent patients may produce long phrases or even sentences. *Comprehension* should be tested by asking patients to perform simple tasks ranging in complexity from simple commands (e.g., "close your eyes") to complex, sequential actions that require grammatical competence (e.g., "After you point to the ceiling, point to the door with your left thumb."). *Repetition* should be assessed by asking patients to repeat utterances that vary across the dimensions of frequency and length; for example, patients may be asked to repeat single, high-frequency words (e.g., dog) to more complex utterances with multiple, low-frequency words (e.g., "The seamstress stitched the wedding gown."). Finally, it is important to have a large sample of language to evaluate; to that end, it is often useful to ask patients to tell a story or elaborate on topics of particular interest to them.

A number of distinct types of aphasia have traditionally been described. Although not all investigators agree that aphasia subtypes are readily distinguished or consistent across patients, they have a venerable history and are clinically useful.

A. Anomic aphasia, the most common type of aphasia, is characterized by difficulty naming objects and concepts with relatively preserved comprehension, fluency, and repetition. It may be caused by lesions anywhere in the left hemisphere but is most frequently observed as a residual effect of more severe aphasias.

B. Conduction aphasia is characterized by impaired repetition and naming but relatively preserved fluency and comprehension. Traditionally it is attributed to lesions of white matter tracts connecting Wernicke and Broca areas, but it is most frequently observed as the residual manifestation of Wernicke aphasia.

C. Transcortical aphasias are characterized by intact repetition with impairments in other language faculties. Transcortical motor and sensory aphasia are associated with deficits in fluency and comprehension, respectively. Mixed transcortical aphasia is associated with impaired comprehension and poor fluency. In these disorders perisylvian tissue, including white matter tracts, is preserved; lesions are often subcortical.

D. Wernicke aphasia (Fig. 5.1) is characterized by fluent speech with impaired comprehension, repetition, and naming. It is associated with lesions involving the posterior portion of the superior temporal gyrus.

E. Broca aphasia (Fig. 5.1) is characterized by non-fluent, effortful speech; naming is poor with frequent failures to respond and sound-based errors. Comprehension is relatively preserved but repetition is impaired. It is associated with lesions that involve the left inferior frontal gyrus and, in most cases, other portions of the lateral frontal lobe and anterior insula.

F. Global aphasia is characterized by impairment in all language functions and is typically seen with large lesions involving much of the perisylvian portion of the left hemisphere.

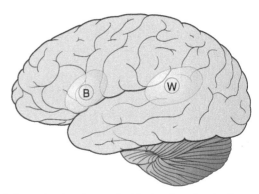

FIG. 5.1 Schematic showing typical lesion location in Broca aphasia *(B)* involving the left inferior frontal gyrus, and in Wernicke aphasia *(W)* involving the posterior portion of the superior temporal gyrus.

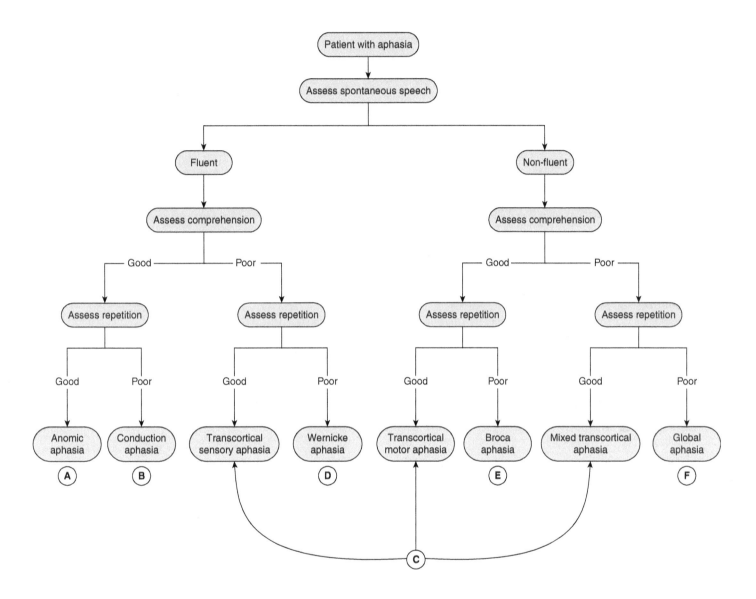

Chronic Cognitive Decline

Murray Grossman

Slowly progressive cognitive decline is seen most often in the elderly, and frequently causes great concern to family members, though the affected patient may be unconcerned or even unaware of the problem. In some cases, gradual behavior change may be the predominant symptom noted by the patient or family, and cognitive impairment may be less obvious. Unfortunately, largely untreatable neurodegenerative diseases (e.g., Alzheimer dementia) are the most common cause. There are, however, some causes of cognitive decline that can be treated with reversal or stabilization of cognitive function; identification of these conditions is thus paramount.

A. In all patients with cognitive deterioration, evaluation should start with a detailed medical history and screening laboratory testing focusing on conditions that may be associated with cognitive decline. Ask about symptoms suggesting hypothyroidism (sensitivity to cold, weight gain, constipation, dry skin, thinning hair), Cushing syndrome (fatty tissue deposits in the abdomen, upper back, and face, fragile skin, slow healing, acne, hirsutism), vitamin B12 deficiency (extremity numbness/tingling due to peripheral neuropathy, dietary idiosyncrasies), obstructive sleep apnea (snoring, daytime sleepiness), and rheumatologic disease (rashes, joint pain). Renal, liver, gastrointestinal, and cardiac disease should be identified. When appropriate, syphilis and HIV infection should be ruled out. Medications, particularly chronic narcotic or sedative use, may contribute to cognitive decline, as may heavy alcohol use. Finally, brain magnetic resonance imaging should be performed to evaluate for structural lesions that might cause cognitive decline.

B. Deficits on detailed neurologic examination may point to specific neurologic diseases associated with cognitive decline. Bedside cognitive screening using a standardized instrument, for instance the Montreal Cognitive Assessment (MOCA), helps to objectively quantify the degree of impairment and can be useful for following progression over time. This may be supplemented by more detailed neuropsychological evaluation.

C. The triad of cognitive decline, unstable gait, and urinary frequency/urgency can be seen with communicating (or normal pressure) hydrocephalus. Brain imaging will show marked ventricular dilatation out of proportion to atrophy. Improvement in gait soon after large-volume lumbar puncture supports the diagnosis. Treatment is surgical placement of a ventriculoperitoneal shunt.

D. Depression can simulate dementia, causing difficulty with memory and apathy. Most patients recognize they are depressed. Treatment may reverse the cognitive symptoms. Note that patients with organic dementia may develop secondary depression, making evaluation of the depressed patient with cognitive impairment complex.

E. Progressive microvascular disease can accumulate insidiously in the context of hypertension, hyperlipidemia, and/or diabetes leading to cognitive impairment. This may be accompanied by unstable gait and urinary frequency/urgency. This can overlap with communicating hydrocephalus and with common neurodegenerative conditions such as Alzheimer disease.

F. Eighty percent of patients with Parkinson disease develop cognitive difficulties over time. The diagnosis of Parkinson disease is usually, but not always, established by the time marked cognitive impairment occurs.

G. With older age, neurodegenerative conditions become increasingly common. The most common of these is Alzheimer disease, marked by disorders of episodic memory, naming, visuospatial processing, and executive functioning. Frontotemporal degeneration is increasingly recognized, particularly in individuals younger than age 65. This condition may present as a disorder of social comportment, behavior, and personality that can resemble some psychiatric conditions as well as some forms of delirium related to medical conditions. Behavioral variant frontotemporal degeneration can be differentiated from these other conditions by its context and the age of onset (psychiatric conditions such as bipolar disorder begin at a much younger age). Frontotemporal degeneration also can present as a disorder of language known as primary progressive aphasia. Lewy body dementia is associated with prominent visual hallucinations. Parkinsonian features are also common. Cognitive symptoms are often preceded by rapid eye movement sleep behavior disorder by years.

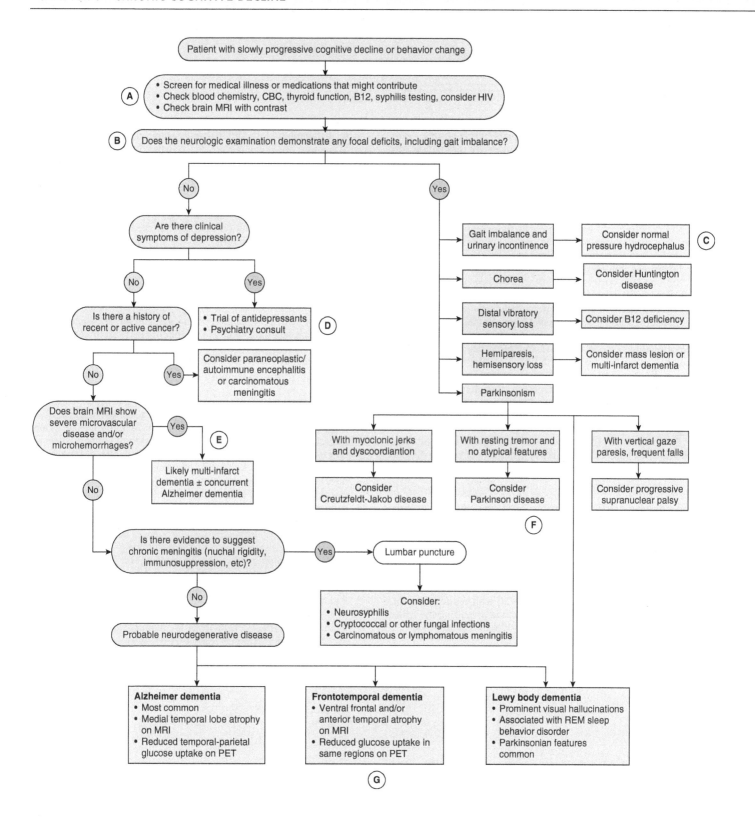

Acute Memory Loss

David Wolk

Abrupt memory loss developing over minutes to days can be a striking clinical picture. Often the symptom is initially mistaken for a confusional state. While some causes of abrupt memory loss may indeed overlap with confusion, others—transient global amnesia being perhaps the best example—are characterized by preserved cognitive function in all domains except memory.

A. Initial evaluation should determine if the symptoms are indeed isolated to memory, or if other neurologic symptoms or signs are present. Special attention should be paid to impairment in level of consciousness (even if mild), witnessed convulsive activity, ataxia, eye movement abnormalities, and visual field defects.

B. If symptoms are isolated to memory loss, the nature of the memory impairment can provide important diagnostic clues. Temporal-limbic memory loss, often involving hippocampal function and its extended network, is marked by an inability to form new episodic memories (anterograde amnesia) and some degree of retrograde memory loss for episodes prior to the presenting event. Retrograde memory loss tends to have a temporal gradient in which memories formed closest to presentation are often more affected than remote ones. If an individual has an isolated retrograde memory loss but is able to form new memories, this generally reflects an underlying psychiatric condition. If there is loss of personal identity, one should consider a dissociative fugue state. Alternatively, if there is intact personal identity, psychogenic amnesia, including conversion disorder, is more likely.

C. If there is alteration of consciousness or the presence of multiple seizures, consider infectious or autoimmune temporal-limbic encephalitis. In these cases, brain magnetic resonance imaging (MRI) with contrast should be performed looking for medial temporal and temporal pole signal abnormality. Herpes simplex virus (HSV) encephalitis is an important consideration, particularly if fever is present; when considered, acyclovir should be started as soon as possible. Lumbar puncture should be performed and cerebrospinal fluid tested with HSV polymerase chain reaction (PCR) with cell count, protein and glucose levels measured; autoimmune/paraneoplastic panels should be considered in the appropriate clinical context.

D. The posterior circulation is the primary source of blood flow to the medial temporal lobe and thalamic regions in the memory network. If memory loss is hyperacute and associated with acute-onset focal neurologic findings such as double vision, visual field deficit, or hemisensory loss, posterior circulation stroke is likely. If present, brain MRI with diffusion weighted imaging will demonstrate infarction and confirm the diagnosis.

E. Memory loss is common following prolonged or multiple seizures, particularly those emanating from the medial temporal lobe. If early recovery to baseline does not occur, electroencephalogram (EEG) monitoring should be pursued to evaluate for nonconvulsive status epilepticus.

F. Relatively rapid memory loss in the setting of confusion or delirium, eye movement abnormalities, or ataxia should prompt consideration of Wernicke encephalopathy. A history of heavy alcohol use is common. Untreated, this can evolve into Korsakoff syndrome, which is associated with more isolated but often more profound amnesia. Immediate treatment with intravenous thiamine is required.

G. The most common cause of isolated sustained anterograde memory loss is transient global amnesia (TGA), a benign though often frightening disorder for patients' families. Memory loss generally lasts several hours, and there is no alteration of consciousness or other neurologic deficits. Due to their rapid rate of forgetting, patients repeatedly ask the same questions over and over, reflecting disorientation to place and time. TGA is often preceded by acute emotional events, strenuous physical activity, or pain. The underlying cause remains uncertain, with seizures, arterial or venous ischemia, and migrainous-type phenomena all proposed as explanations but with little supportive evidence. One should observe these patients to ensure the expected resolution of symptoms within 24 hours. If atypical features are present, brain MRI and EEG should be considered.

H. Patients with recent cardiopulmonary instability, particularly in the intensive care unit setting, may have temporal-limbic memory loss due to the particular sensitivity of the hippocampus to hypoxia.

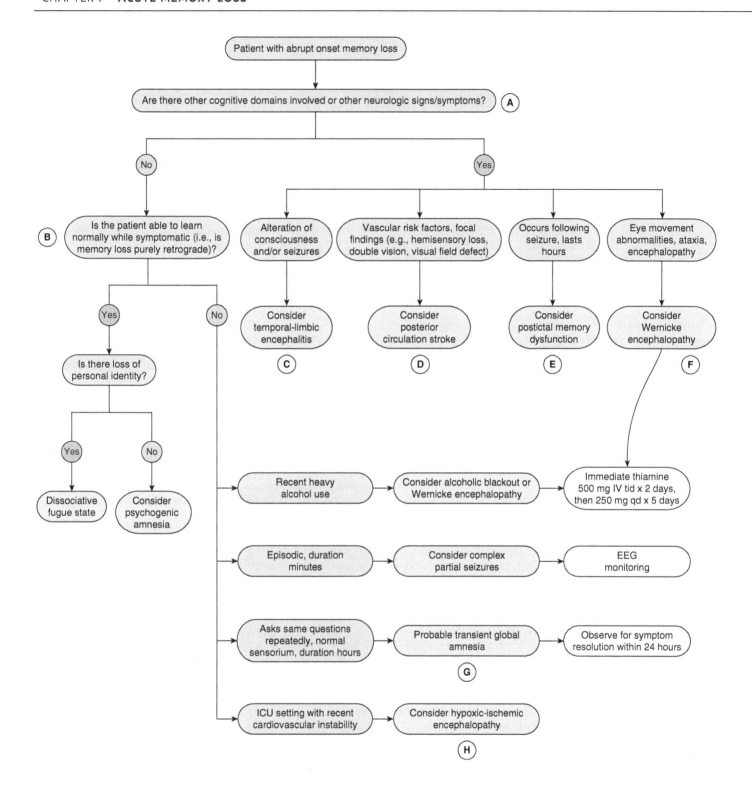

Chronic Memory Loss

David Wolk

Memory loss that develops over several months to years is most commonly seen in older adults and often prompts concern about the possibility of Alzheimer disease. However, other conditions should also be considered; a thorough history should investigate medication use, psychiatric symptoms, sleep disorders, and signs of systemic illness. Focal findings on neurologic examination, or neurologic symptoms beyond just memory loss, should prompt neuroimaging.

A. Memory impairment in older adults is often due to medications that may affect both attention and memory. Anticholinergic medicines, such as meclizine, diphenhydramine, and oxybutynin, can impair memory in otherwise cognitively normal older adults, as may benzodiazepines and other sleep aids. Discontinuation of these medicines and reassessment is appropriate in this context.

B. Depression and anxiety are common causes of memory loss. Both are associated with reductions in attention and concentration, which, in turn, diminish memory encoding and retrieval. At its extreme, depression has been associated with "pseudodementia." Note, however, that even with successful treatment, many such patients go on to experience progressive cognitive decline, suggesting mood disturbances may have "unmasked" an underlying neurodegenerative process. Treatment with antidepressants and antianxiety medications, particularly those without cognitive side effects such as selective serotonin reuptake inhibitors, should be pursued; consider psychiatric consultation depending on the clinical context and response to treatment. Reassess patients for cognitive improvement in the context of improved mood or anxiety. Given the relatively slow time course of improvement in depression or anxiety, psychiatric evaluation and treatment are often done in parallel with workup for other causes of memory loss.

C. Poor sleep is associated with daytime fatigue and also reduces attention and concentration with predictable negative consequences on memory. Sleep, particularly slow wave, is also critical for memory consolidation. Ask patients and their partners about daytime sleepiness and sleep habits. Snoring and gasping for air suggest obstructive sleep apnea, which can be effectively treated with continuous positive airway pressure. Obese patients are at higher risk. Acting out one's dreams, including conversations and physical movements, reflects impaired reduction in muscle tone during rapid eye movement sleep and is a predictor for the presence or development of Lewy body spectrum disorders, including Parkinson disease and Lewy body dementia. Insomnia may have a psychiatric etiology, and such sleep deprivation can also contribute to poor memory. In all cases, an overnight polysomnogram may be necessary for diagnosis.

D. If none of the above potentially reversible causes of memory loss are found, brain magnetic resonance imaging (MRI) should be performed and B12, methylmalonic acid, and thyroid function tested. Suspicion for B12 deficiency should be heightened in the setting of large fiber neuropathy and macrocytic anemia, though cognitive symptoms may exist without these findings. Weight gain, cold intolerance, and cognitive slowing suggest hypothyroidism.

E. Memory loss over weeks to months may be associated with a subdural hematoma, particularly in older adults after a fall. Focal findings are often absent on examination, and memory loss is often driven by poor concentration and executive function. A frontal lobe mass may affect memory encoding and retrieval, and is also often associated with other frontal lobe cognitive manifestations. Brain MRI reliably identifies these abnormalities.

F. Memory impairment associated with a slow, magnetic gait and urinary incontinence suggests normal pressure hydrocephalus. The cognitive profile is typically characterized by slowing of processing speed and memory loss on the basis of poor encoding and retrieval, but normal memory storage (i.e., recall tends to be worse than recognition memory). Brain imaging shows enlarged ventricles. Confirmation of the diagnosis depends on demonstrating clinical improvement after large-volume lumbar puncture.

G. Vascular dementia presents with a cognitive profile similar to normal pressure hydrocephalus (see section F). MRI will show extensive microvascular disease. Note that most with vascular cognitive impairment have a slowly progressive course and not the step-wise progression that is classically described.

H. Prominent and slowly progressive memory loss in a temporal limbic pattern is a hallmark of Alzheimer disease. This form of memory loss reflects a loss of information over time supported by impaired memory recall *and* recognition memory. Other cognitive domains, including executive function, language, and visuospatial processing, tend to be less affected early in the course of disease. MRI demonstrating hippocampal and lateral parietal atrophy supports the diagnosis, though a normal MRI does not exclude Alzheimer disease. In addition to Alzheimer disease, a variety of other neurodegenerative conditions are associated with memory loss, but usually have impairment in other salient nonmemory cognitive domains (e.g., semantic dementia) or other associated neurologic features (e.g., asymmetric dystonia in corticobasal degeneration).

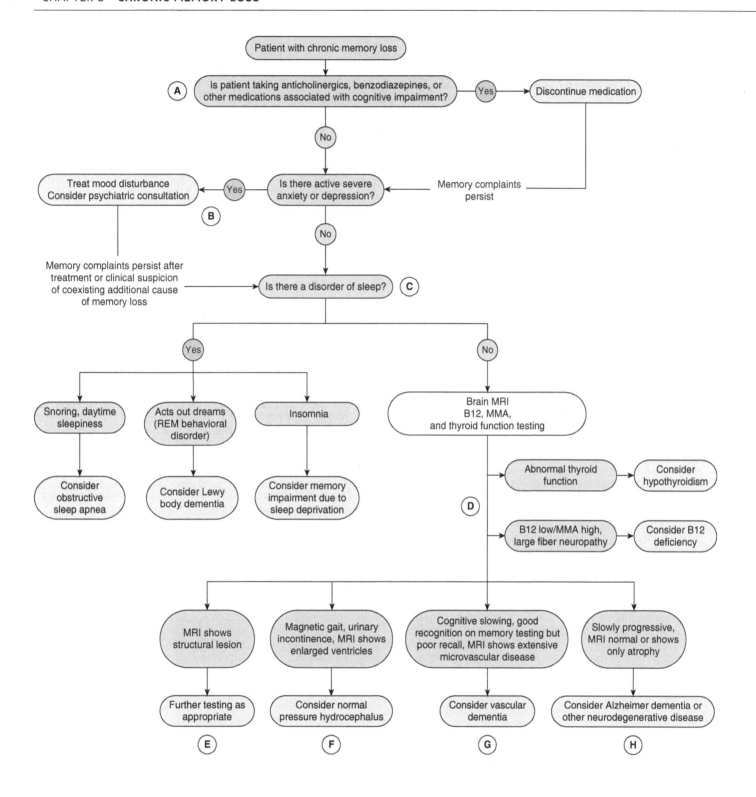

9 Rapidly Progressive Dementia

H. Branch Coslett and Brett L. Cucchiara

Rapidly progressive dementia refers to cognitive and/or behavioral deficits that evolve over weeks to months, much more rapidly than with traditional neurodegenerative diseases such as Alzheimer dementia. Treatable conditions are found in up to 20% of those with rapidly progressive dementia, which is far more often than in patients with more chronically evolving dementia.

A. Obtain a careful history to distinguish between a true rapid decline and a subacute worsening of a preexisting more chronic progressive neurodegenerative disorder. This may require careful focused questioning about the patient's ability to perform specific cognitive tasks (dealing with finances, navigation) over the past few years. Assess medication use with attention to any potential temporal relationship between new medications or changes and the onset of symptoms. Certain toxic exposures (lead, mercury, bismuth) can cause relatively rapid cognitive and behavioral changes. Consider thiamine, niacin, and B12 deficiency. Screen for metabolic derangements, thyroid disease, and syphilis or HIV infection.

B. Limbic encephalitis in the patient with cognitive decline over weeks suggests autoimmune encephalitis (see Chapter 115). Infectious causes tend to progress more rapidly (i.e., over days), though in atypical cases may have a more insidious course.

C. Creutzfeldt-Jakob disease (CJD) is a prion disease causing spongiform encephalopathy. Startle myoclonus and ataxia are frequent clinical findings, as are periodic sharp wave complexes on electroencephalogram (EEG). Early in the disease, brain magnetic resonance imaging (MRI) may be normal; later, characteristic MRI signs appear. Routine cerebrospinal fluid (CSF) studies are often normal. Elevated CSF levels of the 14-3-3 protein support the diagnosis and the real-time quaking-induced conversion (RT-QuIC) assay is confirmatory. Brain biopsy may be necessary in uncertain cases. There is no specific treatment for CJD.

D. Central nervous system (CNS) vasculitis may present with rapidly accumulating infarctions over weeks to months. Headache is a frequent feature, and CSF pleocytosis may be present. As the affected vessels are often small-medium in caliber, noninvasive vessel imaging (magnetic resonance angiogram [MRA]/computed tomography angiogram [CTA]) is often normal, and catheter angiography should be pursued recognizing that even this may be negative if the vasculitis involves only the very small vessels. Brain biopsy is necessary for diagnostic confirmation. Treatment is usually steroids and cyclophosphamide. Intravascular lymphoma may mimic CNS vasculitis clinically and radiographically.

E. It is essential that MRI be performed with susceptibility weighted images (i.e., GRE, SWI) to identify microhemorrhages, which are the cardinal feature of amyloid angiopathy (AA). Patients with AA may have rapid cognitive decline due to accumulation of large numbers of microhemorrhages. Rarely, an inflammatory component may be present (angiitis), resulting in vasogenic edema and in some cases even giving the appearance of a mass lesion. While there is no specific treatment for AA itself, amyloid angiitis is usually highly responsive to steroids.

F. While extremely rare, dural arteriovenous fistulas (dAVFs) can cause rapid cognitive decline. MRI will show parenchymal lesions consistent with venous edema; abnormal flow voids consistent with dilated vessels on T2 images may suggest the diagnosis. Note that dAVFs are often occult on MRA or CTA, such that if the diagnosis is suspected, catheter angiography is required.

G. Thiamine deficiency must be considered in any patient with rapid development of encephalopathy over days to weeks; the presence of eye movement abnormalities (nystagmus or ophthalmoparesis) and ataxia should increase suspicion (Wernicke-Korsakoff syndrome), but neither of these findings are universally present. Chronic alcoholics are particularly susceptible. Clinical suspicion or characteristic MRI findings suggesting Wernicke-Korsakoff syndrome should trigger immediate thiamine administration. A whole blood thiamine level may be sent to confirm the diagnosis, but should not delay treatment.

H. Brain MRI may be normal or show only nonspecific abnormalities in several important causes of rapidly progressive dementia. Hashimoto encephalopathy is a rare condition associated with antithyroid antibodies that may cause rapidly progressive dementia. Concomitant thyroid disease is often but not always present. The condition is extremely steroid responsive. Suspicion for paraneoplastic/autoimmune encephalitis should be raised when the patient has a known malignancy, but certain types often occur without underlying cancer. Accompanying neurologic signs may provide important clues as to which antibody may be mediating the clinical syndrome (see Chapter 115). CJD may occur with a normal brain MRI and routine CSF studies (see section C).

I. Extremely rare causes of rapidly progressive dementia may be suggested by particular accompanying symptoms or signs as outlined in the chart; MRI is usually abnormal in some but not all of these conditions. Prolonged EEG monitoring should be considered to capture the rare patient in nonconvulsive status epilepticus.

J. A variety of other specific causes may be identified on brain MRI, including subdural hematoma, tumors, infection (i.e., focal mass lesions, progressive multifocal leukoencephalopathy), demyelinating disease, inflammatory diseases, and hydrocephalus.

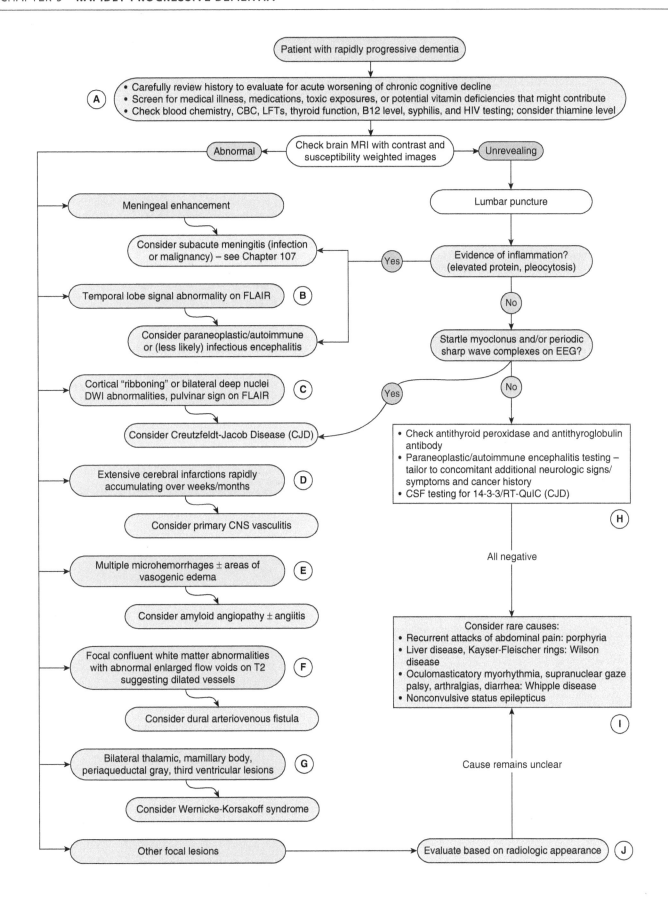

Patient with rapidly progressive dementia

A
- Carefully review history to evaluate for acute worsening of chronic cognitive decline
- Screen for medical illness, medications, toxic exposures, or potential vitamin deficiencies that might contribute
- Check blood chemistry, CBC, LFTs, thyroid function, B12 level, syphilis, and HIV testing; consider thiamine level

Check brain MRI with contrast and susceptibility weighted images

Abnormal ← → Unrevealing

Lumbar puncture

Meningeal enhancement

Consider subacute meningitis (infection or malignancy) – see Chapter 107

← Yes — Evidence of inflammation? (elevated protein, pleocytosis)

No

Temporal lobe signal abnormality on FLAIR B

Consider paraneoplastic/autoimmune or (less likely) infectious encephalitis

Startle myoclonus and/or periodic sharp wave complexes on EEG?

Cortical "ribboning" or bilateral deep nuclei DWI abnormalities, pulvinar sign on FLAIR C

Yes

No

Consider Creutzfeldt-Jacob Disease (CJD)

H
- Check antithyroid peroxidase and antithyroglobulin antibody
- Paraneoplastic/autoimmune encephalitis testing – tailor to concomitant additional neurologic signs/ symptoms and cancer history
- CSF testing for 14-3-3/RT-QuIC (CJD)

Extensive cerebral infarctions rapidly accumulating over weeks/months D

Consider primary CNS vasculitis

All negative

Multiple microhemorrhages ± areas of vasogenic edema E

Consider amyloid angiopathy ± angiitis

I
Consider rare causes:
- Recurrent attacks of abdominal pain: porphyria
- Liver disease, Kayser-Fleischer rings: Wilson disease
- Oculomasticatory myorhythmia, supranuclear gaze palsy, arthralgias, diarrhea: Whipple disease
- Nonconvulsive status epilepticus

Focal confluent white matter abnormalities with abnormal enlarged flow voids on T2 suggesting dilated vessels F

Consider dural arteriovenous fistula

Bilateral thalamic, mamillary body, periaqueductal gray, third ventricular lesions G

Consider Wernicke-Korsakoff syndrome

Cause remains unclear

Other focal lesions

Evaluate based on radiologic appearance J

Delirium

Jon Rosenberg and Brett L. Cucchiara

Delirium refers to an acute impairment in attention that compromises cognitive function; it is often associated with fluctuating arousal. Attention can be easily assessed at the bedside by asking the patient to perform "serial 7s" (subtract 7 from 100 and then repetitively subtracting 7 from each new total) or to repeat a series of numbers forward and then backward. The delirious patient may have periods of seeming lucidity followed by profound agitation and confusion. Hallucinations and combative behavior are common. Delirium is one of the most frequent neurologic conditions encountered in hospitalized patients, and is particularly common in the elderly. Medications commonly used for delirium are presented in Table 10.1 (contained in Appendix 1).

A. Numerous underlying conditions predispose to delirium.[1] The most common risk factors are advanced age, infection, dementia, immobility, electrolyte imbalance, malnutrition, and urinary catheterization. A careful search for underlying causes and reversible risk factors should be undertaken in all patients with delirium. Diagnostic testing should be tailored to the specific clinical scenario, but commonly includes a serum chemistry panel and complete blood count, urinalysis, urine and blood cultures, chest radiography, and toxicology screening. The presence of focal neurologic findings on examination should prompt urgent brain imaging. Electroencephalography and lumbar puncture may be necessary in some cases.

B. In all patients with delirium, a focus on nonpharmacological measures is critical. These include redirection, promoting a normal sleep-wake cycle, removal of unnecessary lines, drains, or catheters, and transfer to a quiet environment whenever possible.

C. Drug intoxication and alcohol withdrawal can mimic delirium. In stimulant intoxication and alcohol withdrawal, patients often have tachycardia, hypertension, diaphoresis, and tremor. Opiate intoxication is usually accompanied by bradycardia, hypotension, hypoventilation, and miosis. Prompt, specific treatment, especially for alcohol withdrawal and opiate overdose, can be life-saving.

D. Alcohol withdrawal is treated with symptom-driven benzodiazepine administration, often using a prespecified protocol such as the Clinical Institute Withdrawal Assessment for Alcohol Scale (CIWA-Ar) to quantify symptom severity and guide dosing.[2] (See the CIWA-Ar protocol in the Appendix.) Patients with severe withdrawal symptoms may require intensive care management. Patients with delirium related to either alcohol intoxication or withdrawal should receive intravenous thiamine as the risk of concomitant thiamine deficiency and thus Wernicke encephalopathy is increased. A typical starting dose is 500 mg IV tid.

E. Delirium may be subdivided into hyperactive, hypoactive, and mixed types. Hyperactive delirium occurs when cognitive impairment is accompanied by agitation and increased motor and speech output, whereas hypoactive delirium is associated with lethargy and decreased motor and speech output. Most patients demonstrate a mixed delirium type. Hypoactive delirium should be treated with nonpharmacological measures alone. For hyperactive and mixed delirium, antipsychotics such as haloperidol are typically used. Atypical antipsychotics or valproic acid should be used if there is a high risk for electrocardiographic QT interval prolongation or for patients at high risk of extrapyramidal side effects (i.e., comorbid Parkinsonism).

REFERENCES

1. Flaherty J, Morely J. Delirium: a call to improve current standards of care. *J Gerontol A Biol Sci Med Sci.* 2004;59(4):341–343.
2. Sullivan JT, Sykora K, Schneiderman J, Naranjo CA, Sellers EM. Assessment of alcohol withdrawal: the revised clinical institute withdrawal assessment for alcohol scale (CIWA-Ar). *Br J Addict.* 1989;84:1353–1357.

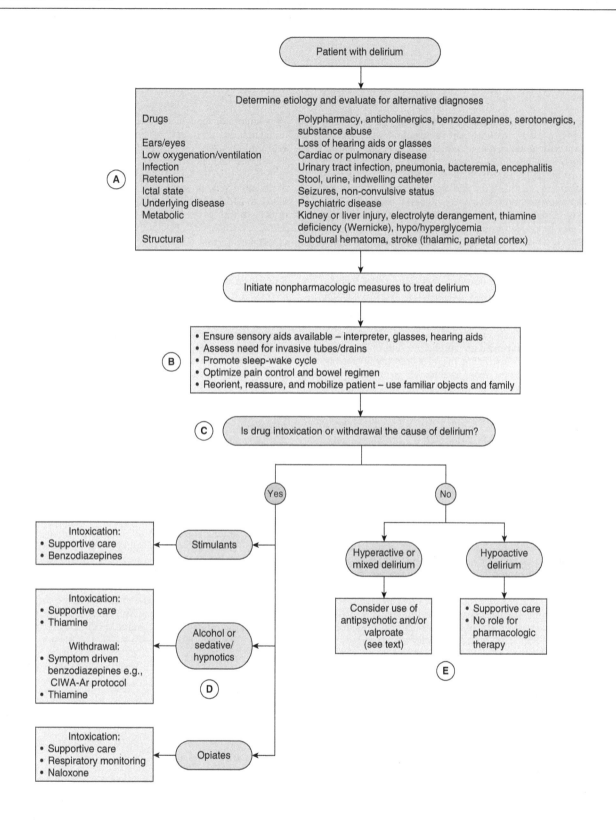

Patient with delirium

Determine etiology and evaluate for alternative diagnoses

(A)

Drugs	Polypharmacy, anticholinergics, benzodiazepines, serotonergics, substance abuse
Ears/eyes	Loss of hearing aids or glasses
Low oxygenation/ventilation	Cardiac or pulmonary disease
Infection	Urinary tract infection, pneumonia, bacteremia, encephalitis
Retention	Stool, urine, indwelling catheter
Ictal state	Seizures, non-convulsive status
Underlying disease	Psychiatric disease
Metabolic	Kidney or liver injury, electrolyte derangement, thiamine deficiency (Wernicke), hypo/hyperglycemia
Structural	Subdural hematoma, stroke (thalamic, parietal cortex)

Initiate nonpharmacologic measures to treat delirium

(B)
- Ensure sensory aids available – interpreter, glasses, hearing aids
- Assess need for invasive tubes/drains
- Promote sleep-wake cycle
- Optimize pain control and bowel regimen
- Reorient, reassure, and mobilize patient – use familiar objects and family

(C) Is drug intoxication or withdrawal the cause of delirium?

Yes / No

Stimulants
Intoxication:
- Supportive care
- Benzodiazepines

Alcohol or sedative/hypnotics
(D)
Intoxication:
- Supportive care
- Thiamine

Withdrawal:
- Symptom driven benzodiazepines e.g., CIWA-Ar protocol
- Thiamine

Opiates
Intoxication:
- Supportive care
- Respiratory monitoring
- Naloxone

Hyperactive or mixed delirium
Consider use of antipsychotic and/or valproate (see text)

Hypoactive delirium
- Supportive care
- No role for pharmacologic therapy
(E)

Coma

Jonathan Ji, Atul Kalanuria, and Joshua M. Levine

The causes of coma are varied and include a number of immediately life-threatening conditions for which emergent intervention is necessary. Close attention to general stabilization measures is necessary for all patients with coma. Simultaneously, laboratory studies should be sent and a brief history obtained from bystanders, family, and emergency medical first responders. At times the etiology of coma is obvious or known, such as traumatic brain injury or witnessed drug overdose. When the cause of coma is unknown, initial therapy is often empiric. Causes of coma may be divided into primary brain disorders and systemic disorders that secondarily cause brain dysfunction. Primary brain disorders may be structural, such as pontine infarction, large intracerebral hemorrhage, or hydrocephalus; or nonstructural, such as seizures or encephalitis. Examples of systemic disorders that cause coma include shock (e.g., from sepsis or hemorrhage), exposure to toxins or drugs (e.g., pesticides, opiates), and severe metabolic derangements (e.g., hypoglycemia).

A. Coma is frequently accompanied by respiratory and/or hemodynamic instability. Initial resuscitation includes securing an airway (usually with an endotracheal tube), mechanical ventilation, and hemodynamic support. Laboratory evaluation includes serum glucose, electrolytes, liver and thyroid function tests, ammonia, osmolality, blood count, arterial blood gas, and toxicology testing.

B. A focused clinical examination includes both a neurologic assessment ("coma exam") and a systemic survey. The coma examination focuses on level of arousal, cranial nerve function—especially the pupils and position of the eyes—and the motor examination with particular attention to motor asymmetry and abnormal reflexive movements (posturing). The goal of the initial neurologic examination is to help determine whether the coma is due to (1) brainstem dysfunction or a large focal hemispheric lesion (in which case a structural lesion is more likely) or (2) to bihemispheric dysfunction (in which case a systemic cause is more likely). Structural lesions may require emergent neurosurgery, whereas systemic causes typically require medical therapy. To facilitate rapid assessment and communication of severity, clinical scales such as the Glasgow Coma Scale are frequently used. A systemic survey should include full exposure of the patient and a search for etiological clues (e.g., the presence of traumatic injuries, skin temperature, needle marks suggesting intravenous drug abuse).

C. When a structural cause is suspected, emergent noncontrast head computed tomography (CT) should be performed. This will identify many intracranial catastrophes leading to coma, such as large intracerebral hemorrhage or other mass lesions leading to herniation and acute hydrocephalus. Diffuse cerebral edema is typically identifiable on head CT, though in a young person the changes may not be as obvious as in older patients. Posterior reversible encephalopathy syndrome sufficient to cause coma is usually apparent on head CT, though better defined on brain magnetic resonance imaging (MRI).

D. Two important though infrequent causes of coma often missed on initial noncontrast head CT are basilar thrombosis and deep cerebral vein thrombosis. In the case of basilar thrombosis, it often takes 12–24 hours for ischemic changes consistent with infarction to be visible in the posterior circulation. Deep cerebral vein thrombosis may cause bi-thalamic venous edema and infarction, but this also may take hours to appear on CT, or the signs may be subtle and symmetric causing them to be unappreciated. CT angiography will rapidly and accurately identify basilar thrombosis, and CT venography deep cerebral vein thrombosis.

E. When coma is of unknown etiology, initial therapy is usually empiric. Empiric measures might include the following: (1) hyperventilation if elevated intracranial pressure is suspected; (2) administration of naloxone (0.4–2 mg SC/IM/IV every 2–3 minutes as needed) to address possible opiate intoxication; (3) gastric lavage with activated charcoal if recent medication overdose is suspected; (4) antibiotic administration if meningitis, encephalitis, or sepsis is suspected; and (5) administration of thiamine (500 mg IV tid × 3 days, then 250 mg IV/IM daily × 5 days) followed by glucose (75 mL of 20% glucose or 150 mL of 10% glucose IV) to treat possible thiamine deficiency and hypoglycemia, respectively. In the setting of significant thiamine depletion, glucose may precipitate acute thiamine deficiency, so thiamine should be given first. Severe thiamine deficiency causes Wernicke encephalopathy, which classically presents with confusion, ataxia, and ophthalmoplegia, but in its extreme form may manifest as coma.

F. The etiology of coma is sometimes known or obvious. Whether neuroimaging is indicated depends on the specific etiology. For example, in the case of traumatic brain injury, neuroimaging is mandatory to determine if the patient requires immediate surgery, whereas in the case of cardiac arrest, neuroimaging might be deferred. When indicated, noncontrast head CT is usually the initial study, given speed of acquisition compared to MRI.

G. Further testing might include lumbar puncture for cerebrospinal fluid analysis, electroencephalography to assess for status epilepticus, or further neuroimaging (e.g., brain MRI).

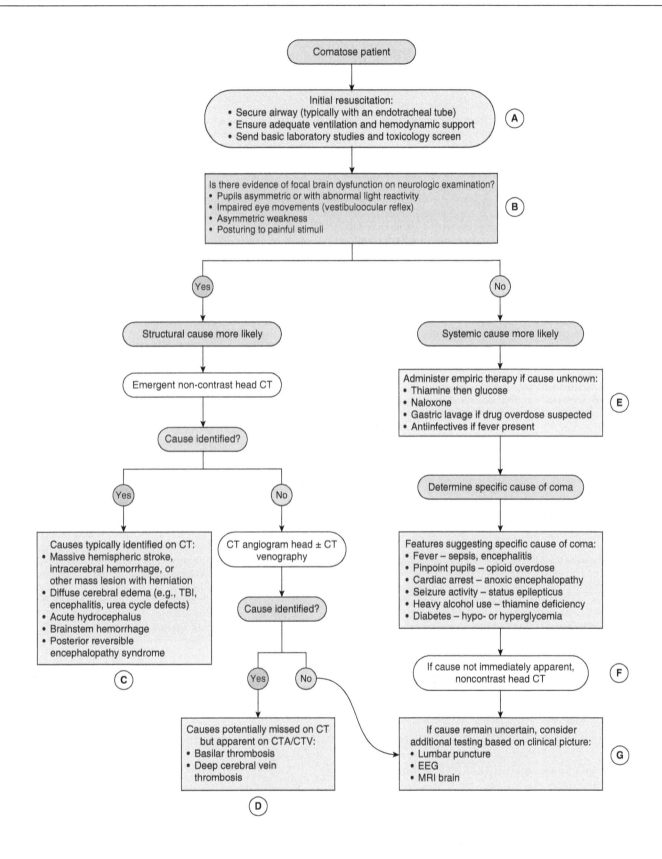

Transient Visual Loss

Ali G. Hamedani

Transient visual loss that has resolved by the time of presentation is often challenging to evaluate, as the examination is often normal, and both benign and dangerous etiologies are possible.

A. A first step is to distinguish between structures that refract and focus light (the cornea and lens) and those that sense light (retina) and carry and process visual information (optic nerves, chiasm, tracts, visual cortex). Ocular surface disease (e.g., corneal dryness, abrasions, or edema) is typically experienced as blurring, haziness, or fogging of vision without overt vision loss. Here, light reaches the retina, but the image projected on the retina is out of focus. In contrast, diseases of the retina, optic nerve, or other visual pathway structures are more likely to be experienced as darkening or loss of vision. Additionally, ocular surface disease usually results in diffuse blurring of vision. A history of distinctly focal visual symptoms such as isolated central, altitudinal, or hemianopic blurring would be atypical for ocular surface disease and increases suspicion for a neurologic process.

B. Uhthoff phenomenon, which refers to fluctuation of neurologic symptoms associated with changes in body temperature in patients with multiple sclerosis, was first described in optic neuritis. An increase in body temperature, such as with a hot shower or exercise, transiently decreases myelin conduction through an affected optic nerve, causing transient visual symptoms.

C. During eye movement, the position of the optic nerve head within the orbit shifts from one side to the other. If there is an intraorbital mass lesion, this movement may cause transient stretching and compression of the optic nerve, which may be experienced as gaze-evoked vision loss. Magnetic resonance imaging (MRI) of the orbits should be performed for evaluation.

D. Transient binocular vision loss can indicate simultaneous bilateral retinal or optic nerve dysfunction or unilateral or bilateral occipital lobe dysfunction. Transient visual obscurations due to papilledema are an example of the former. Retinal and optic nerve perfusion pressure is dependent on both intraocular and intracranial pressure; as either of these increase, retinal and optic nerve perfusion decreases and can be sufficiently impaired to cause transient vision loss. The same principle underlies the vision loss that is experienced during presyncope, which is thought to be due to transient bilateral retinal ischemia caused by a drop in arterial pressure. Rarely, an embolus to the distal basilar artery may obstruct flow to both posterior cerebral arteries, causing transient diffuse visual loss. There are usually other accompanying neurologic symptoms in this scenario.

E. When considering transient visual phenomena of cortical origin, a helpful distinction is between those that cause positive symptoms (photopsias and other visual hallucinations) and those that cause purely negative symptoms (vision loss). Positive visual phenomena are more likely to accompany migraine or occipital lobe seizures, whereas pure loss of vision is more common with occipital lobe ischemia. This distinction is not, however, completely reliable.

F. Retinal migraine is a rare cause of transient monocular visual phenomena, both positive and negative, and is typically associated with headache. The exact mechanism is uncertain, and the diagnosis itself as distinct from classic migraine with aura is somewhat controversial. Often there are multiple recurrent attacks. Carotid dissection can cause retinal ischemia and present with transient monocular visual loss; headache, neck pain, and an ipsilateral Horner syndrome are common symptoms of dissection. Given the risk of potentially catastrophic stroke, a high level of suspicion should exist for this entity. Diagnosis can be made with MRI or computed tomography angiography. Carotid ultrasound is not sufficient to exclude dissection, as it often affects the distal cervical carotid artery, outside the field of view of ultrasound.

G. Giant cell arteritis affects older patients and can cause transient retinal ischemia, though fixed deficits (ischemic optic neuropathy, retinal artery occlusion) are more common. Headache, scalp tenderness, jaw claudication, and constitutional symptoms are often present. The sedimentation rate is usually markedly elevated. Prompt administration of steroids is critical for preventing further vision loss.

H. The term *amaurosis fugax* is synonymous with a transient ischemic attack of the retina, which may be due to carotid stenosis or cardioembolism. Symptoms are often described as being similar to a shade coming down over the eye. Vascular and cardiac imaging should be performed, and appropriate antithrombotic therapy started. If high-grade atherosclerotic carotid stenosis is present, revascularization should be undertaken as soon as feasible. When multiple recurrent attacks of transient monocular visual loss occur with normal cardiac and vascular testing, vasospasm should be considered. These patients often respond to calcium channel blockers.

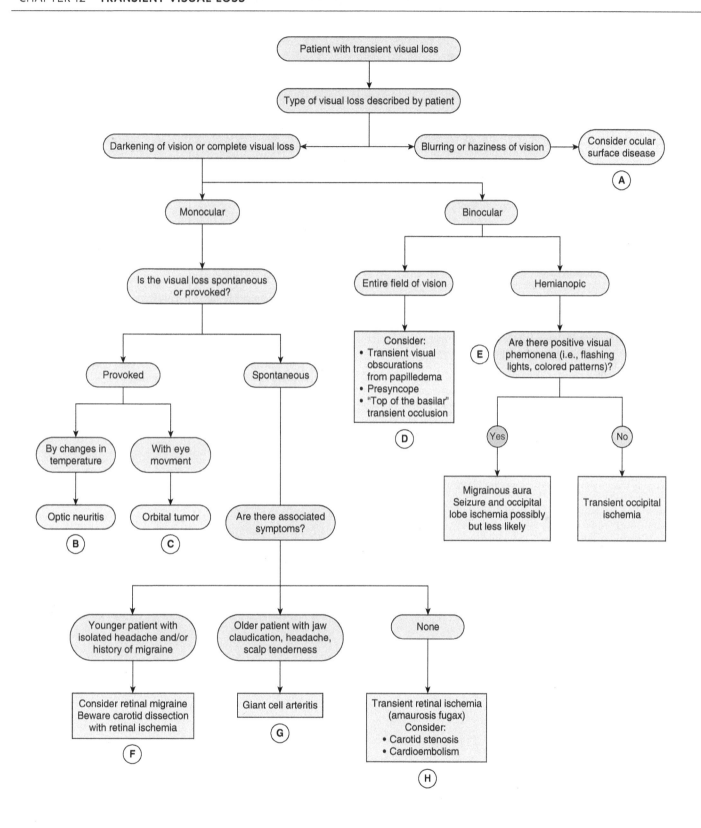

13 Visual Field Loss

Ali G. Hamedani

A. The visual fields for the right and left eye have significant but not complete overlap with one another. Because the temporal visual field for each eye is larger than its nasal field, there is a portion of the visual field at the horizontal extremes—the "temporal crescent"—served by the temporal field of one eye but extending beyond the nasal field of the other eye. An anterior occipital lesion may therefore produce a monocular visual field defect affecting the temporal crescent in the eye contralateral to the lesion.

B. At the optic chiasm, fibers from the nasal aspect of the optic nerves (which subserve the temporal visual fields of each eye) decussate and continue in the contralateral optic tracts. Lesions of the optic chiasm, especially when compressive, tend to affect these crossing fibers at the center of the chiasm first, resulting in a bitemporal hemianopia. Note that because fibers in the superior aspect of the optic nerve and chiasm represent the inferior visual fields and vice versa, compression of the optic chiasm from below produces an upper bitemporal hemianopia (often seen with pituitary adenomas), whereas compression from above produces a lower bitemporal hemianopia (as seen, for instance, with craniopharyngiomas).

C. An afferent pupillary defect may be seen in optic tract lesions, usually ipsilateral to the side of field loss and thus contralateral to the optic tract lesion. The temporal visual field (served by the nasal fibers of the optic nerve) is larger than the nasal visual field (served by the temporal fibers of the optic nerve). This leads to a relative overrepresentation of the nasal optic nerve fibers within the optic tract—that is, since only the nasal fibers decussate at the chiasm, the optic tract contains a greater proportion of nasal fibers from the contralateral eye than it does temporal fibers from the ipsilateral eye. Therefore, in an optic tract lesion, there can be more pupillary constriction when light is shone in the ipsilateral eye (since only the temporal fibers have been affected) than in the contralateral eye (since more nasal fibers have been affected), resulting in a contralateral afferent pupillary defect. Hemianopias due to optic tract lesions also tend to be incongruous (one eye is affected more than the other).

D. Macular sparing is occasionally seen in ischemic stroke affecting the occipital lobe and reflects the fact that blood supply to the occipital pole is variable and may be from branches of either the middle or posterior cerebral arteries. While not always present in hemianopia due to occipital lobe lesions, when present it is highly localizing.

E. Quadrantanopsias due to occipital lobe lesions tend to respect the horizontal meridian, whereas those due to lesions of the temporal radiations typically do not extend fully to the horizontal meridian, and those due to lesions of the parietal radiations can extend past the horizontal meridian.

F. The lateral geniculate nucleus consists of the medial horn, lateral horn, and hilum. The medial and lateral horns are supplied by the anterior choroidal artery (a branch of the internal carotid artery) and the hilum is supplied by the lateral choroidal artery (a branch of the posterior cerebral artery). Anterior choroidal artery infarctions can result in a quadruple quadrantanopsia, and lateral choroidal artery infarctions in a horizontal sectoranopia.

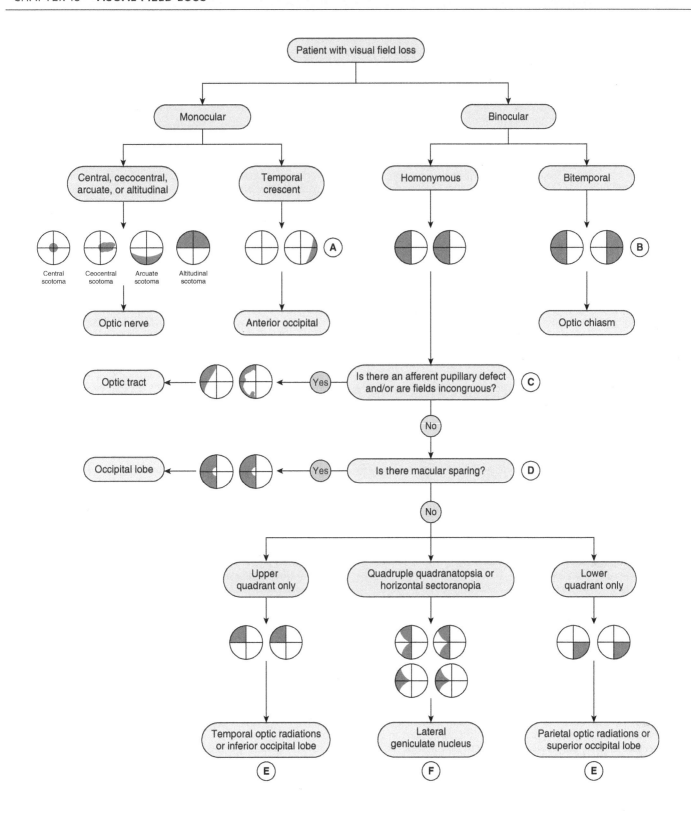

Visual Hallucinations

Ali G. Hamedani

A. While technically not a hallucination but rather a distortion of an otherwise real image, metamorphopsia is a particular type of visual disturbance characterized by wavy or warped vision. It is tested using an Amsler grid, during which patients are asked if a grid with straight lines appears wavy or distorted. Metamorphopsia most commonly localizes to the macula (e.g., age-related macular degeneration, central serous chorioretinopathy, epiretinal membrane) but can also occur transiently in migraine.

B. Scheerer's phenomenon is experienced as small bright dots arcing across the visual field, often temporally to nasally. They are most often experienced when looking against a light background, for instance a clear blue sky, and are thought to represent leukocytes traveling through the retinal circulation. Purkinje figures are generated by the retinal vasculature casting a shadow on the photoreceptor layer of the retina in response to bright light. Flick and pressure phosphenes are brief flashes of light that arise due to mechanical stimulation of the outer retina, either by eye movement or manual pressure on the globes, respectively.

C. Pathologic photopsias commonly occur in vitreoretinal disease due to mechanical irritation or inflammation of the outer retina, which causes signals to be transmitted to the optic nerve in the absence of direct stimulation by light. As such, a sudden increase in flashes or floaters, especially if monocular, is concerning for retinal detachment and should always be evaluated with dilated fundus examination. When severe eye pain is present, acute angle-closure glaucoma should also be considered and is also an ophthalmic emergency; it may be precipitated by medications commonly prescribed by neurologists, such as topiramate. Acute idiopathic blind spot enlargement comprises a group of autoimmune retinopathies characterized by enlargement of the physiologic blind spot, which may be accompanied by mild optic disc edema. It is distinguished from optic neuritis and other optic neuropathies by prominent symptoms of photopsias out of proportion to vision loss.

D. Release hallucinations refer to visual hallucinations that occur in the context of vision loss, due to either ocular, pregeniculate, or retrogeniculate visual pathway lesions. While the genesis of hallucinations is complex and incompletely understood, one hypothesis is that they represent an imbalance between internal and external visual stimuli. Under normal conditions, the brain relies on external visual stimulation to suppress internal (cortically generated) visual percepts. When vision loss occurs, external stimulation is decreased, and internal visual stimuli fill in those areas in which vision is lacking. Charles Bonnet syndrome refers to visual hallucinations occurring in older individuals with ophthalmic disease, often age-related macular degeneration. They are classically thought to have normal cognition and insight into the unreal nature of their hallucinations, though some of these traditional diagnostic criteria have been questioned.

E. Peduncular hallucinosis occurs due to midbrain lesions, often ischemic and with associated ocular motor abnormalities. The patient typically experiences vivid, complex imagery and may or may not have insight into their unreal nature. The mechanism of peduncular hallucinosis is unclear but is thought to represent abnormal regulation of rapid eye movement (REM) sleep centers in the reticular activating system—essentially, dream-like imagery from REM sleep intruding into wakefulness. Cognitive and sleep disturbances may also be present.

F. Palinopsia refers to the persistence of a visual percept after its object is no longer present. Examples include continuing to see a person even though he or she has already left the room, seeing a string of objects behind an object that is moving, and superimposing part of one image (e.g., a man's beard) onto other images (e.g., the face of a person who has no beard). Central polyopia is the multiplication of objects within an image. It is the rare cause of monocular diplopia due to neurologic disease. Both occur in the setting of parietooccipital lesions or hallucinogenic drug exposure and likely exist on a similar spectrum.

G. The content of formed visual hallucinations in neuropsychiatric disease does not readily distinguish between specific etiologies, but the presence of accompanying symptoms and signs is of great diagnostic value. For example, parkinsonism or cognitive impairment would suggest an underlying neurodegenerative disorder such as Lewy body disease or Alzheimer disease, whereas delusions and disordered thought would be more consistent with a primary psychotic disorder. Note that in Parkinson disease and Lewy body disease, visual hallucinations may initially occur in the relative absence of overt cognitive impairment and with preserved insight; they may also be triggered or exacerbated by dopaminergic therapy such as dopamine agonists. Visual hallucinations in narcolepsy typically occur as the patient is falling asleep (hypnagogic hallucinations) or awakening from sleep (hypnapompic hallucinations); there may also be a history of sleep paralysis or cataplexy. Multiple drugs may precipitate visual hallucinations, particularly illicit drugs such as LSD, psilocybin, and mescaline; hallucinations are also seen with drug and alcohol withdrawal.

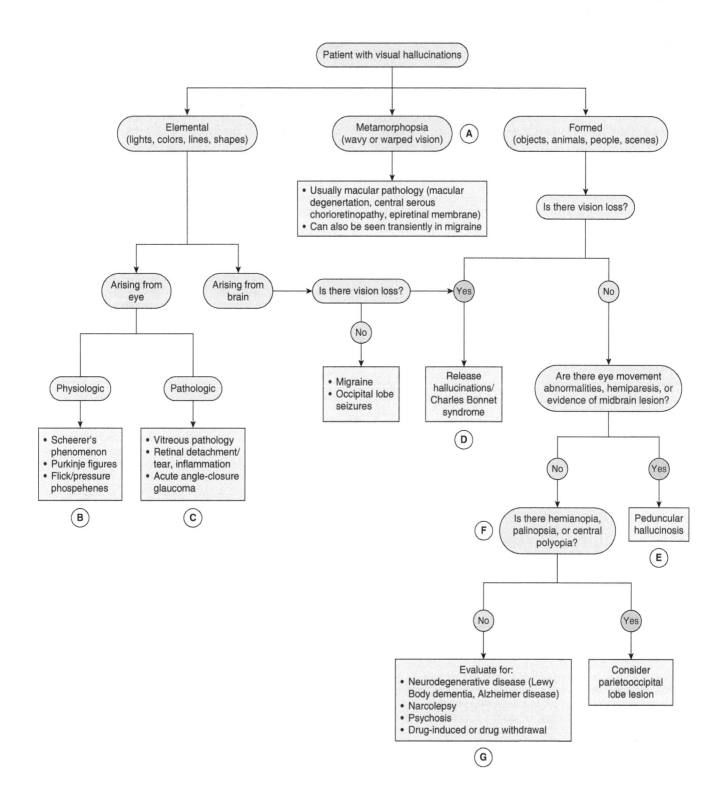

Ptosis

Ali G. Hamedani

The primary muscle of eyelid elevation is the levator palpebrae (LP), which is innervated by the oculomotor nerve. A secondary muscle (the superior tarsal) is innervated by oculosympathetic nerve fibers arising from the superior cervical ganglion and produces a small amount of eyelid opening that varies with level of arousal and sympathetic tone. The primary muscle of eyelid closure is the orbicularis oculi, which is innervated by the facial nerve.

A. Initial evaluation should focus on determining if the patient has true ptosis or a ptosis mimic. Eyelid edema and anatomical variants of eye position can give the erroneous impression of ptosis. Facial weakness, such as that seen with Bell palsy, results in an abnormally widened palpebral fissure due to orbicularis weakness. This can give the mistaken impression of contralateral ptosis. Conversely, orbicularis overaction, such as that seen with hemifacial spasm, causes narrowing of the palpebral fissure, but this is not considered ptosis, as the eyelid closure is active, not passive. Eyelid-opening apraxia is a disorder of voluntary eyelid opening of supranuclear origin often seen in progressive supranuclear palsy and other neurodegenerative disorders. Reflexive eyelid opening is normal, and patients can often sustain eyelid opening after briefly elevating their eyelids manually, distinguishing this from true ptosis. A similar phenomenon can be seen with nondominant hemispheric stroke. Hering's law of equal innervation refers to the fact that an increase in activity of one levator muscle is accompanied by an obligatory increase in activity of the other levator muscle. This is explained by the fact that both muscles are innervated by a single midbrain nucleus. In cases of unilateral primary eyelid retraction (e.g., thyroid eye disease, dorsal midbrain syndrome), eyelid opening decreases in order to minimize eyelid retraction, but because both LP muscles relax, contralateral pseudoptosis occurs. Hering's law also underlies the phenomena of curtaining (with manual lifting of one eyelid, the other lid comes down or "curtains").

B. Eyelid excursion is the distance the upper eyelid margin travels between downgaze and upgaze. It reflects LP function. Reduced eyelid excursion (<12 mm) indicates levator weakness due to a neurogenic, myogenic, or neuromuscular junction process. In contrast, preserved eyelid excursion (≥12 mm) suggests that levator function is normal and that ptosis is due to other causes.

C. Levator dehiscence-disinsertion is the most common cause of acquired ptosis in adults. It occurs when the LP dehisces from its attachment on the upper eyelid and reinserts more proximally. The lid crease, visualized as a horizontal skin crease on the upper eyelid in downgaze, is defined by the insertion of the LP on the upper eyelid. When the levator dehisces and reinserts more proximally, the lid crease is heightened. Because the levator muscle itself is otherwise normal, eyelid excursion is preserved. Levator dehiscence-disinsertion commonly occurs with advancing age but can be accelerated by repetitive eyelid trauma (e.g., eye rubbing, contact lens wear).

D. Orbicularis strength can be tested by asking the patient to forcefully close their eyes while the examiner attempts to manually open them.

E. Horner syndrome is caused by lesions of the oculosympathetic pathway extending from the hypothalamus to the lower cervical and upper thoracic spinal cord, chain, superior cervical ganglion, and internal carotid artery. Causes include brainstem (e.g., lateral medullary infarction) and spinal cord lesions, apical lung tumors (Pancoast syndrome), and carotid dissection. Ptosis in Horner syndrome is mild and accompanied by miosis (pupillary constriction) and anhidrosis.

F. In addition to the LP, the oculomotor nerve also innervates multiple extraocular muscles (superior, inferior, and medial recti and inferior oblique) and the pupillary sphincter. Therefore, ptosis due to a third nerve palsy is typically accompanied by ophthalmoparesis and sometimes pupillary dilation. Pupillary involvement in a third nerve palsy is more frequently seen in compressive etiologies because the pupillary fibers are located more superficially than the oculomotor fibers and are thus the first to be affected in extrinsic compression. Myasthenia gravis does not affect pupillary function but does cause ophthalmoparesis and can do so in a pattern that may mimic any cranial nerve, nuclear, or internuclear eye movement disorder. Thus, myasthenia gravis should be considered in the differential diagnosis of a pupil-sparing third nerve palsy.

G. Myasthenia gravis is an autoimmune disorder of neuromuscular transmission. Ptosis and diplopia are extremely common symptoms, classically occurring later in the day with fatigue. About half of patients present with purely ocular symptoms. Of patients presenting with ocular disease, over half will eventually develop axial and limb weakness, usually within 2–3 years of diagnosis. Acetylcholine receptor antibodies are present in only about half of patients with ocular myasthenia gravis, so nerve conduction studies with repetitive stimulation or single fiber electromyography may be needed to confirm the diagnosis. Most inherited and acquired myopathies spare the eyelids due to histologic differences in the extraocular muscles compared to other skeletal muscles. Notable exceptions include mitochondrial disease (chronic progressive external ophthalmoplegia), myotonic dystrophy, and oculopharyngeal muscular dystrophy. Ptosis in myopathies is almost always symmetric, whereas in myasthenia it may be symmetric or asymmetric.

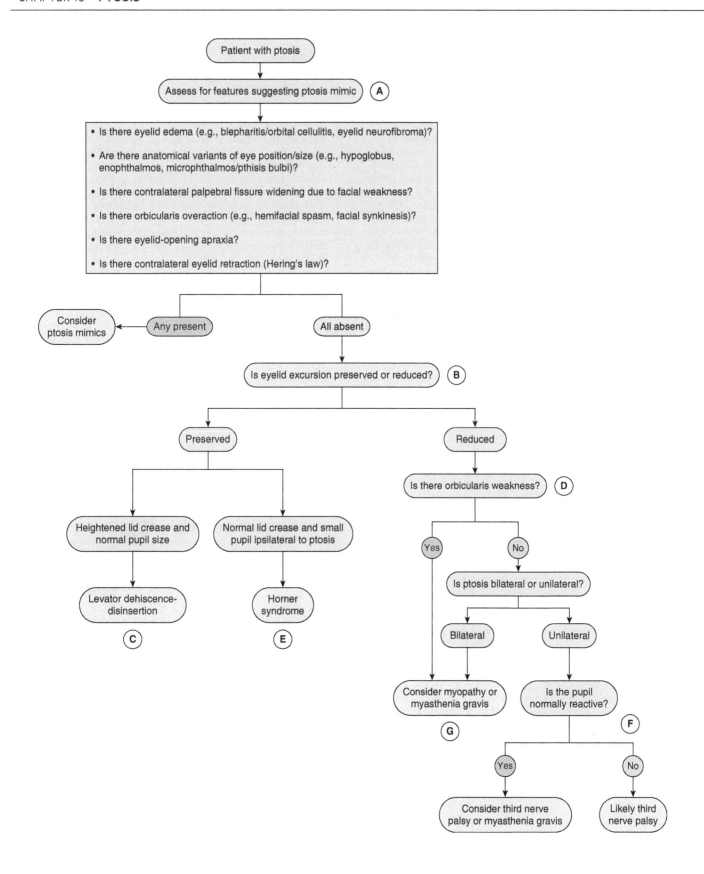

Pupillary Asymmetry (Anisocoria)

Ali G. Hamedani

Anisocoria refers to asymmetry in pupillary diameter between the two eyes. When pathologic, anisocoria indicates a disorder of pupillary constriction or dilation. If the disorder is of pupillary constriction, the larger pupil is abnormal, since it does not constrict as well to light. If the problem is of pupillary dilation, the smaller pupil is abnormal, as it has dilated less than the other pupil. To distinguish between these, the size of the pupils should be assessed in both dark and light. If the size difference between the pupils increases in dark, it suggests that the smaller pupil did not adequately dilate, since maximal dilation should occur in dark. However, if anisocoria is more prominent in light, it indicates that the larger pupil did not adequately constrict to light. If the difference in pupillary diameter is equal in both light and dark, it indicates physiologic anisocoria, which is a normally occurring phenomenon. Note that an afferent visual process (e.g., optic neuropathy) should not cause anisocoria when both pupils are observed under the same degree of lighting.

A. Horner syndrome is caused by lesions of the oculosympathetic pathway extending from the hypothalamus to the lower cervical and upper thoracic spinal cord, sympathetic chain, superior cervical ganglion, and along the internal carotid artery. Because sympathetic fibers innervate the iris dilator and result in pupillary dilation, Horner syndrome causes a pupil that dilates incompletely in dark, resulting in anisocoria that is greater in dark than light, with the smaller, constricted pupil being the abnormal one. The oculosympathetic pathway also innervates the tarsal muscles of the eyelid, and thus ptosis is also typically present in Horner syndrome. Diagnosis can be confirmed by apraclonidine or cocaine eyedrop testing. Apraclonidine is a weak sympathomimetic, but in Horner syndrome there is upregulation of postsynaptic receptors on the iris dilator resulting in denervation hypersensitivity; therefore, apraclonidine will dilate a Horner pupil more than a normal pupil, thus reversing the anisocoria. In contrast, cocaine is a norepinephrine reuptake inhibitor and dilates a normal pupil but not a Horner pupil, thereby accentuating the anisocoria.

B. The pupils constrict under two circumstances: (1) when light enters the eye (pupillary light reflex), and (2) when attempting to view a target at near, such as when reading (near response). Light-near dissociation refers to a pupil that does not constrict to light but does constrict to near. Tonic pupil is the most common cause of unilateral light-near dissociation (see section C). Other causes of light-near dissociation include severe retinal or optic nerve disease (differentiated pupil), dorsal midbrain lesions (Parinaud syndrome), aberrant regeneration of a third nerve palsy (pupillary sphincter becomes reinnervated by oculomotor rather than pupillomotor fibers and constricts during attempted adduction rather than to light), and Argyll-Robertson pupils (classically described in syphilis but also seen in diabetes).

C. Tonic pupil is caused by a lesion of the ciliary ganglion. Because the fibers for the pupillary light reflex synapse at the ciliary ganglion whereas the fibers for the near response pass through but do not synapse in it, tonic pupil is often characterized by light-near dissociation. There is also delayed redilation following pupillary constriction to near. Tonic pupil is typically idiopathic and thought to be postviral or autoimmune. When bilateral and accompanied by areflexia, it is termed Adie syndrome. Other causes include local orbital processes and autonomic neuropathy (e.g., diabetes, amyloidosis, multiple systems atrophy). Over time, a tonic pupil may become smaller than the unaffected pupil.

D. Pupillary involvement is more likely to occur with compressive rather than vasculopathic or other intrinsic processes affecting the oculomotor nerve because the parasympathetic fibers responsible for pupillary constriction are located superficially along the outside of the nerve, whereas the fibers that innervate the levator palpebrae and extraocular muscles are located more internally. Potential causes include an ipsilateral mass lesion (e.g., tumor, aneurysm) or uncal herniation.

E. Pharmacologic pupillary dilation (mydriasis) occurs most commonly due to antimuscarinic agents that block the neuromuscular junction at the pupillary sphincter. Sympathomimetics also cause mydriasis. This may be intentional due to the instillation of mydriatic eyedrops or unintentional due to accidental ocular contact with anticholinergics (e.g., inhaled ipratropium, scopolamine patch). Mechanical causes of impaired pupillary constriction include iris trauma or tears, adhesions between the iris and cornea (anterior synechiae) or lens (posterior synechiae), and acute angle-closure glaucoma; these are associated with other abnormalities on slit lamp biomicroscopy.

Tonic pupil, third nerve palsy, and pharmacologic pupil can also be distinguished using eyedrop testing with pilocarpine, a muscarinic agonist. One drop of dilute pilocarpine (0.125%) is instilled in each eye. The normal response is to not constrict, as this concentration is too low to cause physiologic pupillary constriction. However, if the larger pupil constricts, it indicates a tonic pupil that has experienced denervation hypersensitivity (upregulation of postsynaptic receptors) and is therefore able to constrict in response to small amounts of pilocarpine. If there is no constriction to low-dose pilocarpine, then one drop of high-dose (1%) pilocarpine is used. If the larger pupil constricts, it indicates a third nerve palsy. If there is no constriction, it indicates a pharmacologic or mechanical pupil that is incapable of constriction due to saturation of postsynaptic receptors by a muscarinic antagonist or a structural abnormality of the pupillary sphincter.

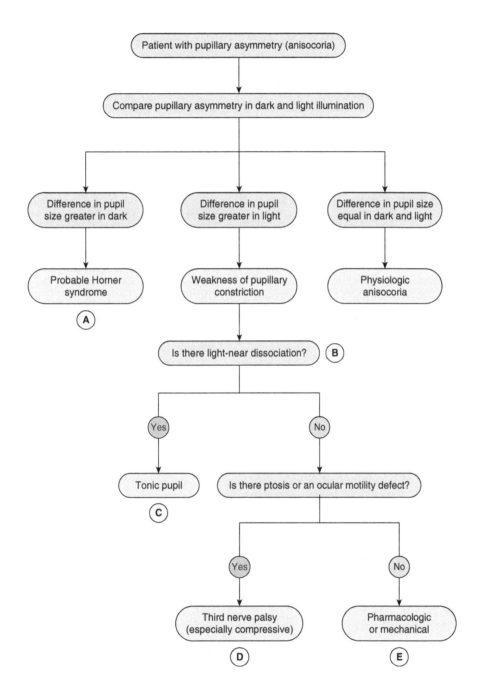

Diplopia

Ali G. Hamedani

A. Diplopia is the visual symptom of "double vision," in which a single object appears as two separate images. With the exception of central polyopia, which is exceedingly rare, diplopia due to neurologic disease is always binocular. Due to ocular misalignment from brainstem, cranial nerve, neuromuscular junction, or extraocular muscle disease, the two eyes are pointed at different targets and thus see two different images, which are perceived as double vision. These symptoms resolve when either eye is covered, as with only one eye open there is only one image to see. Very subtle ocular misalignment can cause two images to overlap so much that they are not perceived as discrete images but rather as a single blurry image that resolves when either eye is covered (binocular blur). In contrast, diplopia due to ophthalmic disease persists when the unaffected eye is covered and represents an intrinsic ocular process that is causing two images to be projected onto the same retina.

B. Ocular motor function can be evaluated by assessing ocular motility and ocular alignment. Ocular motility assesses eye movement in different directions of gaze. If movement is clearly limited in one or more directions, the lesion can often be localized based on the pattern of extraocular muscles that are affected. However, a patient with binocular diplopia may appear to have full extraocular motility, either because the degree of extraocular muscle weakness is very subtle or because the disorder is one of gaze-holding, whereby the eyes are misaligned but the extraocular muscles themselves function normally. In this case, testing ocular alignment is helpful, most commonly with the alternating eye cover test. The patient is asked to fixate on a single target as the examiner alternates covering either eye. If the eyes are normally aligned, each remains steadily fixated on the target, and there are no refixation eye movements. If the eyes are misaligned, refixation movements will be observed during alternate eye covering.

C. If ocular misalignment worsens in one direction of gaze and improves in the other, it is referred to as *incomitant*. This suggests subtle specific extraocular muscle weakness. In contrast, if ocular misalignment is *comitant*, that is, equal in different directions of gaze, this argues against weakness of any particular extraocular muscle and suggests decompensation of a congenital strabismus or an acquired gaze-holding disorder.

D. The primary function of the superior oblique muscle, innervated by the fourth cranial nerve, is incyclorotation of the eye (rotation of the globe inward such that the superior aspect becomes displaced nasally and the inferior aspect rotates temporally), and its secondary function is depression. Because it is a relatively weak depressor, fourth nerve palsies are generally characterized by full ocular motility, and alignment testing is important for diagnosis. Vertical misalignment in a fourth nerve palsy (where the affected eye is the higher eye) increases in contralateral gaze and with ipsilateral head tilt. Many patients with fourth nerve palsy will have a visible contralateral head tilt as a means to correct for the ocular misalignment.

E. Third nerve palsies may be complete or partial, affecting some muscles more than others. A vertical misalignment that changes in upgaze and downgaze (one eye is lower than the other in upgaze but higher than the other in downgaze), even with full ocular motility, can indicate a third nerve palsy. Pupillary involvement may be present or absent and is more likely to occur with compressive lesions due to the somatotopic organization of the oculomotor nerve. Not all third nerve palsies need be "down and out."

F. A skew deviation refers to a vertical misalignment due to an intrinsic brainstem lesion in the pathway responsible for maintaining tonic vertical eye position in response to head tilt. The localization of a skew deviation follows the "high-high, low-low" rule: if one eye is higher than the other, the lesion may be higher (midbrain) on the side of the high eye, or lower (pontomedullary junction) on the side of the low eye. Skew deviations are distinguished from fourth nerve palsies by their comitance (since no one cranial nerve nucleus is affected, the misalignment is generally equal in different directions of gaze).

G. Decompensated exotropia and esotropias are horizontal misalignments that present early in life. Their precise cause is unknown, but they are thought to represent abnormal development of binocularity and gaze-holding in the brain.

H. Myasthenia gravis and thyroid eye disease can present with isolated motility defects that can mimic any nuclear or internuclear eye movement abnormality. They should be suspected if there is a history of variable symptoms or if there are associated external and eyelid findings on examination (ptosis or orbicularis weakness for myasthenia gravis; eyelid retraction, proptosis, and periorbital edema for thyroid eye disease).

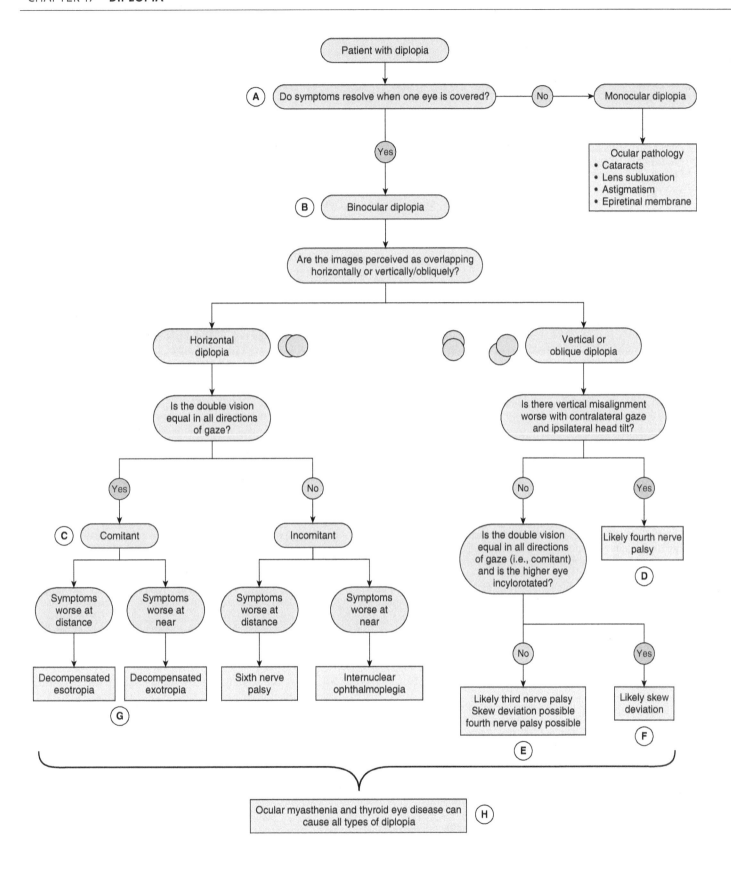

Nystagmus

Ali G. Hamedani and Raymond S. Price

A. Nystagmus is a rhythmic, biphasic, oscillatory eye movement consisting of a slow phase in one direction followed by either a fast phase (jerk nystagmus) or another slow phase (pendular nystagmus) in the opposite direction. Jerk nystagmus is named for the direction of its fast phase. For example, upbeat nystagmus refers to a pattern of slow downward drift followed by a quick upbeat saccade. Not all abnormal oscillatory eye movements are nystagmus. Some consist only of fast eye movements (e.g., opsoclonus), and others are less rhythmic than nystagmus (e.g., ocular bobbing); these are collectively known as nystagmoid eye movements.

B. The Heimann-Bielschowsky phenomenon refers to pendular vertical oscillation of one eye associated with severe vision loss in the same eye. It usually affects children or young adults with severe unilateral optic nerve disease or amblyopia but generally does not occur in older adults with acquired vision loss.

C. Dissociated abducting nystagmus is present in one eye (the abducting eye) but not the other adducting eye when the patient is looking to one side. It indicates a contralateral internuclear ophthalmoplegia (INO). For example, if the left eye has abducting nystagmus in left gaze, it is due to a right INO, and one should look for incomplete adduction of the right eye.

D. Oculopalatal tremor/myoclonus is caused by brainstem lesions, specifically within the area between the red nucleus, dentate nucleus of the cerebellum, and inferior olive (i.e., Mollaret triangle).

E. Congenital nystagmus consists of large amplitude pendular horizontal nystagmus in primary gaze and jerk nystagmus in lateral gaze. It retains a horizontal vector in upgaze, unlike most acquired forms of nystagmus (e.g., gaze-evoked nystagmus), which either disappear or acquire an upbeat waveform in upgaze. It usually presents between 2–4 months of age and can occur with or without vision loss.

F. Oculomasticatory myorrhythmia consists of slow (1–2 Hz) pendular convergent-divergent eye movements with synchronous jaw movement. It is pathognomonic for Whipple disease.

G. Seesaw nystagmus consists of repetitive cycles in which one eye elevates and intorts and the other eye depresses and extorts. Both phases may be of equal velocity, or one may be faster than the other. It localizes to the midbrain or the parasellar region.

H. Opsoclonus ("dancing eyes") refers to multidirectional fast phase (saccades) conjugate eye movements without an intersaccadic interval (a pause between individual eye movements). It is seen with the opsoclonus-myoclonus-ataxia syndrome, which is associated with viral encephalitis (e.g., West Nile virus), as an autoimmune process, or as a paraneoplastic syndrome associated with neuroblastoma in childhood and various malignancies (e.g., breast cancer, associated with anti-Ri antibodies) in adulthood.

I. Ocular bobbing is a nonrhythmic movement with a quick, large amplitude, downward ocular deviation followed by a pause and then a slow upward drift. The reverse, known as ocular dipping, can also occur. These are seen in diffuse bihemispheric dysfunction (e.g., severe toxic-metabolic encephalopathy) or large pontine lesions.

J. Convergence-retraction "nystagmus" (technically not true nystagmus, as it lacks a slow phase) occurs with dorsal midbrain lesions (i.e., Parinaud syndrome) and is typically accompanied by other pretectal signs such as pupillary light-near dissociation, vertical gaze paresis, and eyelid retraction. Co-contraction of the medial recti with other extraocular muscles results in retraction of the globes into the orbits.

K. Square-wave jerks are small horizontal saccadic intrusions that occur in primary gaze and are separated by a brief pause between each conjugate eye movement (an intersaccadic interval). More than 10–15 per minute are associated with neurodegenerative diseases such as progressive supranuclear palsy. When similar movements are variable in amplitude and occur following a visually guided saccade, consider macrosaccadic oscillations—essentially, an extreme form of the hypermetric saccades seen in cerebellar disease. Ocular flutter is distinguished by the lack of an intersaccadic interval, and has clinical implications similar to opsoclonus.

L. Nystagmus that has a rotary component without a corresponding unidirectional horizontal component (e.g., purely rotary, mixed vertical-rotary) is broadly known as central vestibular nystagmus and indicates dysfunction of the brainstem vestibular system.

M. Downbeat nystagmus, best seen in lateral gaze, typically indicates a lesion at the cervicomedullary junction. Chiari malformations are a common cause. It can also be seen in cerebellar degeneration. Upbeat nystagmus can be seen in brainstem, particularly midbrain, and cerebellar lesions.

N. A mixed horizontal-rotary jerk nystagmus typically indicates peripheral vestibular dysfunction (semicircular canals, vestibulocochlear nerve), though can be seen on occasion with lesions of the vestibular nuclei. It is unidirectional with the fast phase beating away from the affected side, retains a horizontal waveform in up and downgaze, increases when looking in the direction of the fast phase, and decreases when looking in the direction of the slow phase.

O. Periodic alternating nystagmus changes direction in cycles of 45–90 seconds. It indicates a lesion of the cerebellum and its projections to the dorsal medulla.

P. The most common type of nystagmus encountered in clinical practice is physiologic nystagmus, which is a normal finding. It consists of small amplitude horizontal nystagmus present only in extreme gaze that beats left in left gaze and right in right gaze, and extinguishes after several beats. Larger amplitude nystagmus present in both maximal and submaximal gaze that does not extinguish is gaze-evoked (sometimes called "direction-changing") nystagmus and indicates a lesion in the brainstem or cerebellum. It can also be seen with some medications (e.g., phenytoin).

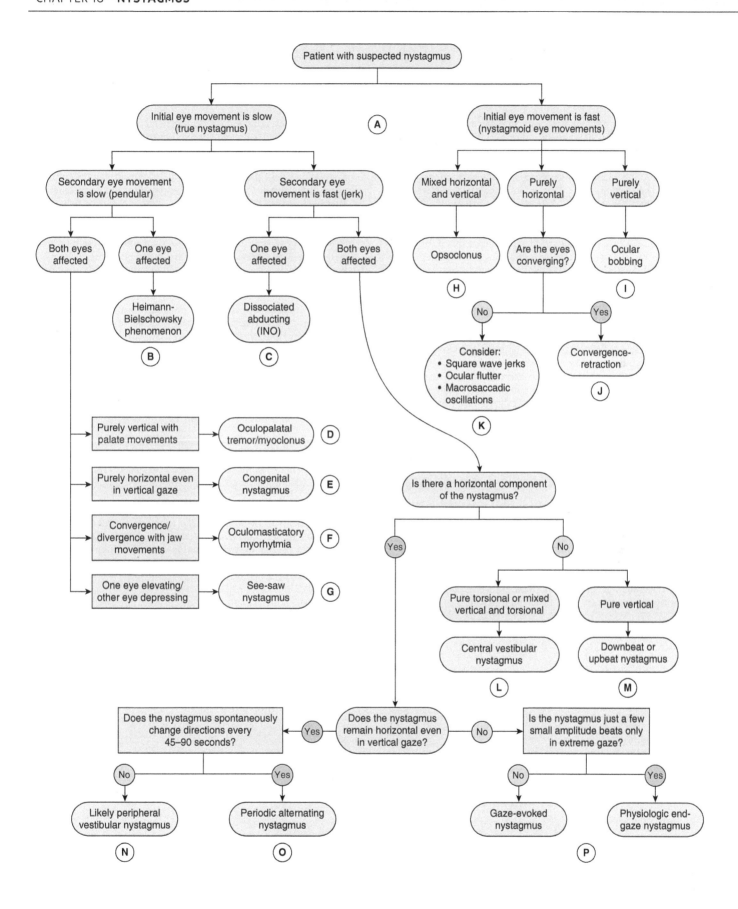

Facial Weakness

Raymond S. Price

A. The upper motor neurons that innervate the face (corticobulbar tract) originate from the primary motor cortex in the frontal lobe and travel through corona radiata and genu of the internal capsule, entering the brainstem through the cerebral peduncle and descending to the pons where they cross to synapse on the facial motor nucleus. The portion of the facial motor nucleus that elevates the forehead receives bilateral corticobulbar innervation, but the remainder of the facial motor nucleus, which controls the lower face, receives only contralateral corticobulbar innervation. This important, and clinically useful, anatomic feature means that a corticobulbar lesion on one side of the brain will cause contralateral facial weakness of the lower face, but preserved ability to elevate the forehead due to intact innervation from the ipsilateral corticobulbar tract. This defines the so-called "central" seventh nerve palsy. When present, brain imaging with magnetic resonance imaging (MRI) should be performed to identify the underlying lesion.

B. Unilateral facial weakness that involves both the lower and upper face (i.e., including the inability to elevate the forehead) is frequently referred to as a "peripheral" seventh nerve palsy, implying a lesion to the facial nerve after exiting the brainstem. Bell's palsy is the prototypical example. Note, however, that a "peripheral" seventh nerve palsy can in fact be seen with brainstem lesions that involve the ipsilateral facial motor nucleus or the axons of the facial nerve prior to exiting the brainstem (the fascicle). Given its compact organization, brainstem lesions that cause "peripheral" facial weakness are almost always associated with additional focal neurologic findings, such as hemiparesis or eye movement abnormalities.

C. All nerve roots and cranial nerves except for the olfactory nerve travel through the subarachnoid space. Therefore, any process causing inflammation in the cerebrospinal fluid contained within the subarachnoid space can lead to multiple cranial neuropathies and/or radiculopathies. Examples include infections such as Lyme disease, autoimmune diseases such as sarcoidosis, and carcinomatous meningitis. Diagnosis is made by lumbar puncture and analysis of cerebrospinal fluid.

D. Bell's palsy is an acute idiopathic peripheral facial palsy, and is by far the most common cause of peripheral facial weakness. The weakness typically develops over hours to one day. A slower onset of symptoms or continued worsening beyond 3 weeks is inconsistent with Bell's palsy and should prompt brain MRI. Infrequently, an identifiable cause of facial palsy may be found in patients with a presentations otherwise consistent with Bell's palsy. These include varicella zoster infection, Lyme disease, human immunodeficiency virus (HIV) seroconversion, syphilis, and autoimmune conditions such as sarcoidosis or Sjögren syndrome. Laboratory testing for these should be considered in the appropriate clinical scenario (see sections E and F). Acute peripheral facial palsy should be treated empirically with prednisone 60 mg daily for 5 days followed by a taper of 10 mg/day for 5 days, starting as soon as possible and ideally within 3 days of symptom onset to increase the likelihood of complete facial recovery and reduce the time to recovery. Treatment should not be delayed while awaiting any laboratory tests for known causes of an acute peripheral facial palsy. Antivirals (acyclovir and valacyclovir) do not appear to improve outcome and, unless there is suspicion for zoster, should be avoided. One consequence of peripheral facial weakness is difficulty closing the affected eye, which can lead to corneal injury. Eye care should include artificial tears and ointments at night as needed and protective glasses or a patch for patients without full eye closure.

E. Ramsay Hunt syndrome is the combination of an acute peripheral facial palsy, ear pain, and a vesicular rash on the ear, in the external auditory canal, or in the oropharynx due to zoster. Treatment is valacyclovir 1000 mg three times daily for 10 days in addition to prednisone as with Bell palsy.

F. Lyme disease can cause acute facial palsy and is an important consideration in endemic areas. Patients should be asked about tick exposure and rash, and Lyme testing done when appropriate. Provided neurologic involvement is limited to facial palsy, treatment with oral doxycycline for 14 days is reasonable.

G. Substantial, though not always complete, early improvement is seen in the vast majority of patients with Bell's palsy. If there is no improvement in the facial weakness on follow-up 4 months after onset, consider the possibility of a mass lesion and perform brain MRI.

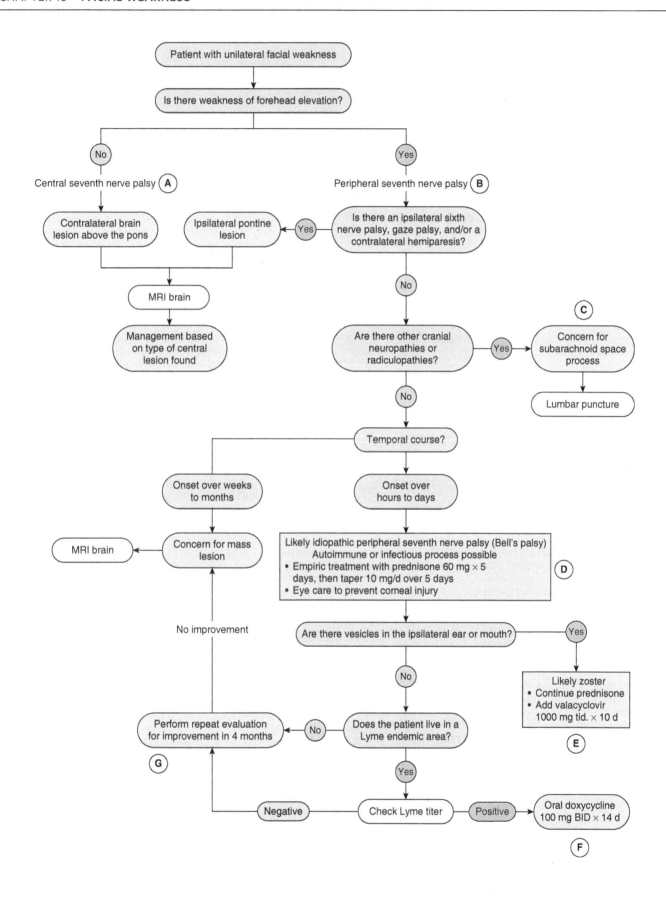

Acute Vertigo

Raymond S. Price

A. Acute continuous vertigo, with onset over seconds to hours, is a common symptom. It is often associated with nausea, vomiting, gait unsteadiness, head motion intolerance, and nystagmus. The main diagnostic distinction is between central lesions affecting the brainstem/cerebellum, such as potentially life-threatening posterior circulation stroke, and peripheral lesions, such as vestibular neuritis, which affect the vestibulocochlear nerve. Central lesions require further diagnostic evaluation and directed management of the underlying etiology. Vestibular neuritis (also referred to as vestibular neuronitis or, when associated with hearing loss, labyrinthitis) is thought due to idiopathic inflammation of the vestibular nerve, possibly related to a viral infection. Symptoms typically resolve spontaneously over time, and additional diagnostic testing is generally not necessary.

B. Distinguishing between recurrent episodes of transient vertigo and persistent, continuous vertigo requires careful, focused questioning of the patient. Patients often misunderstand this question and incorrectly report persistent symptoms either because (1) the vertigo recurs every time they move their head or (2) because between discrete attacks of vertigo they retain a vague persistent feeling of ill-defined incomplete recovery. Both these scenarios are common in benign paroxysmal positional vertigo, the most common cause of transient episodic vertigo.

C. The presence of abnormalities on the general neurologic examination may indicate involvement of brainstem structures outside of the vestibular system. Critically, it should be recognized that the general neurologic examination has poor sensitivity for identifying a central cause of vertigo; it is often normal even in patients with brainstem or cerebellar lesions.

D. In contrast to the general neurologic examination, a series of specific bedside tests of eye movement (referred to the "HINTS" examination for head impulse-nystagmus-test of skew) is highly sensitive for identification of central causes of vertigo, possibly even more sensitive than brain magnetic resonance imaging.[1] The three components of the "HINTS" examination are (1) the head impulse test (oculocephalic reflex), (2) assessing the direction of horizontal nystagmus, and (3) testing for vertical ocular alignment.

E. The classic finding in vestibular neuritis is a mixed horizontal/torsional nystagmus that beats away from the affected ear. The direction of this nystagmus remains the same regardless of which direction the eyes move. In contrast, the classic finding of a horizontal cerebellar nystagmus is nystagmus that beats in the direction of gaze, meaning there is right-beating nystagmus when the patient looks to the right and left-beating nystagmus when the patient looks to the left. This "direction changing" nystagmus thus indicates a central lesion is likely present.

F. The head impulse test assesses the horizontal oculocephalic reflex. To perform a head impulse test, the patient is asked to fixate on a target like the examiner's nose and the patient's head is rapidly moved to the right or left. A patient with an intact oculocephalic reflex will reflexively move their eyes in the opposite direction of head movement to maintain fixation. In a patient with an impaired oculocephalic reflex, their eyes will move with their head. To move their eyes back on the target, they will have a catch-up saccade in the opposite direction of the head movement. An abnormal head impulse test suggests an ipsilateral lesion in the horizontal semicircular canal, eighth cranial nerve, or the vestibular nuclei. An abnormal head impulse test is thus usually but not universally indicative of a peripheral lesion, whereas a normal head impulse test suggests a central lesion.

G. Vertical misalignment of the eyes in the setting of acute vertigo suggests a skew deviation. When the head is tilted in one direction, the eye in the direction of the head tilt must elevate and the contralateral eye must depress to maintain vertical alignment. In addition, both eyes rotate in the opposite direction of the head tilt. An injury to the peripheral or central vestibular pathway can result in a skew deviation in which the eyes are reflexively positioned as if the head is tilted even though the head is not tilted. A skew deviation is usually but not universally indicative of a central lesion.

H. The combination of normal vertical ocular alignment, direction-fixed nystagmus, and an abnormal head impulse test is considered a "benign" HINTS bedside examination, as it is consistent with a peripheral lesion such as vestibular neuritis.

I. Treatment of vestibular neuritis consists primarily of supportive care, as symptoms typically improve spontaneously. Patients with acute vestibular neuritis are often markedly uncomfortable due to vertigo, nausea, and vomiting. Benzodiazepines (such as lorazepam) or antihistamines (such as meclizine or dimenhydrinate) can be used for symptomatic relief but should generally only be used for 24–48 hours as longer use may interfere with vestibular recovery. A program of vestibular rehabilitation exercises may be beneficial for some patients. A short-course of corticosteroids is recommended by some experts to speed time to recovery, though no clear benefit has been shown in randomized trials.[2]

REFERENCES

1. Kattah JC, Talkad AV, Wang DZ, Hsieh YH, Newman-Toker DE. HINTS to diagnose stroke in the acute vestibular syndrome: three-step bedside oculomotor examination more sensitive than early MRI diffusion-weighted imaging. *Stroke.* 2009;40(11):3504–3510.
2. Fishman JM, Burgess C, Waddell A. Corticosteroids for the treatment of idiopathic acute vestibular dysfunction. *Cochrane Database Syst Rev.* 2011;5: CD008607.

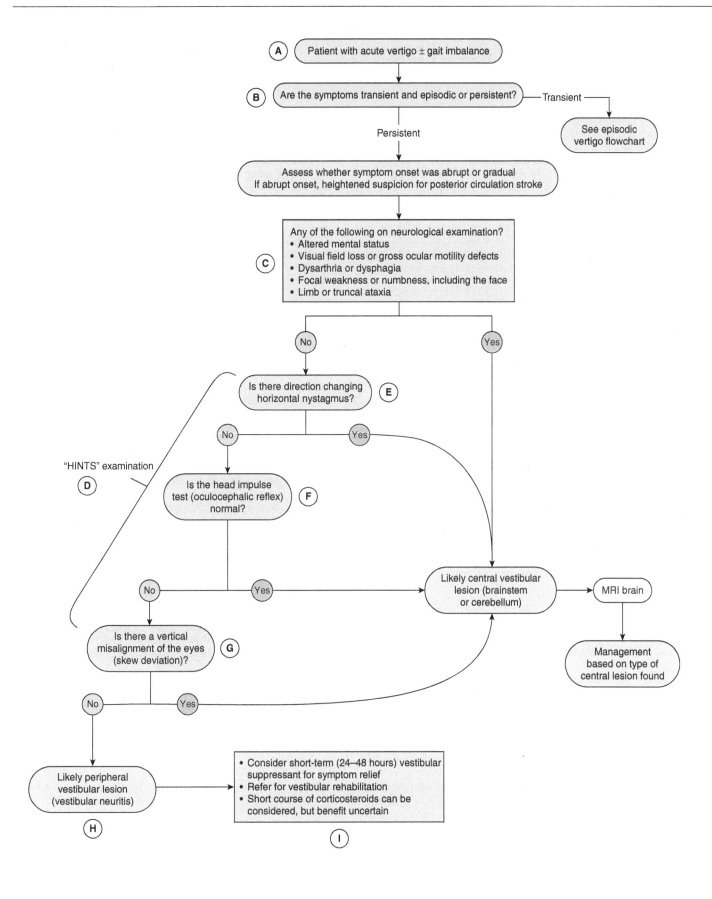

Recurrent Episodic Dizziness

Raymond S. Price and Brett L. Cucchiara

Patients use the term "dizziness" to refer to many qualitatively different symptoms. Lightheadedness, such as is seen with presyncope, gait imbalance, true vertigo, and, not uncommonly, generalized weakness or mental slowing, may all be described as dizziness. While an attempt should be made to classify a patient's complaint into one of these more precise categories, this is not always successful; patients frequently endorse more than one category or change categories on repeated questioning. Given this, when a patient reports episodic dizziness it is often more informative to ask what triggers the episodes and how long they last, as this information tends to be more reliable and is diagnostically useful. This chapter describes the approach to the patient with discrete episodes of dizziness which are consistent with vertigo, i.e., the sensation that the patient or their surrounding are moving when they are not.

A. The presence of abnormalities on the standard neurologic examination raises concern for a brainstem or cerebellar lesion or a more diffuse central nervous system process, and brain magnetic resonance imaging (MRI) is warranted. If the patient reports the presence of any transient focal neurologic symptoms concurrent with their episodes of dizziness, this is particularly concerning for posterior circulation transient ischemic attack (TIA) and imaging of the posterior circulation with MR angiography should be considered. Importantly, the neurologic examination can be normal even in patients with brainstem or cerebellar lesions, and episodic vertigo with no other associated symptoms can occur with posterior circulation TIA. A high level of vigilance is thus required.

B. The most common cause of brief (<1 minute) episodes of vertigo triggered by positional change is benign paroxysmal positional vertigo (BPPV), which is particularly common in the elderly, though can affect those of any age. In BPPV, the discrete attacks of severe vertigo rarely last longer than 30 seconds; however, patients are often left with a vague sense of imbalance and very subtle vertigo that persists for much longer. When categorizing the duration of the episodes, the period of time during which symptoms were obvious and severe should be used.

C. At some time in life, most people have experienced sudden lightheadedness (often interpreted as dizziness) due to orthostatic hypotension on rising suddenly from a recumbent position. A careful history establishing that episodes only occur when moving to an upright position indicates that orthostatic hypotension is the likely diagnosis. Note that many medications can contribute to this, particularly in older patients. Near immediate relief when returning to recumbency further establishes the diagnosis. As BPPV is also triggered by positional change, at times the distinction between BPPV and orthostatic hypotension can be challenging. Asking whether episodes *ever* occur with changes in head position not related to moving upright (e.g., rolling over in bed), and about the quality of the symptoms (i.e., lightheadedness versus true vertigo) may be useful. Very rarely, a patient with severe vertebral or basilar artery stenosis will experience TIAs triggered by reduced perfusion pressure when rising suddenly.

D. The Dix-Hallpike maneuver is easily performed at the bedside; a positive test triggers the patient's vertigo and causes torsional nystagmus with a brief latency and fatiguability. When these conditions are met, it is diagnostic for BPPV, which is caused by otoliths that have been displaced from the utricle into the semicircular canals. Otolith repositioning, also called the Epley maneuver, will cure about 80% of patients. Unfortunately, a negative Dix-Hallpike does not exclude the diagnosis of BPPV, and is in fact not at all uncommon in those with BPPV.

E. Ménière disease is a chronic condition thought to be due to excessive accumulation of endolymph within the inner ear. It is characterized by repeated spontaneous attacks of vertigo, each lasting 20 min to 12 hours, low- to medium-frequency sensorineural hearing loss in the affected ear, and fluctuating aural symptoms such as tinnitus or a sense of fullness or pressure in the affected ear.[1] Long-term treatment generally consists of a low sodium diet and thiazide diuretics.

F. The head impulse test assesses the horizontal oculocephalic reflex. The patient is asked to fixate on a target like the examiner's nose and while their head is rapidly moved to the right or left. A patient with an intact oculocephalic reflex will reflexively move their eyes in the opposite direction of head movement to maintain fixation. In a patient with an impaired oculocephalic reflex, their eyes will move with their head. To move their eyes back on the target, they will have a catch-up saccade in the opposite direction of the head movement. An abnormal head impulse test is usually but not universally indicative of an ipsilateral peripheral lesion, and in a patient with recurrent brief attacks of vertigo suggests a chronic, fixed peripheral vestibular lesion with breakdown of compensatory recovery under conditions of sudden position change. An example might be someone with prior vestibular neuritis and incomplete recovery.

G. When the examination is normal despite provoking maneuvers, the cause of brief episodes of positional vertigo often remains elusive. BPPV is probably the most common cause, but any cause of chronic vestibular dysfunction may present this way.

H. Vertigo associated with migraine (vestibular migraine) is probably an underappreciated cause of episodic vertigo.[2] Headache is not always present concurrent with the attacks of vertigo, making diagnosis challenging. Prophylactic treatment is the same as for migraine in general. See Chapter 2.

I. Dizziness, unsteadiness or lightheadedness is seen in about 20% of patients with panic attacks, and is common in anxiety disorders in general. Dangerous causes, such as posterior circulation TIA, must be excluded before entertaining this diagnosis.

REFERENCES

1. Lopez-Escamez JA, Carey J, Chung WH, et al. Diagnostic criteria for Ménière's disease. *J Vestib Res.* 2015;25:1–7.
2. Furman JM, Marcus DA, Balaban CD. Vestibular migraine: clinical aspects and pathophysiology. *Lancet Neurol.* 2013;12:706–715.

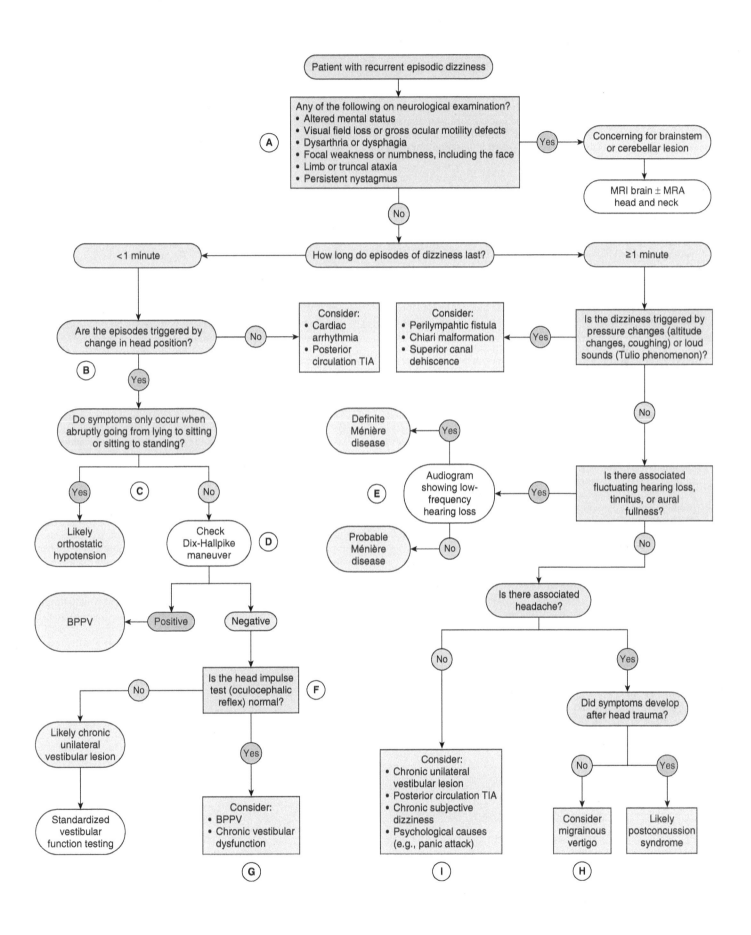

Hearing Loss

Neena Cherayil and Brett L. Cucchiara

Evaluation of hearing loss begins with determining whether one or both ears are involved. With bilateral symmetric hearing loss, symptoms are almost always slowly progressive over time. Unilateral hearing loss may be acute or chronic, a distinction with important implications for determining the underlying cause.

A. Sound enters the external auditory canal and vibrates the tympanic membrane (TM) first, then the ossicular chain in the air-filled middle ear, both of which amplify the sound. It is then transmitted to the inner ear where the cochlea resides. Disruption along this pathway by trauma (perforated TM), obstruction (cerumen, otosclerosis, neoplasm, serous middle ear effusion), or infection (otitis media) will cause conductive hearing loss. The Rinne and Weber tests rely on the principle that sound transmitted via bone bypasses the external and middle ear conductive system entirely and stimulates the cochlea directly. In the Rinne test, a vibrating 512-Hz tuning fork is placed on the mastoid bone and then moved to the ear canal, and sound perception compared between the two. Normally, sound from air conduction via the ear canal should be heard much longer than that via bone conduction. Conductive pathology will cause sound transmitted via bone to be detected longer than sound transmitted through air. Patients with sensorineural hearing loss (SNHL) will typically perceive air conduction longer than bone conduction. The Weber test can help lateralize asymmetric hearing loss. A vibrating tuning fork is placed midline on the forehead, and the patient is asked if sound is heard louder in one ear. With conductive pathology, the sound will be louder or lateralized to the affected ear. In SNHL, the sound will lateralize to the unaffected ear. Note that the reliability of both tests is questioned by many experts.

B. Ménière disease is a chronic condition characterized by multiple, recurrent hours-long episodes of fluctuating SNHL, vertigo, and tinnitus or aural fullness. It is thought to be caused by distortion of the endolymph system within the inner ear.

C. Lesions of the brainstem and cerebellopontine angle (CPA) can involve the eighth cranial nerve (CN VIII) or its nuclei. Brainstem lesions affecting this area can be due to stroke, demyelination, or neoplasm; additional focal neurologic findings are usually present. The most common CPA lesion is acoustic neuroma (also known as vestibular schwannoma), a benign tumor that arises from CN VIII and typically causes progressive unilateral SNHL. Other common symptoms include tinnitus and disequilibrium/gait imbalance; facial numbness and peripheral facial weakness or twitching can also be seen due to involvement of CN V and CN VII respectively. Brain magnetic resonance imaging (MRI) with contrast is the diagnostic test of choice.

D. Sudden onset or rapidly progressive unilateral hearing loss should be assessed with brain MRI with contrast. The labyrinthine or auditory artery is the main arterial supply to the cochlea and vestibular system, and is a branch of the anterior inferior cerebellar artery (AICA), though it can originate anomalously from the vertebral or basilar artery. Stroke in the territory of these arteries can cause sudden-onset unilateral SNHL. However, stroke affecting only the labyrinthine artery is uncommon, so *isolated* acute onset hearing loss as a result of AICA infarction is rare. Even rarer are cases where a single AICA anomalously supplies bilateral AICA territories. Cortical deafness occurs with bilateral infarcts affecting the auditory cortex in the temporal lobes. This is also exceedingly rare. Other focal brain lesions may also present with rapidly progressive hearing loss, and management obviously depends on the specific lesion identified.

E. The vestibular nerve innervates the semicircular canals and otolith organs and courses together with the cochlear nerve to form CN VIII. Vestibular neuritis is an inflammation of the vestibular division of CN VIII that presents with acute-onset persistent vertigo; it is generally a benign, self-limited infectious or postinfectious phenomenon. When accompanied by hearing loss, which implies involvement of the cochlear nerve, it is known as labyrinthitis.

F. Idiopathic sudden-onset SNHL is an otherwise unexplained hearing loss that develops over less than 3 days. Oral or intratympanic glucocorticoids are often used in the acute period, though evidence for benefit is limited. A majority of patients with this condition will recover hearing though those with more severe deficits at onset are less likely to recover. These patients should be referred for formal audiologic evaluation and treatment by otorhinolaryngology.

G. Slowly progressive chronic SNHL is most often due to age-related loss of hair cells; exposure to loud noise or ototoxic medications can also damage hair cells. Less commonly, progressive bilateral SNHL can be caused by syphilis, systemic autoimmune disease, mitochondrial disease, or severe hypothyroidism, but these etiologies typically have other clinically apparent sequelae in addition to hearing loss. Lyme disease is an unusual cause of hearing loss but an important consideration in endemic areas.

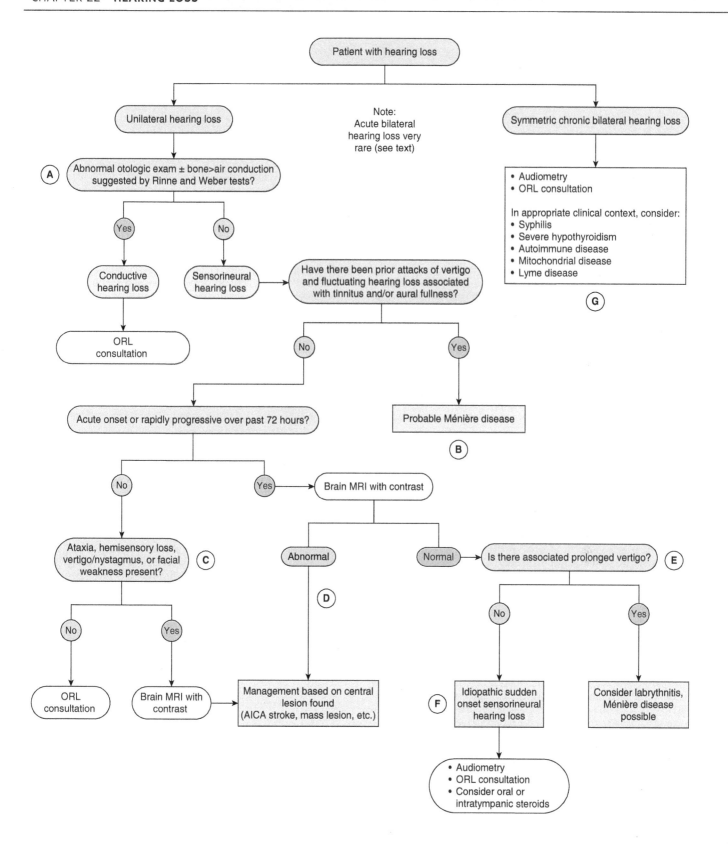

23 | Pulsatile Tinnitus

Jose Torres and Brett L. Cucchiara

Pulsatile tinnitus refers to a perception of sound that coincides with the heartbeat. It may arise from a vascular lesion causing disruption of laminar flow, leading to turbulence that produces a bruit audible to the patient, or from normal sounds that are perceived as more intense because of proximity of vascular and auditory structures. Both venous and arterial anomalies may cause pulsatile tinnitus. Occasionally patients perceive intermittent clicking or pulsing sensations in their ear that are not consistently synchronized with the heartbeat and thus not true pulsatile tinnitus. These may be due to myoclonus of the muscles of the middle ear, and are seen in those with prior brainstem stroke or multiple sclerosis.

A. High-output cardiac states, such as thyrotoxicosis, severe anemia, or pregnancy, may cause pulsatile tinnitus, which will typically resolve along with the underlying condition.

B. Examine for an audible bruit, taking into consideration the patient's description of the location from which they perceive the sound coming. If the patient notes the sound is enhanced with specific maneuvers or positions, be certain to auscultate under these conditions. Be sure to note if the patient perceives the pulsatile tinnitus during the examination. Objective pulsatile tinnitus (i.e., a bruit is audible to the examiner) is more likely to be associated with an identifiable underlying vascular abnormality.

C. An audible bruit over the posterior neck suggests vertebral artery disease such as atherosclerotic stenosis or dissection. Bruits may be transmitted from the intracranial circulation as well.

D. Cranial bruits indicate a high likelihood of significant and potentially dangerous pathology. Both brain and vascular imaging with magnetic resonance imaging/angiography (MRI/MRA) is indicated. Note that dural arteriovenous fistulas, an important cause of pulsatile tinnitus associated with a cranial bruit, may be occult on MRA or computed tomography angiography (CTA); catheter angiography is often necessary for diagnosis.

E. Anterior cervical bruits typically rise from either the carotid arteries or jugular veins. If the bruit disappears with gentle neck compression, a Valsalva maneuver, or change in position such as turning of the head, it is likely venous.

F. Carotid stenosis is the most common cause of an arterial bruit in the neck, most often due to atherosclerotic disease, which typically occurs at the carotid bifurcation and is usually easily diagnosed with carotid ultrasonography. Arterial dissection and segmental irregularity due to fibromuscular dysplasia may also cause pulsatile tinnitus but are not well-imaged by ultrasound. A very rare cause of pulsatile tinnitus is a carotid paraganglioma, a tumor of the carotid body. In these latter cases, MR or CT angiography is necessary for diagnosis.

G. Venous bruits in the neck most often represent a benign venous hum. However, abnormalities of venous drainage of the brain can cause pulsatile tinnitus, and cervical venous bruits are audible on occasion. Look for signs or symptoms suggestive of increased intracranial pressure; if present, MRI and MR venography of the brain is indicated. Lumbar puncture should be performed if MRI is normal and idiopathic intracranial hypertension (pseudotumor cerebri) is a consideration.

H. Otologic abnormalities may cause pulsatile tinnitus audible to the patient but not the examiner (subjective pulsatile tinnitus). If a middle ear effusion is present and the onset of symptoms coincides with a middle ear infection, capillary hyperemia from otitis media may be responsible. A visible retrotympanic mass on examination may indicate a paraganglioma (typically a red, pulsatile mass) or an anomalous vessel.

I. Autophony refers to an enhanced perception of bodily sounds, typically the patient's own voice and breathing. Patients complaining of audible breathing or increased resonance of their own voice may have a persistently open or patulous Eustachian tube, allowing for excessive communication between the middle ear and the nasopharynx. In superior semicircular canal dehiscence syndrome there is thinning in the bony structures overlying the superior semicircular canal; patient's may describe hearing their own eye movements, and in some cases may have vertigo triggered by loud noises (Tullio phenomenon).

J. Many patients with subjective pulsatile tinnitus have no obvious clinical diagnostic clues to point to a specific etiology, and thus deciding whether to pursue neuroimaging can be difficult. Duration of symptoms, associated systemic or neurologic symptoms, and medical history should all be considered. While most identified causes in these patients (e.g., anomalous or aberrant vessels, thinning of bony structures between vessels and inner ear) do not require specific treatment, this is not universally the case. Osseous abnormalities of the temporal bone, such as Paget disease and otosclerosis, invasive highly vascular tumors, dural arteriovenous fistulas, and vascular stenosis may all be important conditions to identify.

REFERENCES

1. Hofmann E, Behr R, Neumann-Haefelin T, Schwager K. Pulsatile tinnitus: imaging and differential diagnosis. *Dtsch Arztebl Int.* 2013;110(26):451–458.
2. Pegge SAH, Steens SCA, Kunst HPM, Meijer FJA. Pulsatile tinnitus: differential diagnosis and radiological work-up. *Curr Radiol Rep.* 2017;5(1):5.

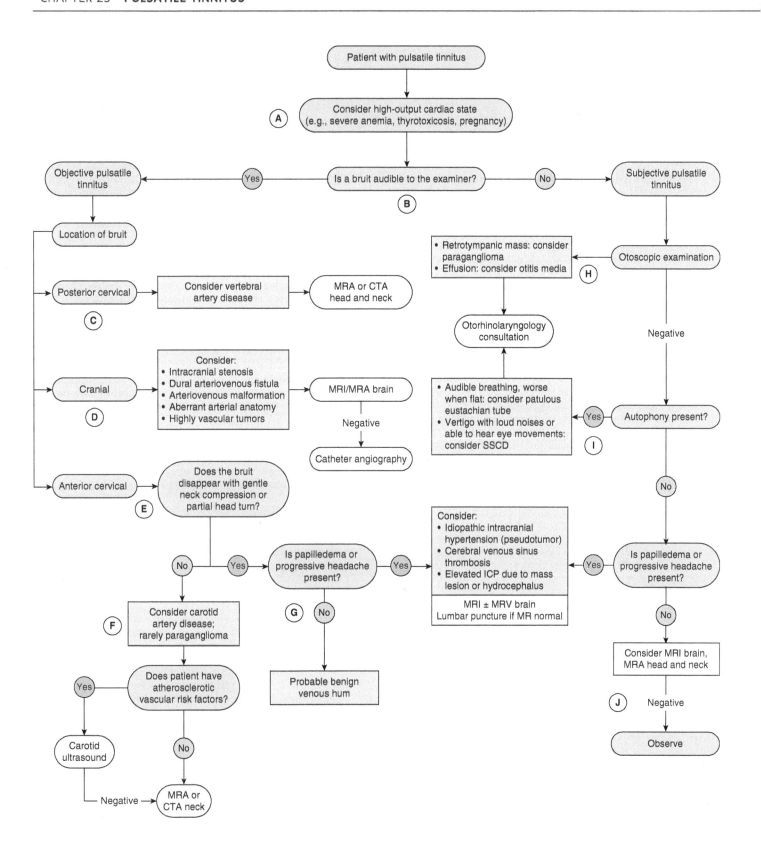

Dysarthria

Stephen Aradi and Brett L. Cucchiara

A. Dysarthria refers to abnormal phonic characteristics of speech production due to impairment of the motor processes of speech. This contrasts with aphasia, in which abnormalities of language underlie impaired communication. The neurologic pathways involved in speech articulation include upper motor neurons in the primary motor cortex and other associated regions of cortex, the basal ganglia, the cerebellum, cranial nerves (CN) V, VII, IX, X, and XII, the neuromuscular junction, and the oropharyngeal muscles of speech; disruption anywhere along these pathways can lead to dysarthria. Dysarthria can be categorized based on its particular phonic characteristic, although this can be challenging to assess in routine practice:
  - Spastic: Typically caused by bilateral dysfunction of the corticobulbar pathways innervating the cranial nerves mentioned above, as may be seen with bilateral strokes, demyelinating disease, or motor neuron disease. Features can include a strained hoarseness with slow and imprecise articulation.
  - Hypo/hyperkinetic: In Parkinsonism, speech is quiet and often slow, but sometimes rapid and mumbling. Spasmodic dysphonia causes a choked-sounding speech. Vocal tremor is a feature of essential tremor. Irregular rate and volume of speech occur in hyperkinetic disorders such as Huntington disease.
  - Ataxic: "Scanning" speech, with irregular intonation, pitch, volume, and speed, can be seen with cerebellar lesions.
  - Flaccid: There may be specific parts of the oropharyngeal musculature affected, identified by eliciting syllables of "ka", "la", and "ma", which involves CN IX/X, XII, and VII, respectively. Fasciculations in these muscles, but especially the tongue, suggests motor neuron disease.
  - Mixed: More complicated patterns involving features of two or more of the above types.

B. Ischemic stroke is a frequent cause of acute onset dysarthria, especially if other focal neurologic signs and symptoms are present. Rapid neuroimaging and triage for possible reperfusion therapy are indicated.

C. Dysarthria without other focal neurologic symptoms in the setting of altered mentation suggests intoxication, with alcohol being the most common offender. Toxic-metabolic encephalopathy is also common in susceptible hospitalized patients with underlying infections, acute kidney injury, or other metabolic derangements.

D. Acute inflammatory polyneuropathies can affect the cranial nerves in addition to nerve roots and peripheral nerves, causing rapidly progressing bulbar symptoms. This is most common in the Miller-Fisher variant of Guillain-Barré syndrome (GBS), but classic GBS and other variants can also feature prominent bulbar symptoms. Clues to the diagnosis include areflexia (though reflexes may remain early in the disease course) and, particularly with Miller-Fisher syndrome, weakness of the extraocular muscles manifesting as double vision.

E. Signs of raised intracranial pressure (positional headache, nausea, and vomiting) with or without other progressive deficits may suggest an enlarging mass lesion. Demyelinating disease should be considered especially if there is a history of prior, recurrent attacks of focal neurologic symptoms.

F. Because all spinal nerve roots and cranial nerves except the olfactory and optic nerves traverse the subarachnoid space, processes involving inflammation within or infiltration of the subarachnoid space or the leptomeninges can cause multiple cranial neuropathies and/or radiculopathies; atypical infections, leptomeningeal carcinomatosis, and inflammatory diseases such as neurosarcoidosis should be considered.

G. If dysarthria is episodic and fluctuating, neuromuscular junction disorders such as myasthenia gravis should be considered. Other features of fatigable weakness including ptosis with curtaining, double vision, and limb weakness should be sought. If detected, testing for acetylcholine receptor antibodies and electromyography with repetitive stimulation should be done (see Chapter 97).

H. Very rarely, recurrent brief episodes of isolated dysarthria may occur with transient ischemic attack, usually when there is a large vessel stenosis. Diagnosis typically requires computed tomography or magnetic resonance angiography. While atypical, isolated fluctuating dysarthria can also be due to myasthenia gravis.

I. Motor neuron disease should be suspected when there is evidence of upper and lower motor neuron signs on examination in addition to dysarthria (see Chapter 96).

J. Slowly progressive dysarthria can be a feature of numerous neurodegenerative and/or hereditary conditions, such as Parkinson disease, atypical Parkinsonian syndromes, hereditary or acquired ataxias, vocal tremor (as in essential tremor), spasmodic dysphonia, and paraneoplastic cerebellar degeneration. Associated features on examination can suggest further workup, including structural and functional neuroimaging and laboratory testing.

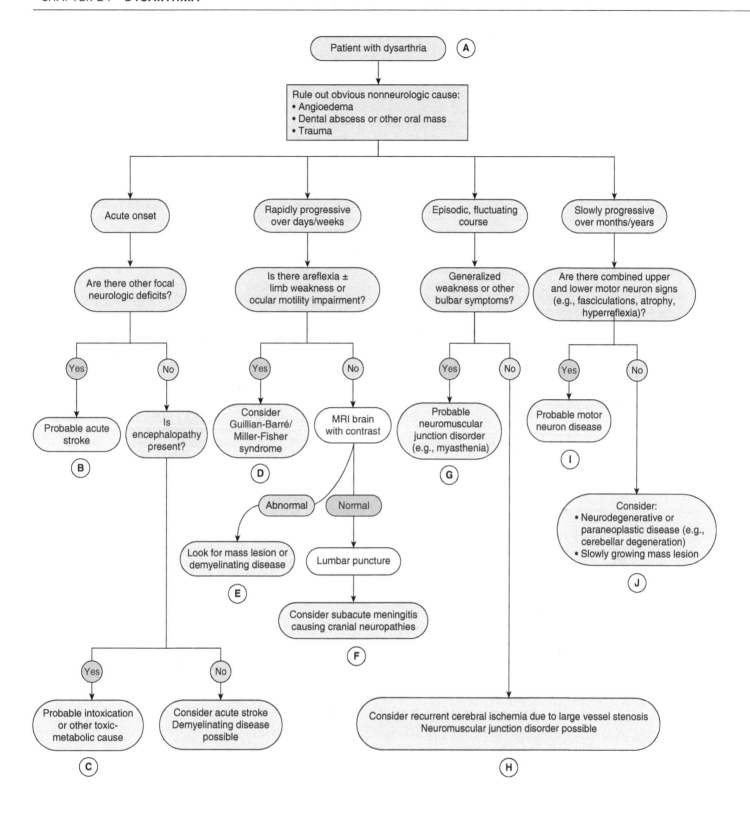

Patient with dysarthria — A

Rule out obvious nonneurologic cause:
• Angioedema
• Dental abscess or other oral mass
• Trauma

Acute onset

Rapidly progressive over days/weeks

Episodic, fluctuating course

Slowly progressive over months/years

Are there other focal neurologic deficits?

Is there areflexia ± limb weakness or ocular motility impairment?

Generalized weakness or other bulbar symptoms?

Are there combined upper and lower motor neuron signs (e.g., fasciculations, atrophy, hyperreflexia)?

Yes | No | Yes | No | Yes | No | Yes | No

Probable acute stroke — B

Is encephalopathy present?

Consider Guillian-Barré/Miller-Fisher syndrome — D

MRI brain with contrast

Probable neuromuscular junction disorder (e.g., myasthenia) — G

Probable motor neuron disease — I

Abnormal | Normal

Look for mass lesion or demyelinating disease — E

Lumbar puncture

Consider:
• Neurodegenerative or paraneoplastic disease (e.g., cerebellar degeneration)
• Slowly growing mass lesion — J

Consider subacute meningitis causing cranial neuropathies — F

Yes | No

Probable intoxication or other toxic-metabolic cause — C

Consider acute stroke Demyelinating disease possible

Consider recurrent cerebral ischemia due to large vessel stenosis Neuromuscular junction disorder possible — H

25 Proximal Weakness

Hannah Machemehl and Colin Quinn

Symmetric proximal weakness is most commonly associated with primary muscle disease (myopathy). However, diseases of the neuromuscular junction, neuropathies, spinal cord disease, and very rarely cerebral infarction can produce similar symptoms. Patients with symmetric proximal weakness commonly describe difficulty rising from a chair, climbing stairs, and combing their hair.

A. Myelopathy and lumbar radiculopathies from spinal canal stenosis typically cause asymmetric weakness; however, unusual presentations of these common conditions do occur. For instance, while rare, symmetric isolated involvement of the L2/L3 nerve roots causes weakness of hip flexion and knee extension along with a reduced or absent patellar reflex. Cervical or thoracic myelopathy with corticospinal tract involvement classically causes a pattern of prominent weakness of hip flexion, knee flexion, and ankle dorsiflexion. If the ankle dorsiflexion weakness is subtle, it may not be appreciated on examination giving the impression of proximal weakness alone. If myelopathy is suspected, magnetic resonance imaging (MRI) of the cervical and thoracic spine should be performed.

B. Several unique conditions should be considered in patients with isolated symmetric proximal arm weakness. Acute, proximal arm weakness with preservation of hand and leg strength ("man in a barrel" syndrome) may be seen with bilateral cerebral infarctions in the anterior watershed zones, typically as a consequence of hypoperfusion. Brain MRI is diagnostic, and vessel imaging should be performed, as large vessel stenosis is commonly present. Cervical spine syrinx classically causes symmetric bilateral arm or hand weakness, as well as loss of pain and temperature sensation with preservation of vibration sensation in the back and neck in a "cape-like" distribution. MRI of the cervical spine will identify a syrinx; if present, brain MRI should also be performed, as associated Chiari malformations can be present. Cervical myelopathy affecting the upper cervical spinal cord at C5/C6 can cause prominent proximal arm weakness. In this case, upper motor neuron abnormalities (i.e., brisk reflexes) are usually present below the level of injury.

C. Chronic inflammatory demyelinating polyneuropathy often causes a distinct pattern of distal numbness with proximal weakness. Patients often reports paresthesias and loss of sensation in their feet while at the same time reporting greater difficulty getting out of a chair or going up stairs (see Chapter 90).

D. Serum creatine kinase (CK) is helpful in distinguishing myopathic from non-myopathic disease. However, one should approach modest levels of CK elevation with caution, as this may also be seen in neuropathic or motor neuron disease. In a patient with nonfluctuating, symmetric proximal weakness without numbness and a CK level >1500 U/L, myopathy is the likely cause. In patients with lower CK levels and electromyography (EMG) demonstrating small motor units with early recruitment, myopathy is also the likely diagnosis. In some instances of chronic myopathies, the small motor units expected on EMG may not be present and a more neurogenic pattern may be seen. In these instances, muscle biopsy may be helpful to distinguish these entities (see Chapter 99).

E. Myasthenia gravis (MG) is an autoimmune disorder caused by antibodies directed against the postsynaptic neuromuscular junction of skeletal muscle. MG is characterized by fluctuating weakness that worsens with activity and improves with rest. In generalized MG, weakness may involve the limb muscles, respiratory muscles, pharyngeal muscles, extraocular muscles, and levator palpebrae (see Chapters 97 and 98).

F. In a patient with proximal weakness without numbness and diffuse chronic denervation on needle EMG, motor neuron diseases such as amyotrophic lateral sclerosis (ALS), Kennedy disease (spinal-bulbar muscular atrophy), or spinal muscular atrophy are most likely. Symmetric weakness is an uncommon initial presentation of ALS, as it usually begins with asymmetric weakness (see Chapter 96).

G. Lambert-Eaton myasthenic syndrome is an autoimmune disease associated with antibodies against the voltage-gated calcium channel (VGCC). Weakness is commonly seen in the proximal limbs, particularly in the legs, mimicking a myopathic process. Other symptoms include dysarthria, dysphagia, and dysautonomia (e.g., dry mouth or dry eyes). CK levels are usually normal. Diagnosis is based on nerve conduction studies/electromyography and the presence of serum VGCC antibodies (see Chapter 97).

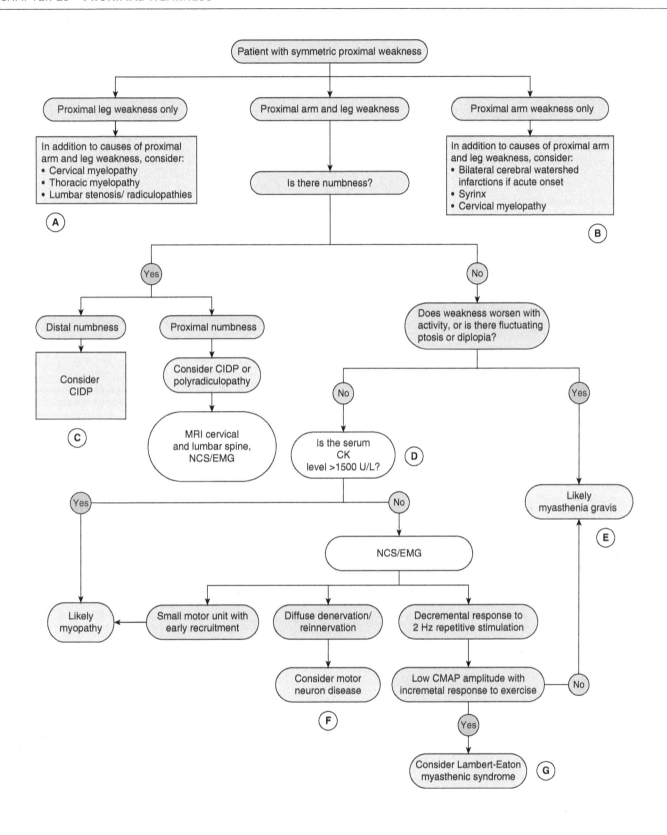

Patient with symmetric proximal weakness

Proximal leg weakness only

In addition to causes of proximal arm and leg weakness, consider:
• Cervical myelopathy
• Thoracic myelopathy
• Lumbar stenosis/ radiculopathies

(A)

Proximal arm and leg weakness

Is there numbness?

Proximal arm weakness only

In addition to causes of proximal arm and leg weakness, consider:
• Bilateral cerebral watershed infarctions if acute onset
• Syrinx
• Cervical myelopathy

(B)

Yes

Distal numbness

Consider CIDP

(C)

Proximal numbness

Consider CIDP or polyradiculopathy

MRI cervical and lumbar spine, NCS/EMG

No

Does weakness worsen with activity, or is there fluctuating ptosis or diplopia?

No

Is the serum CK level >1500 U/L?

(D)

Yes

Likely myasthenia gravis

(E)

Yes

NCS/EMG

Likely myopathy

Small motor unit with early recruitment

Diffuse denervation/ reinnervation

Consider motor neuron disease

(F)

No

Decremental response to 2 Hz repetitive stimulation

Low CMAP amplitude with incremetal response to exercise

No

Yes

Consider Lambert-Eaton myasthenic syndrome

(G)

Wrist Drop

Raymond S. Price

Wrist drop refers to an impairment in hand extension at the wrist. There is usually concurrent finger extension weakness ("finger drop"). The most common localizations are peripheral processes, such as a C7 radiculopathy or radial nerve compression at the spiral groove ("Saturday night palsy").

A. The rapidity of onset and the duration of weakness should be assessed. Primary motor cortex has significant representation of hand movement, and abrupt onset wrist drop and hand weakness can be seen with cerebral infarction or hemorrhage affecting the contralateral frontal lobe ("hand knob"). When concurrent new-onset neck or radicular pain is present, a C7 radiculopathy is most likely.

B. On clinical examination, a C7 radiculopathy cannot be distinguished from a middle trunk plexopathy, as both have a combination of wrist extension, arm extension, and forearm pronation weakness and numbness of the middle finger. In this instance, nerve conduction studies and needle electromyography (NCS/EMG) are indicated. NCS should demonstrate normal sensory responses in the setting of radiculopathy. In a middle trunk plexopathy, the radial sensory response should be abnormal.

C. A radial neuropathy with arm extension weakness indicates that the lesion must be in the axilla, which is proximal to the innervation of the triceps muscle. A radial neuropathy that spares the triceps is most commonly seen as part of a Saturday night palsy, in which the patient experienced prolonged compression of the radial nerve at or near the spinal groove, distal to the innervation of the triceps. This results in numbness of the dorsal forearm and hand, and weakness of the wrist and finger extensors and the brachioradialis muscle; elbow extension is spared. The radial nerve divides into a superficial radial sensory nerve that conveys sensation on the dorsal lateral hand, and the posterior interosseous nerve, which innervates wrist and finger extensors. The brachioradialis muscle is innervated prior to this division, thus a patient with finger extension and wrist extension weakness without weakness of either arm extension (triceps) or elbow flexion when the forearm is half pronated (brachioradialis) likely has a posterior interosseous neuropathy.

D. A posterior cord plexopathy is a rare cause of wrist drop and can be easily confused with a radial neuropathy at the axilla as both cause weakness of arm extension, elbow flexion when the forearm is half pronated, wrist and finger extension and numbness of the dorsal forearm and lateral hand. A posterior cord plexopathy should be suspected when there is also arm abduction weakness, since the axillary nerve also arises from the posterior cord.

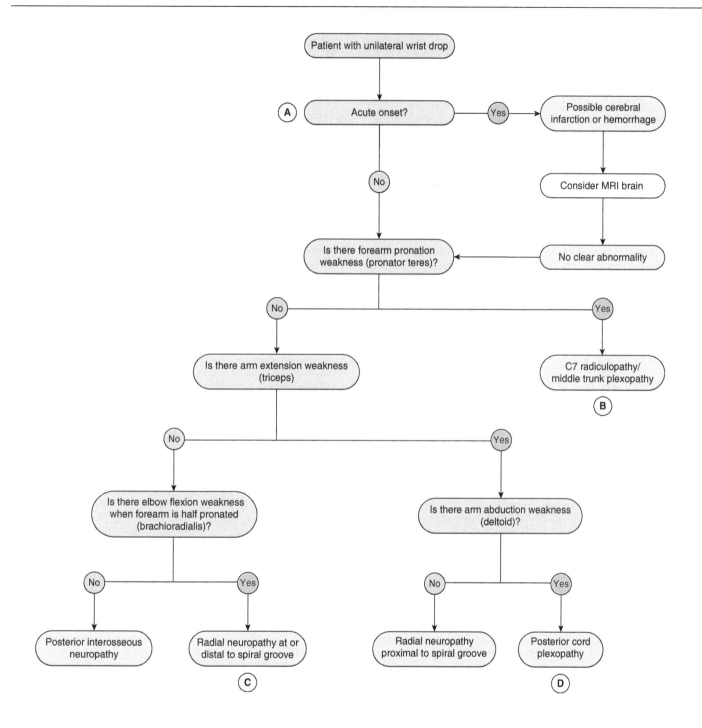

27 Unilateral Hand Weakness

Raymond S. Price

Careful examination of the anatomical pattern of unilateral hand weakness helps identify the most likely location of the causative lesion. In some cases, clinical weakness is subtle and the pattern of weakness is more easily identified on needle electromyography (EMG) examination of these muscles.

A. The rapidity of onset and the duration of weakness should be assessed. Primary motor cortex has significant representation of hand movement, and abrupt-onset isolated hand weakness can be seen with cerebral infarction or hemorrhage affecting the contralateral frontal lobe ("hand knob"). There are often, but not always, other associated neurologic symptoms or signs in this scenario. When concurrent neck or radicular pain is present, cervical radiculopathy should be considered.

B. Ulnar neuropathy occurs most frequently at the elbow as the ulnar nerve travels through the cubital tunnel, but can also occur at the wrist or even in the hand. Ulnar neuropathy must be proximal to the wrist if there is weakness of medial wrist flexion, since the flexor carpi ulnaris muscle is innervated proximal to the wrist. Similarly, an ulnar neuropathy must be proximal to the wrist if there is sensory loss of the dorsal palm, ring finger, and small finger because the dorsal ulnar cutaneous sensory nerve leaves the ulnar nerve prior to the wrist.

C. A radial neuropathy with arm extension weakness indicates that the lesion must be in the axilla, which is proximal to the innervation of the triceps muscle. A radial neuropathy that spares the triceps is most commonly seen as part of a "Saturday night palsy," in which the patient experienced prolonged compression of the radial nerve at or near the spinal groove, distal to the innervation of the triceps. This results in numbness of the dorsal forearm and dorsal lateral hand and weakness of the wrist and finger extensors but spares elbow extension. The radial nerve terminates into a superficial radial sensory nerve, which conveys sensation on the dorsal lateral hand, and the posterior interosseous nerve, which innervates wrist and finger extensors. A patient with finger extension and wrist extension weakness without dorsal lateral hand numbness likely has a posterior interosseous neuropathy, although a predominantly motor process such as motor neuron disease, brachial neuritis, or multifocal motor neuropathy should also be considered in the appropriate clinical context.

D. A medial cord plexopathy is a rare cause of hand weakness and can be easily confused with a C8/T1 radiculopathy clinically. Both cause median and ulnar hand weakness as well as numbness of the ring and small finger and medial hand (since the ulnar sensory fibers arise from the medial cord) and medial forearm (due to involvement of the medial antebrachial cutaneous sensory nerve). A medial cord plexopathy should be suspected when there is a combination of median and ulnar hand weakness but finger extension strength is preserved.

E. On clinical examination, a C8/T1 radiculopathy cannot be distinguished from a lower trunk plexopathy, as both cause a combination of median and ulnar hand weakness, finger extension weakness, and numbness of the medial forearm, hand, and ring and small fingers. In this instance, nerve conduction studies (NCS) and EMG are indicated. NCS should demonstrate normal sensory responses in the setting of radiculopathy. In a lower trunk plexopathy, the ulnar and medial antebrachial sensory responses should be abnormal.

F. The anterior interosseous nerve is a branch of the median nerve in the forearm that innervates the pronator quadratus, flexor pollicis longus, and flexor digitorum profundus. There is no sensory component to the anterior interosseous nerve. Weakness of these muscles causes difficulty flexing the distal thumb and index finger. When trying to grasp objects between the thumb and index finger, patients compensate for this weakness by adducting these two digits. A patient with distal thumb and index finger flexion weakness likely has an anterior interosseous neuropathy, although a predominantly motor process, such as motor neuron disease, brachial neuritis, or multifocal motor neuropathy, should also be considered in the appropriate clinical context.

G. Median neuropathy most frequently occurs at the wrist (carpal tunnel syndrome) but can rarely occur in the forearm. The presence of weakness of median-innervated forearm muscles such as the pronator teres or flexor carpi radialis would not be consistent with carpal tunnel syndrome and indicates a proximal median neuropathy.

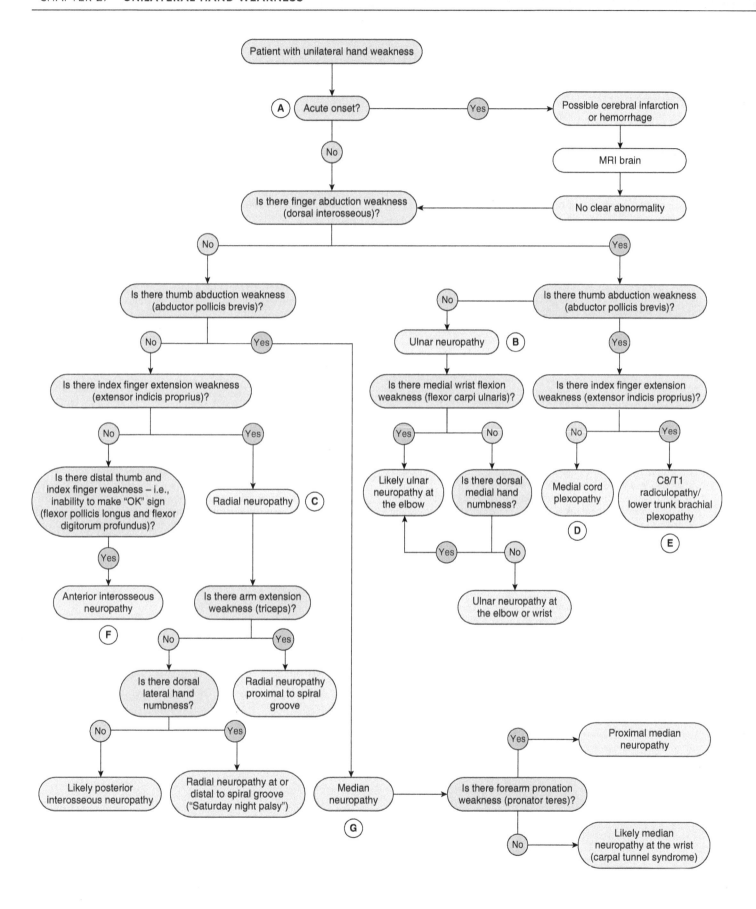

Unilateral Hand Numbness

Raymond S. Price and Colin Quinn

Unilateral hand numbness is a common complaint with multiple potential causes. Careful examination of the anatomical pattern of the numbness helps identify the most likely location of the causative lesion.

A. The rapidity of onset and the duration of numbness should be assessed. Primary sensory cortex has significant representation of hand sensation, and abrupt-onset isolated hand numbness can be seen with cerebral infarction or hemorrhage affecting the contralateral parietal lobe. There are usually, but not always, other associated neurologic symptoms or signs in this scenario. When concurrent neck or radicular pain is present, cervical radiculopathy is the most likely diagnosis.

B. In the setting of abrupt-onset hand numbness with negative brain and cervical spine imaging, acute peripheral nervous system injury should be considered. Examples include compressive nerve injuries or trauma.

C. Dorsal hand numbness is less common than numbness of the palmar surface. If a patient is unable to precisely localize the pattern of dorsal hand numbness, then radial and ulnar neuropathies and lower cervical radiculopathies (C6/C7/C8) are all possible.

D. Many patients are unable to localize the distribution of their hand numbness; they may state that their "whole hand" is numb when in fact a mononeuropathy or single radiculopathy accounts for their symptoms. It is useful to ask the patient to compare the degree of numbness present in the medial compared to lateral portions of the hand, as often this leads to recognition of a more localized sensory disturbance. If the pattern of sensory loss remains unclear, one should proceed to test for muscle weakness as outlined here, as this may still help identify the lesion location.

E. In a patient with isolated ring and small finger numbness, ulnar neuropathy is the most common cause, but a C8 radiculopathy or, even less likely, a brachial plexopathy is possible. Ask about neck pain and radicular symptoms, but in the absence of weakness or hyporeflexia, the clinical examination cannot precisely localize the source of their symptoms. In this instance, nerve conduction studies and needle electromyography (NCS/EMG) are indicated.

F. A radial neuropathy that spares the triceps is most commonly seen as part of a "Saturday night palsy," in which the patient experienced prolonged compression of the radial nerve at or near the spinal groove, distal to the innervation of the triceps. This results in numbness of the dorsal forearm and hand and weakness of the wrist and finger extensors but spares elbow extension.

G. In a patient with numbness of the lateral hand without weakness, carpal tunnel syndrome is the most common cause, although a C6 or C7 lesion is also possible. Ask about neck pain and radicular symptoms, but NCS/EMG is needed to conclusively determine the affected location.

H. In a patient with lateral hand numbness and biceps or triceps weakness, a C6 or C7 radiculopathy is most likely but a brachial plexopathy is possible. This is more easily distinguished on NCS/EMG. NCS should demonstrate normal sensory responses in the setting of radiculopathy. In an upper trunk or lateral cord injury, the median and lateral antebrachial sensory responses should be abnormal.

I. In a patient with medial hand numbness and weakness of the first dorsal interosseous, abductor digiti minimi, abductor pollicis brevis, and extensor indicis proprius muscles, a C8 or T1 radiculopathy is most likely but a brachial plexopathy is possible. NCS should demonstrate normal sensory responses in the setting of radiculopathy. In a brachial plexus injury the ulnar and medial antebrachial sensory responses should be abnormal.

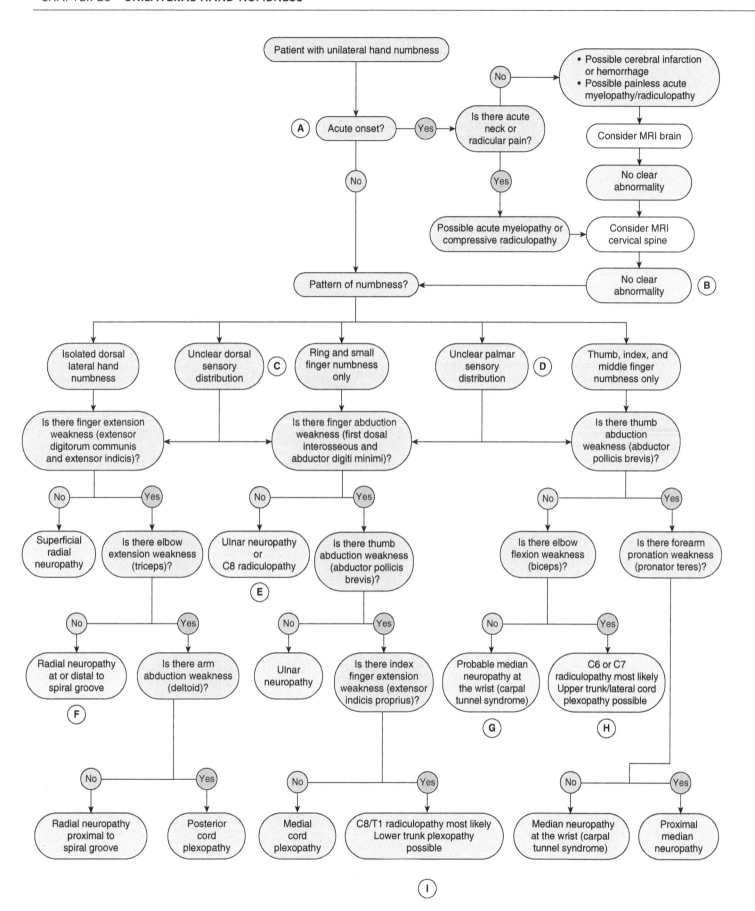

Knee Extension Weakness

Raymond S. Price

The quadriceps muscles in the anterior thigh extend the knee and are innervated by the femoral nerve, which arises from the lumbar plexus. The L2, L3, and L4 nerve roots provide axons to the femoral nerve. The quadriceps muscles are primarily innervated by axons from L3 and L4 roots. The axons from the L2 root in the femoral nerve innervate the iliopsoas muscle, which flexes the leg at the hip. Knee extension weakness will typically present with difficulty rising from a seated position, climbing stairs, or with falls secondary to the knee buckling when walking. Careful examination of the anatomical pattern of the weakness helps identify the most likely location of the causative lesion. In some cases, clinical weakness is subtle and the pattern of weakness is more easily identified on needle electromyography (EMG) examination of these muscles.

A. Symmetric knee extension weakness is commonly seen in myopathies and can also be seen in neuromuscular junction disorders, particularly Lambert-Eaton myasthenic syndrome. However, unilateral knee weakness is primarily caused by neuropathic lesions. One exception to this is sporadic inclusion body myositis, which, unlike most myopathies, is frequently asymmetric. The pattern of muscle involvement in sporadic inclusion body myositis is also atypical for most myopathies, with a predilection for the deep finger flexor muscles of the anterior forearm in addition to the quadriceps. If finger flexor weakness is present in a patient with quadriceps weakness, consider inclusion body myositis.

B. In a patient with unilateral knee extension weakness, next assess for weakness with hip adduction, tested by asking the patient to squeeze the thighs together. The muscles that adduct the hip are innervated by the obturator nerve, which also arises from the lumbar plexus and receives axons from the L2, L3, and L4 nerve roots.

C. The combination of hip adduction weakness and knee extension weakness indicates either a L3/4 radiculopathy or lumbar plexopathy, with the former being much more common. A lumbar plexus lesion should be considered in a diabetic patient with weight loss and pain (diabetic amyotrophy). Patients with either lumbar plexopathy or L3/4 radiculopathy will typically also have numbness over the lateral thigh. Magnetic resonance imaging (MRI) of the lumbar spine without contrast should be the initial diagnostic test in patients with the combination of hip adduction weakness and knee extension weakness. MRI of the lumbar plexus and EMG can be considered if the lumbar spine MRI is nondiagnostic.

D. In the absence of clinical or EMG evidence of hip adduction weakness, unilateral knee extension weakness is likely due to femoral neuropathy. A lesion of the femoral nerve can be further localized based on whether the lesion is proximal or distal to the innervation of the iliopsoas muscle, which flexes the leg at the hip. The branch to the iliopsoas comes off above the inguinal ligament. Injury to the femoral nerve proximal to the inguinal ligament typically occurs in abdominal surgeries due to retraction. Injury to the femoral nerve at or distal to the inguinal ligament, which spares hip flexion, typically occurs secondary to a hematoma from catheterization of the femoral artery or vein or from prolonged flexion and external rotation of the leg as seen in pelvic surgery or labor and delivery.

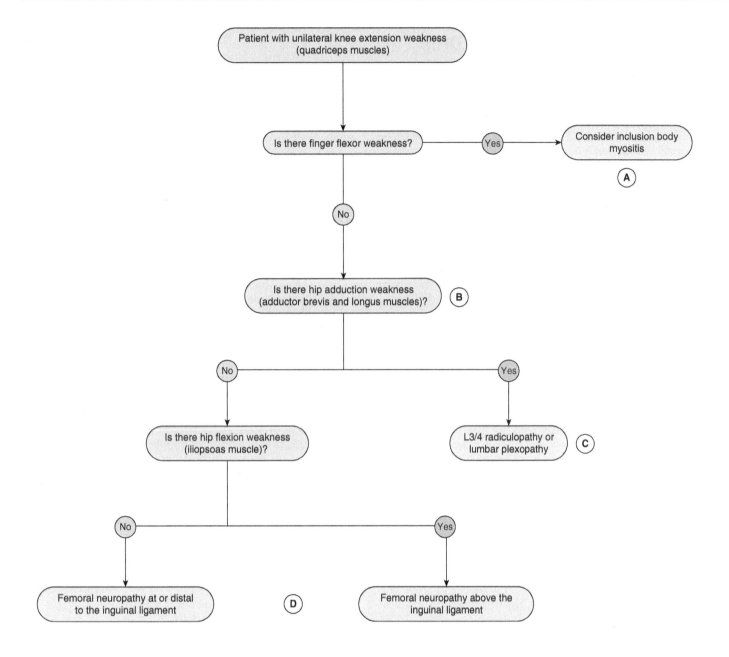

Unilateral Foot Drop

Raymond S. Price

Unilateral foot drop is a common complaint. Careful examination of the anatomical pattern of the weakness helps identify the most likely location of the causative lesion. In some cases, clinical weakness is subtle and the pattern of weakness is more easily identified on needle electromyography (EMG) examination of these muscles.

A. A corticospinal tract lesion can present with preferential weakness of unilateral hip flexion, knee flexion, and ankle dorsiflexion because the extensor muscles of the legs also receive innervation from the lateral vestibulospinal tract. While this weakness is not consistent with an isolated foot drop, the ankle dorsiflexion weakness may be the primary symptom noticed by the patient. In addition to assessing for subtle hip flexion and knee flexion weakness, a careful examination for other upper motor neuron signs such as spasticity and hyperreflexia should be performed.

B. In a patient with foot drop, the first movements to assess for weakness are ankle eversion and inversion. These movements need to be performed with the foot in a neutral or dorsiflexed position, which usually requires the examiner to dorsiflex the foot. If the foot remains plantarflexed, the gastrocnemius muscle can participate in eversion or inversion, potentially causing the examiner to mislocalize the lesion.

C. The common peroneal (fibular) nerve bifurcates into the deep peroneal and superficial peroneal nerves. The superficial peroneal nerve innervates the peroneus longus, which everts the foot and carries sensory information from the lower lateral leg and the dorsum of the foot. In this context, a patient with a deep peroneal neuropathy would have a foot drop without ankle eversion weakness or obvious sensory loss. The only sensory fibers carried by the deep peroneal nerve convey sensation between the great and second toe, and thus this sensory distribution would need to be carefully assessed in a patient with foot drop but preserved eversion.

D. A common peroneal (fibular) neuropathy is a frequent cause of foot drop. The typical location of the lesion is where the common peroneal nerve crosses the head of the fibula. This frequently occurs in the context of excessive crossing of the legs, particularly in patients who have recently lost a significant amount of weight. A patient with a common peroneal neuropathy will have numbness over the lower lateral leg and the dorsum of the foot and weakness of ankle dorsiflexion and eversion, but inversion will be normal because the tibialis posterior muscle, which inverts the ankle, is innervated by the tibial nerve.

E. An L5 radiculopathy is the other frequent cause of foot drop. The presence of radicular back pain suggests an L5 radiculopathy. On examination, the presence of ankle inversion weakness distinguishes an L5 radiculopathy from a common peroneal neuropathy.

F. Sciatic neuropathy is a rare cause of foot drop (note that the term "sciatica" usually refers to an L5 radiculopathy and not a sciatic neuropathy). The sciatic nerve bifurcates into the tibial and common peroneal nerves. A sciatic neuropathy can involve the fibers that will travel in both of these nerves or preferentially involve the common peroneal nerve fibers. When both the tibial and common peroneal fibers in the sciatic nerve are affected, there is ankle plantarflexion (gastrocnemius muscle) weakness due to tibial nerve involvement, which would not be expected in a common peroneal neuropathy. Involvement of the gastrocnemius muscle is also not seen with an L5 radiculopathy, since the gastrocnemius muscle is innervated by the S1 nerve root. More difficult is distinguishing a sciatic neuropathy with preferential involvement of the common peroneal fibers from a common peroneal neuropathy. In this case, the key factor is that the common peroneal nerve fibers contained within the sciatic nerve innervate the short head of the biceps femoris, part of the hamstring muscle. Involvement of this muscle, therefore, implicates the sciatic nerve and is inconsistent with a common peroneal neuropathy. Because the hamstring is a very strong muscle, the examiner may not be able to appreciate weakness of this muscle on examination. The presence of denervation of the short head of the biceps femoris on needle EMG will make the distinction.

G. A sciatic neuropathy with involvement of tibial and common peroneal fibers needs to be distinguished from a lumbosacral plexopathy. The superior gluteal nerve, which innervates the gluteus medius (responsible for leg abduction) and tensor fascia lata muscles, arises from the lumbosacral plexus but not the sciatic nerve. Similarly, the inferior gluteal nerve, which innervates the gluteus maximums (responsible for leg extension), arises from the lumbosacral plexus but not the sciatic nerve. The presence of either hip abduction weakness or hip extension weakness in a patient with ankle dorsiflexion and ankle plantarflexion weakness indicates a lumbosacral plexopathy instead of a sciatic neuropathy.

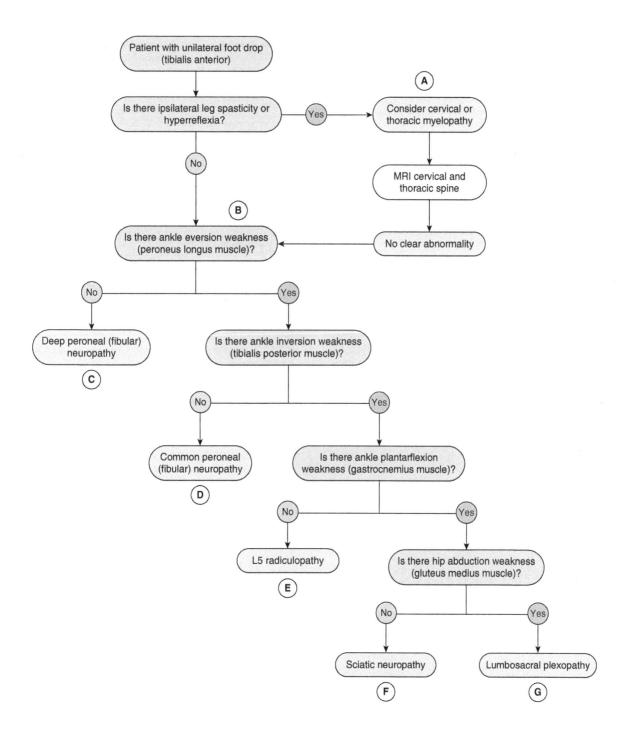

Fasciculations

Colin Quinn and Raymond S. Price

Fasciculations are caused by spontaneous depolarization of lower motor neurons, which results in contraction of the muscle fibers in the associated motor unit. Clinically this manifests as a visible twitch of the muscle beneath the skin. In most instances this twitching is not sufficient to cause joint movement, though this can be seen in late-stage motor neuron diseases in which a single motor unit may innervate a large territory within the muscle. Patients often become quite concerned by fasciculations due to their association with amyotrophic lateral sclerosis (ALS); however, unless weakness and/or hyperreflexia are present, more benign causes of fasciculations are substantially more likely.

A. Evaluation of fasciculations should include a careful examination of all body regions including the limbs, trunk, and bulbar regions. Patients should be examined with limited clothing to avoid obstructing the view of proximal fasciculations. Many patients describe muscle twitching that is not visible to the examiner despite a careful search of all body regions. In these instances, provided the remainder of the neurologic examination is unremarkable, reassure patients that a dangerous neurologic condition is unlikely and reexamine in 6 months to be sure there is no clinical change. It is quite unusual for these patients to progress to manifest a clinically discernable neurologic condition.

B. Fasciculations that occur repetitively in a single muscle are typically less concerning for ALS than more diffuse fasciculations. Electromyography and nerve conduction studies (EMG/NCS) are helpful for identifying nerve or nerve root injury which may explain the presence of focal fasciculations.

C. Diffuse fasciculations are substantially more concerning, as they are more likely to be related to a systemic or diffuse motor neuron/nerve root process.

D. Myokymia is due to the repetitive involuntary firing of multiple motor units in concert (grouped fasciculations). Limb myokymia is most commonly associated with a delayed radiation therapy effect, though it can occur rarely secondary to a radiculopathy or mononeuropathy in the absence of radiation exposure. Facial myokymia can be seen in multiple sclerosis or mass lesions; in such cases, a magnetic resonance image (MRI) of the brain should be performed.

E. Isaac syndrome is a disorder of motor neuron hyperactivity characterized by fasciculations, cramps, and impaired muscle relaxation. Issac syndrome is caused by autoantibodies usually directed against CASPR2 and less frequently LGI1. If the patient also has dysautonomia and a limbic encephalitis, then it is referred to as Morvan syndrome. During the needle EMG study of a patient with motor neuron hyperactivity, neuromyotonia may be seen. Neuromyotonia is characterized by very-high-frequency (>100 Hz) spontaneous motor unit discharges that tend to rapidly dissipate. Issac syndrome can occur as an isolated autoimmune syndrome, in the setting of other disorders of autoimmunity (e.g., myasthenia gravis), or as a paraneoplastic process. Cancers most commonly associated with Isaac syndrome are thymoma, lung cancer, and lymphoma. Symptomatic treatment of fasciculations, cramps, and impaired muscle relaxation can be achieved with sodium channel antagonists, such as phenytoin or carbamazepine. Definitive treatment is immunosuppression with intravenous immunoglobulin (IVIG) or plasmapheresis. In paraneoplastic cases, treatment must also be directed at the underlying malignancy.

F. Rarely, hypocalcemia or hypomagnesemia may cause benign fasciculations; measurement of serum electrolytes can be considered in patients with risk factors for such abnormalities.

G. Diffuse fasciculations combined with diffuse weakness in the absence of numbness is highly concerning for a motor neuron disorder, such as ALS. Look for evidence of upper motor neuron dysfunction (i.e., brisk reflexes) to support this diagnosis. A thorough evaluation should be performed to exclude ALS mimics (see Chapter 96).

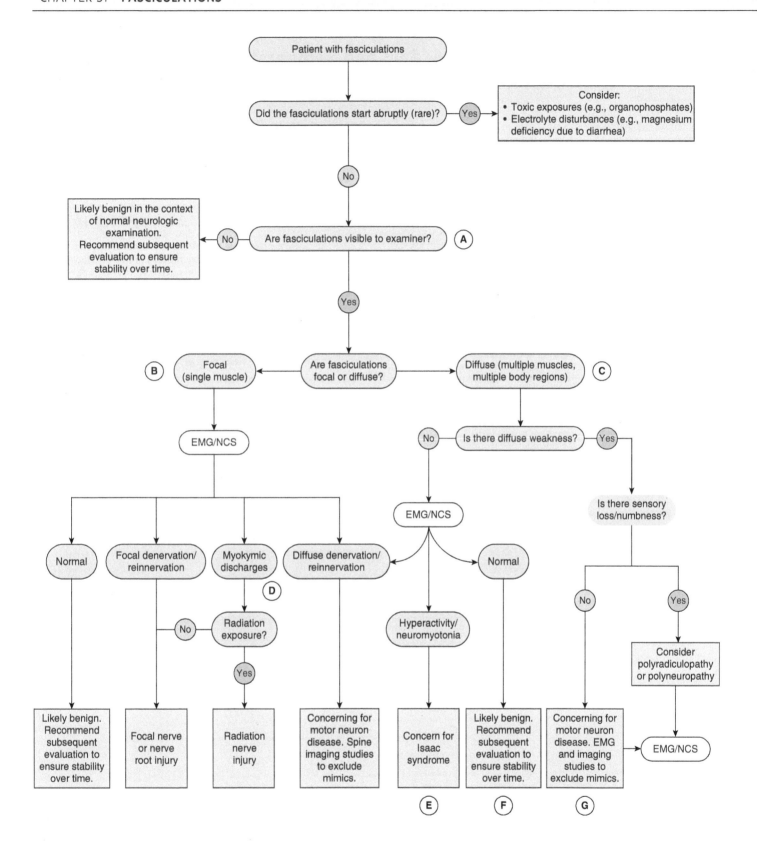

32 Sensory Disturbance: Pain and Temperature

Raymond S. Price

Temperature and pain sensations are conveyed via small myelinated and unmyelinated nerve fibers. These enter the spinal cord via the dorsal spinal root and synapse in the dorsal horn at the level of entry or ascend or descend ipsilaterally one to two spinal levels and then synapse in the dorsal horn. The second-order neurons then decussate at that level in the anterior commissure and ascend contralaterally through the spinal cord and brainstem to the thalamus. The third-order neurons from the thalamus synapse mainly in primary sensory cortex in the parietal lobe.

Clinically, pain sensation is assessed by gently applying a sharp stimulus, such as a pin, to the patient's skin. Temperature sensation is usually assessed by applying a cold stimulus, such as the metal of the tuning fork, to the patient's skin. When assessing temperature or pain sensation, it is important to assess for asymmetry and to compare proximal and distal sites.

A. A lesion involving the anterior commissure will cause bilateral reduction of pain and temperature sensation at that level due to disruption of the second-order neurons decussating through the anterior commissure. Pinprick and temperature sensation below the level of the anterior commissure lesion is spared, creating a so-called "suspended sensory level." This differentiates it from bilateral anterolateral system lesions in which pinprick and temperature sensation are reduced at the level of the lesion and below. The most common cause of an anterior commissure lesion is hydromyelia, which is a cystic lesion involving the central canal, or syringomyelia (syrinx), which is a cystic lesion not connected to the central canal. A midline intrinsic spinal cord tumor such as an ependymoma or demyelination from multiple sclerosis can also involve the anterior commissure. If the sensory loss is over the neck or arms, a magnetic resonance image (MRI) of the cervical spine is indicated. If the sensory loss if over the abdomen, an MRI of the thoracic spine is indicated.

B. Since the second-order axons carrying pain and temperature sensations decussate in the spinal cord and the axons carrying proprioception and vibration sensations and the upper motor neurons decussate in the medulla, the combination of loss of pinprick and temperature sensations on one side and either loss of vibration and proprioception or upper motor neuron signs on the other side is diagnostic of a spinal cord lesion. When all three are present, the patient has a hemicord (Brown-Sequard) syndrome.

C. In addition to carrying pain and temperature sensations, small myelinated and unmyelinated peripheral nerves carry autonomic fibers. Patients with a small fiber dysfunction typically present with length-dependent burning and shooting pain, autonomic dysfunction such as decreased or increased sweating, dry eyes or mouth, orthostasis, urinary retention, constipation or gastroparesis, or a combination of both. Patients can have polyneuropathy with a combination of small and large fiber dysfunction or polyneuropathy with preferential involvement of the small fibers (i.e., small fiber polyneuropathy). Patients with a small fiber polyneuropathy will not have weakness or loss of vibration sensation above the toes or loss of reflexes above the ankles. Nerve conduction studies and electromyography (EMG) do not assess small fiber nerve function and thus are normal in small fiber polyneuropathy. Small fiber polyneuropathy is often diagnosed based on clinical findings; additional testing if there is diagnostic uncertainty can include assessing intraepidermal nerve fiber density on skin biopsy of the distal leg at the ankle, quantitative sensory testing, or autonomic testing. Common causes of small fiber polyneuropathy include diabetes, amyloidosis, HIV, and autoimmune disease such as systemic lupus erythematosus or Sjögren syndrome. About 30%–50% of small fiber polyneuropathy cases are idiopathic with a relatively stable course.

D. In the setting of unilateral focal loss of pain and temperature sensations, an attempt should be made to map this loss to the known sensory distribution of a nerve (e.g., lateral anterior thigh in meralgia paresthetica) or a dermatome. If this can be mapped to a particular nerve or nerve root and the patient does not have weakness, further diagnostic testing is usually not necessary. However, in many patients with mononeuropathies or radiculopathies the description of the distribution of numbness cannot be definitively ascribed to a single nerve or dermatome. In these cases, further diagnostic testing such as nerve conduction studies and EMG can be helpful.

E. Hemisensory pain and temperature disturbance affecting the face and body on the same side suggests a central (brain) lesion above the level of the medulla. Crossed sensory symptoms, with the face affected on one side and the body on the other, localize to the lateral medulla.

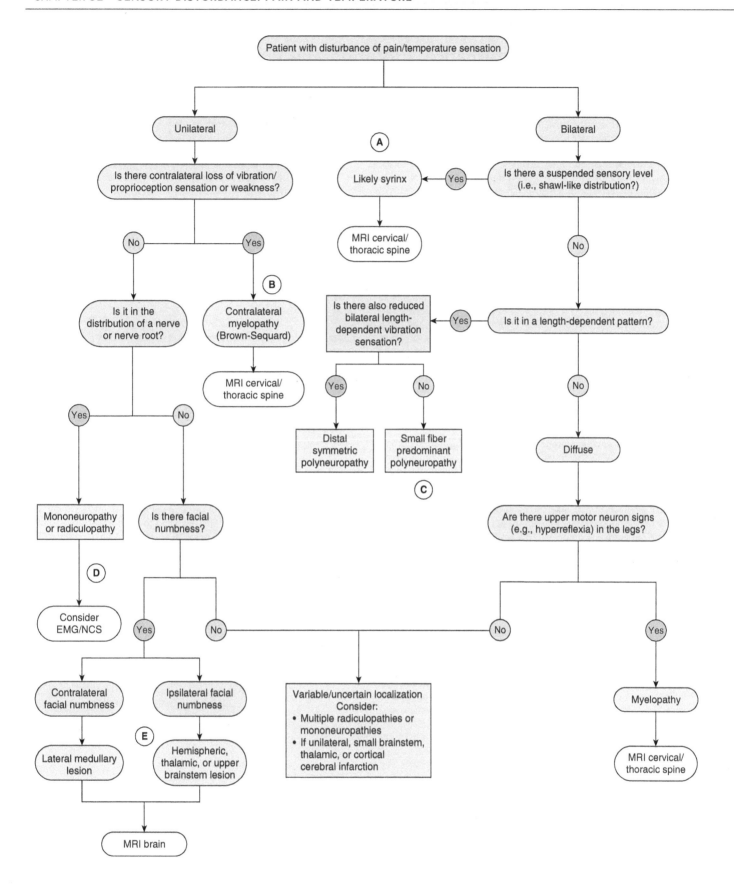

33 | Sensory Disturbance: Vibration and Proprioception

Raymond S. Price

Vibration and proprioception sensations are conveyed via large myelinated nerve fibers. These enter the spinal cord via the dorsal spinal root; the majority of these fibers then ascend ipsilaterally in the spinal cord in the dorsal (posterior) column. They then synapse in the medulla in the nucleus gracillis for axons from the leg and nucleus cuneatus for axons from the arms. The second-order neurons from those nuclei decussate in the medulla and ascend contralaterally in the medial lemniscus to synapse at the ventral posterior nucleus of the thalamus. Third-order axons from the thalamus synapse mainly in primary sensory cortex in the parietal lobe.

Clinically, proprioception is tested by holding the medial and lateral aspects of a body part, such as the great toe, and moving it up or down across the distal joint while asking the patient (with eyes closed) to indicate which direction it was moved. Both large- and small-amplitude movements should be tested. Vibration sensation is usually assessed with a 128-Hz tuning fork placed on a bony prominence such as the distal interphalangeal joint of the great toe or internal ankle. The presence or absence of vibration sensation as well as a subjective assessment of reduced but present vibration sensation is assessed. Alternatively, a graduated 64-Hz tuning fork can be used to quantitatively assess reduced vibration sensation with published normal values based on age. When assessing vibration or proprioception, it is important to assess for asymmetry and to compare proximal and distal sites.

A. Since the axons carrying proprioception and vibration sensation ascend ipsilaterally in the spinal cord and the second-order axons carrying pain and temperature sensations decussate in the spinal cord, the combination of loss of pain and temperature sensations on one side and loss of vibration and proprioception sensations on the other side is diagnostic of a spinal cord lesion. When these findings are present in combination with ipsilateral upper motor neuron signs, the patient has a hemicord (Brown-Sequard) syndrome.

B. In the setting of unilateral reduction of vibration or proprioception without contralateral loss of pain or temperature sensation, the causative lesion can be anywhere along the path of the ipsilateral dorsal columns or the contralateral brainstem, thalamus, or parietal lobe.

C. Since the axons carrying vibration and proprioception sensations from the arms enter the central nervous system in the cervical spinal cord and ascend to the brain, the presence of arm signs or symptoms indicates a lesion cannot be in the thoracic spinal cord. However, the absence of arm signs or symptoms does not exclude a cervical spinal cord process, and thus patients with isolated leg signs and symptoms suggestive of myelopathy require imaging of both the cervical and thoracic spinal cord.

D. Patients with non–length-dependent proprioception sensory loss typically present with sensory ataxia. In severe cases, patients may have pseudoathetosis of their fingers and toes due to proprioceptive loss. These patients may be misclassified as having weakness due to their difficulty in performing the motor examination secondary to proprioceptive loss. Weakness can be excluded by performing a motor examination with the patient visually focused on the requested movement. Non–length-dependent proprioceptive sensory loss can be caused by lesions of the dorsal root ganglia. Typical causes include autoimmune conditions such as Sjögren syndrome, paraneoplastic syndromes such as anti-HU and anti-CV2, platinum-based chemotherapies, and excess intake of vitamin B6. It can also be caused by multifocal lesions affecting sensory nerves, such as is seen with sensory-predominant chronic inflammatory demyelinating polyneuropathy (CIDP).

E. Isolated length-dependent proprioception and vibration loss can be caused by injury to the large myelinated axons in the peripheral nervous system or from a process involving the axons as they ascend in the dorsal columns of the spinal cord. The afferent limb of the deep tendon reflexes is also carried in the peripheral nervous system by large sensory axons. The reduction or absence of ankle jerks thus suggests a peripheral nervous system process such as a distal symmetric polyneuropathy, whereas the preservation of reflexes suggests a dorsal column process.

F. Vitamin B12 deficiency (including when secondary to nitrous oxide exposure), copper deficiency, and syphilis (tabes dorsalis) cause dorsal column lesions. When such a lesion is suspected, magnetic resonance imaging of the cervical and thoracic spine should be performed to assess for T2 hyperintensity restricted to the dorsal columns. Note that serum nontreponemal tests (e.g., rapid plasma reagin, RPR) may be negative in tabes dorsalis; treponemal tests (e.g., microhemagglutination assay for treponema pallidum antibodies, MHA-TP; fluorescent treponemal antibody absorption test, FTA-ABS) should be performed instead.

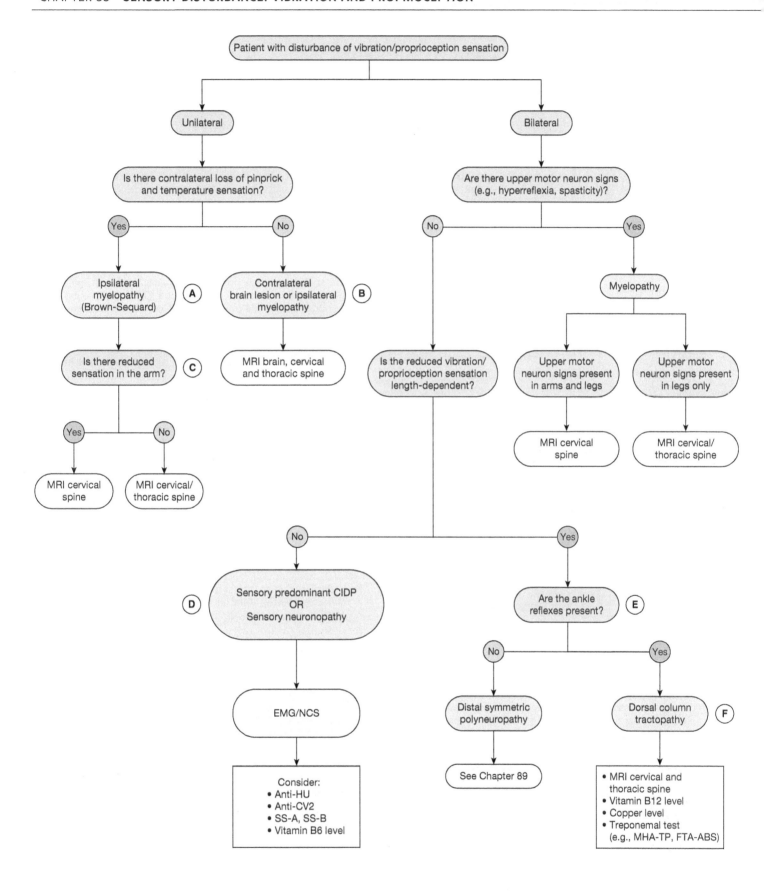

34 Hyperreflexia and Hyporeflexia

Raymond S. Price and Brett L. Cucchiara

The muscle stretch, or "deep tendon," reflex is the product of a segmental reflex arc involving specific spinal cord or brainstem regions; this makes testing reflexes useful for anatomic localization. Table 34.1 shows the most commonly tested reflexes and the segmental arc involved. When assessing reflexes, the muscle should be in midposition and relaxed. Grading of reflexes is shown in Table 34.2. Consider the amount of force required to elicit the reflex and the amplitude of the reflex when determining how to grade the response. Asymmetry is particularly important to note, more so than the absolute intensity of the response as this may vary widely across normal subjects. An anxious, thin person may often have brisk reflexes, and even a few beats of clonus, despite being neurologically normal; likewise, diffusely symmetric hypoactive reflexes are also often normal.

TABLE 34.1 REFLEX LOCALIZATION

Reflex	Segmental arc
Jaw jerk	Cranial nerve V
Biceps reflex	5th and 6th cervical root (C5–C6)
Brachioradialis reflex	5th and 6th cervical root (C5–C6)
Triceps reflex	Primarily 7th cervical root (C7)
Patellar (knee) reflex	3rd and 4th lumbar root (L3–L4)
Achilles (ankle) reflex	1st sacral root (S1)

TABLE 34.2 GRADING REFLEXES

Response	Grade	Description
Absent	0	No reflex despite a large amount of force
Hypoactive	1+	Small amplitude reflex generated by a large amount of force
Normal	2+	Normal amplitude reflex generated by a normal amount of force
Hyperactive (brisk)	3+	Large amplitude reflex generated by a small amount of force
Sustained clonus	4+	Repetitive or continuous reflex response with steady stretching pressure applied

Hyporeflexia

A. Hyporeflexia indicates dysfunction of the peripheral nervous system, and may be due to disruption of either sensory or motor pathways. Disruption of the sensory pathway (the afferent arc of the reflex) is much more common, and is signaled by the absence of weakness or hyporeflexia out of proportion to weakness. In the case of disruption of the motor pathway, hyporeflexia is considered a lower motor neuron sign along with muscle atrophy and decreased tone, and the reduction in the reflex is directly proportional to the coexisting muscle weakness. The causative lesion can be anywhere along the path of the lower motor neuron (anterior horn cell, spinal nerve root, plexus, nerve, neuromuscular junction, or muscle).

B. The most common pattern of hyporeflexia is bilateral, symmetric, and length dependent (meaning distal reflexes are more affected than proximal reflexes) and is seen in distal symmetric polyneuropathy such as diabetic polyneuropathy. The cell bodies of sensory neurons reside in the dorsal ganglia of each spinal nerve at that spinal level. Those that innervate the feet are the longest cells in the body, which makes them particularly susceptible to metabolic derangements, nutritional deficiencies, or other toxic exposures. Since the Achilles (ankle) reflexes are the most distal reflexes, they are the first affected in distal symmetric polyneuropathy, and symptoms gradually ascend from distal to proximal.

C. The triceps muscle is primarily innervated by the C7 spinal nerve (with some contributions from C6 and C8) via axons that run in the radial nerve. The proximal radial nerve innervates the triceps, then wraps around the humerus at the spiral groove and supplies the brachioradialis muscle more distally. Isolated unilateral triceps hyporeflexia (without involvement of the brachioradialis) suggests a C7 radiculopathy instead of a radial neuropathy because brachioradialis hyporeflexia should also be present in the, latter case.

D. The biceps muscle is innervated primarily by C5 and C6 spinal nerves via axons that run in the upper trunk and lateral cord of the brachial plexus, and in the musculocutaneous nerve. The brachioradialis muscle is innervated primarily by C5 and C6 spinal nerves via axons that run in the upper trunk and posterior cord of the brachial plexus, and in the radial nerve. Therefore, the combination of biceps and brachioradialis hyporeflexia is suggestive of either a C5/C6 radiculopathy or less likely an upper trunk plexopathy.

E. Isolated unilateral biceps hyporeflexia is suggestive of a musculocutaneous neuropathy instead of a C5/C6 radiculopathy or upper trunk plexopathy, because the latter lesions should also cause brachioradialis hyporeflexia.

F. Isolated unilateral brachioradialis hyporeflexia is suggestive of a radial neuropathy distal to the spiral groove, because a proximal radial neuropathy will also cause triceps hyporeflexia.

G. In acquired demyelinating polyneuropathies, such as Guillain-Barré syndrome or chronic inflammatory demyelinating polyneuropathy (CIDP), there is typically diffuse hyporeflexia.

H. A tonic pupil refers to a dilated pupil that does not constrict significantly to light but does constrict to a near stimulus. In reaction to a near stimulus, the pupil will constrict more than the other pupil and will dilate slowly when the stimulus is removed. The combination of a tonic pupils and areflexia is termed Adie syndrome. The etiology of this syndrome is usually unknown, and pathology has demonstrated neuronal loss in the peripheral sensory and parasympathetic ganglia.

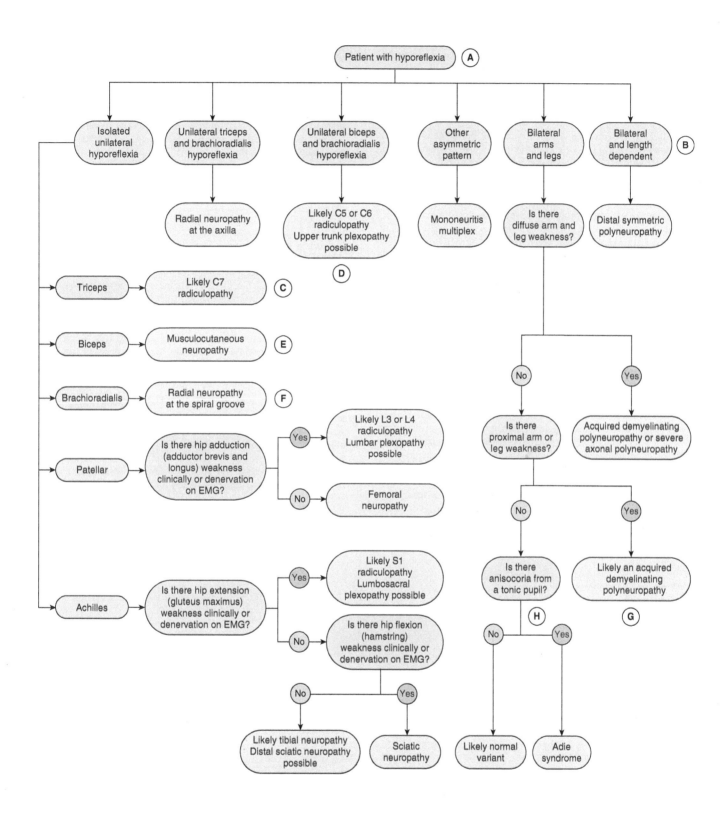

Hyperreflexia

A. Hyperreflexia indicates an upper motor neuron lesion, and reflects a loss of inhibitory modulation of the motor pathways. It is often associated with increased muscle tone (spasticity). The causative lesion may be anywhere along the pathway of the upper motor neuron in the corticospinal tract, including primary motor cortex, subcortical motor pathways, ventral brainstem, and the lateral column of the spinal cord. Common causes of hyperreflexia include focal brain lesions (typically causing unilateral hyperreflexia), cervical myelopathy, and motor neuron disease (amyotrophic lateral sclerosis, ALS). The latter is characterized by a combination of upper and lower motor neuron findings. This combination is also frequently seen in patients with cervical myelopathy and coexistent radiculopathy.

B. The first step in evaluation of the patient with hyperreflexia is to determine if other neurologic findings are present that would indicate cortical or brainstem dysfunction such as aphasia, neglect, hemianopia, or cranial neuropathies; if so, this strongly suggests a focal brain or brainstem lesion, and brain magnetic resonance imaging (MRI) is indicated for evaluation. A brisk jaw jerk also suggests a lesion above the cervical cord, and should focus attention on brain and brainstem processes.

C. The combination of hyperreflexia and lower motor neuron signs of atrophy and/or fasciculations suggests either multifocal spine disease involving both myelopathy (causing the hyperreflexia) and radiculopathy (causing the lower motor neuron signs) or ALS. The anatomic pattern of findings should be evaluated. A cervical cord lesion that involves the anterior horn cell will present with lower motor findings at the level of the lesion and upper motor neuron signs (i.e., hyperreflexia) below the lesion. For example, a C6 cord lesion involving the anterior horn cell might cause biceps atrophy and fasciculations and ipsilateral triceps and leg hyperreflexia. In this setting, MRI of the cervical spine identifying the lesion would be diagnostic. Similarly, coexistent cervical myelopathy and lumbosacral radiculopathy might present with arm and leg hyperreflexia with atrophy and fasciculations in the leg. Unremarkable spine imaging in these scenarios suggests ALS.

D. Unilateral hyperreflexia suggests a contralateral brain or ipsilateral cervical spinal cord lesion. Cerebral infarction would be a common cause of the former, and a demyelinating lesion from multiple sclerosis of the latter.

E. Note that small spinal cord lesions may not be well demonstrated on initial MRI. If there is high clinical suspicion, serial MRI may be necessary.

F. Myelopathy is most commonly compressive due to disc disease or central canal narrowing, and is also frequently caused by demyelinating disease or inflammation which will demonstrate hyperintense cord lesions on MRI. However, less common causes of myelopathy should be considered as well. Human T-lymphotropic virus (HTLV)-associated myelopathy typically shows nonspecific atrophy on MRI, though edema or longitudinally extensive hyperintense cord lesions can be seen. Vitamin B12 deficiency and copper deficiency classically demonstrate longitudinally extensive hyperintensity in the dorsal columns on MRI. However, these findings are not seen in all cases. Given the treatable nature of these conditions, any patient with an unexplained myelopathy should have serum vitamin B12, methylmalonic acid, copper, and ceruloplasmin studies. Nitrous oxide exposure causes irreversible inactivation of vitamin B12 that can lead to a presentation identical to vitamin B12 deficiency. Hereditary spastic paraplegia primarily involves the lower extremities, as neurodegeneration is most pronounced in the terminal segments of the longest axons such as the lumbar cortical spinal tract and cervical dorsal columns. Despite the name, arm involvement can occur but is typically milder than in the legs.

G. Occasionally, bilateral hyperreflexia can be seen with diffuse subcortical white matter disease (leukoencephalopathy), such as in advanced small vessel ischemic disease and multiple sclerosis. Rarely, a bilateral medial frontal lobe process, such as a large midline meningioma, can cause bilateral leg hyperreflexia and weakness.

H. Primary lateral sclerosis is a variant of ALS in which degeneration affects only the upper motor neurons. It typically presents with slowly progressive symmetric hyperreflexia and spasticity, which affects the legs initially, then progresses to involve the arms. Urinary urgency and diffuse mild weakness also occur as the disease progresses. Some patients will go on to develop lower motor neuron findings and meet diagnostic criteria for ALS.

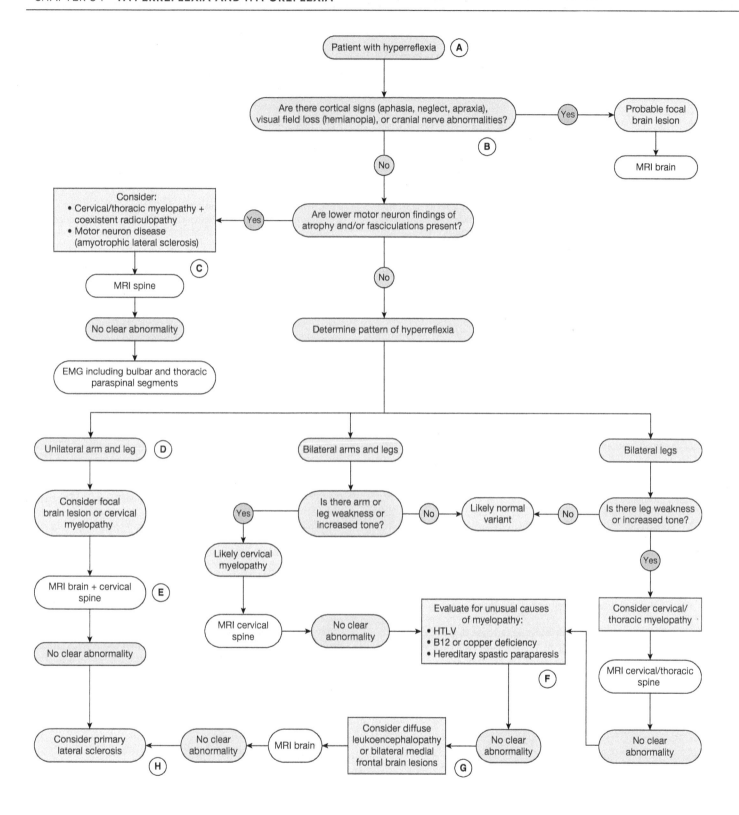

Multiple Cranial Neuropathies

Raymond S. Price

Aside from the olfactory cranial nerve (CN I) and the optic nerve (CN II), the remaining cranial nerves (CN III–XII) have nuclei in the brainstem. These then have axons extending through the brainstem (the fascicle), exiting into the subarachnoid space, and on to individual paths to exit the skull. Since some cranial nerves run near each other either in the brainstem or as they exit the skull, particular combinations of cranial neuropathies can suggest a precise anatomic localization. Similarly, the combination of cranial nerve dysfunction and either long tract dysfunction (hemiparesis, hemibody sensory loss) or cerebellar dysfunction strongly suggests a brainstem lesion. When a combination of motor cranial neuropathies does not suggest a precise anatomic localization, then myasthenia gravis should be considered and, less commonly, the Miller Fisher variant of Guillain-Barré syndrome, botulism, or a subarachnoid space process. When a combination of motor and sensory cranial neuropathies does not suggest a precise anatomic localization, a subarachnoid space process is likely.

A. The oculomotor (CN III), trochlear (CN IV), and abducens (CN VI) nerves and the ophthalmic (V1 segment of CN V) and maxillary divisions of the trigeminal nerve (V2 segment of CN V) all run through the cavernous sinus. Pathology there can subsequently affect any combination of these nerves. After passing though the cavernous sinus, the maxillary division of the trigeminal nerve (V2 segment of CN V), which receives sensation from the upper lip to the bridge of the nose, exits the skull through the foramen rotundum. CN III, IV, VI, and the V1 segment of V (which receives sensation from the bridge of the nose to the forehead and posterior scalp) continue on through the superior orbital fissure to enter the orbital apex. Therefore, superior orbital fissure pathology can affect CN III, IV, VI, and the V1 segment of CN V, but not the V2 segment of CN V. The optic nerve travels through the optic canal to enter the orbital apex, where it is in close proximity to CN III, IV, VI, and the V1 segment of CN V. The optic nerve does not run through the superior orbital fissure or the cavernous sinus. Therefore, optic nerve involvement, such as monocular vision loss or an afferent pupillary defect, in conjunction with eye movement abnormalities from CN III, IV, or VI dysfunction, implicates orbital apex pathology.

B. Note that numbness from the bridge of the nose to the forehead and posterior scalp (V1 segment of CN V) may also be present with orbital apex pathology.

C. Neurologic findings of eye movement abnormalities or dysarthria/dysphagia in myasthenia gravis may mimic cranial neuropathies, but are actually due to the more diffuse process of impaired function at the neuromuscular junction.

D. The fascicle of CN VI travels ventrally in the pons exiting near the corticospinal tract. The facial nerve (CN VII) exits the ventral and lateral pons. A lesion of the ventral lateral pons will cause horizontal diplopia from an ipsilateral abduction deficit, ipsilateral facial weakness involving the forehead, and a contralateral hemiparesis (Millard-Gubler syndrome).

E. A dorsal lateral medullary (Wallenberg) syndrome usually involves the nucleus ambiguous, which provides motor axons to the glossopharyngeal (CN IX) and vagus (CN X) nerves, and the cranial portion of the spinal accessory (CN XI) nerve. These axons innervate most of the muscles of the palate, pharynx, and larynx, and a lesion of the nucleus ambiguous or its axons produces dysarthria and dysphagia. A dorsal lateral medullary syndrome can also involve the inferior and medial vestibular nuclei, which can lead to vertigo; the spinal nucleus of the trigeminal nerve, which mediates pinprick and temperature sensation from the ipsilateral face; and the ascending spinothalamic tract, which mediates pinprick and temperature sensation from the contralateral body. The descending sympathetic neurons can also be involved, resulting in an ipsilateral Horner syndrome.

F. The glossopharyngeal (CN IX), vagus (CN X), and spinal accessory (CN XI) nerves exit the skull through the jugular foramen. The hypoglossal nerve (CN XII) exits the skull through the hypoglossal canal. These four cranial nerves then run together in the retroparotid space, as does the carotid artery. In this context, the combination of dysarthria and dysphagia, weakness of contralateral head turn, and ipsilateral trapezius elevation can occur with lesions in either the jugular foramen or the retroparotid space. The presence of ipsilateral tongue weakness (which causes deviation away from the affected side) secondary to hypoglossal nerve dysfunction or a Horner syndrome from a lesion involving the ascending sympathetic neurons on the carotid artery localizes the lesion to the retroparotid space. For the reasons previously stated, a jugular foramen syndrome would be considered in a patient with dysarthria, dysphagia, weakness of contralateral head turn, and ipsilateral trapezius elevation without tongue weakness or a Horner syndrome.

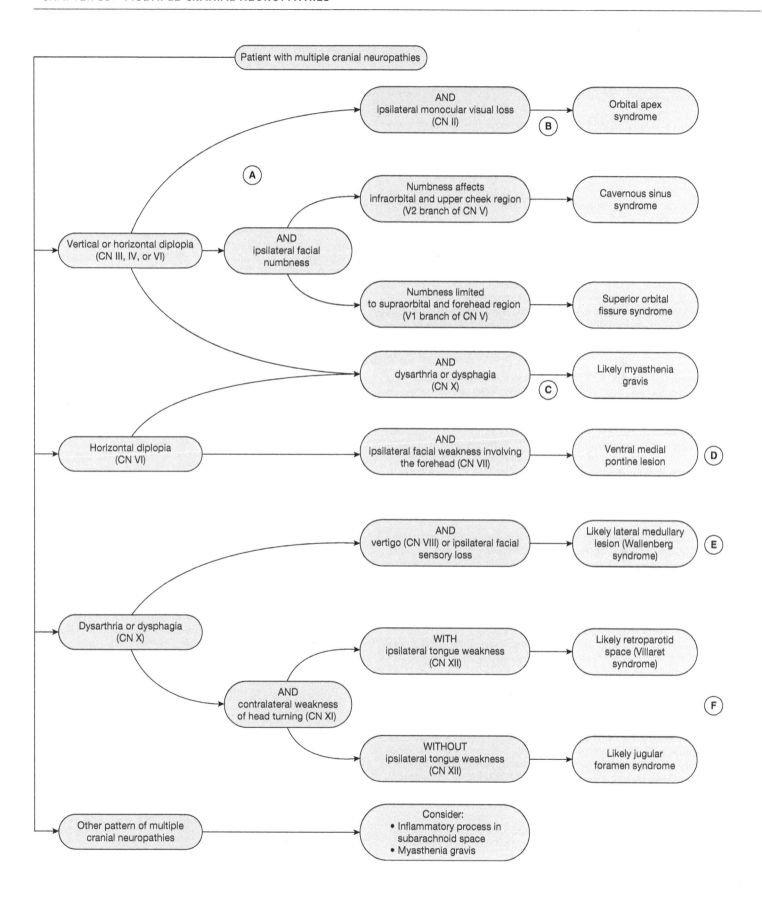

36 Ataxia

David Coughlin and Andres Deik

A. Initial evaluation should determine whether ataxia appears sensory or cerebellar. Profoundly decreased sensation and hyporeflexia in the absence of dysarthria or oculomotor findings make sensory ataxia more likely. Nystagmus, ocular dysmetria, and dysarthria suggest a cerebellar etiology.

B. In some conditions (like Friedrich ataxia), sensory and cerebellar ataxia may coexist.

C. Patients with cerebellar ataxia should undergo brain imaging to exclude causative structural lesions. Certain ataxias have specific magnetic resonance imaging (MRI) changes that facilitate recognition; examples include restricted diffusion in patients with Creutzfeldt-Jakob disease (CJD), pontine hypomyelination in autosomal recessive spastic ataxia of Charlevoix-Saguenay (ARSACS), and middle cerebellar peduncle (MCP) signs in multiple systems atrophy (MSA) or fragile-X tremor ataxia syndrome (FXTAS).

D. Common causes of acute ataxia include toxic ingestions and Wernicke encephalopathy. Immune-mediated causes are an important consideration in patients with ataxia for less than 2 years. Antibodies recognized to cause autoimmune cerebellar degeneration include anti-Yo, anti-Hu, anti-Ri, and anti-TR. The opsoclonus-myoclonus-ataxia syndrome is associated with neuroblastoma in children and most often small cell lung cancer in adults. Other autoimmune causes include Hashimoto encephalopathy (associated with anti-TPO and anti-TG antibodies), anti-GAD65 cerebellar degeneration (which is also associated with stiff person syndrome), and gluten ataxia in celiac disease.

E. While a detailed family history is critical in the evaluation of patients with chronic ataxia, absence of a family history does not exclude a genetic cause. Nonpaternity, *de novo* mutations, and anticipation in triplet repeat disorders are common reasons a family history may be absent. Genetic testing should be performed in conjunction with genetic counseling to ensure patients understand the ramifications of positive, negative, unclear, or unexpected results. Knowledge of a patient's genetic status can allow them to make decisions regarding family planning, avoid unnecessary diagnostic testing, and inform eligibility for clinical trials.

F. Identifying specific associated neurologic signs in autosomal dominant cerebellar ataxias narrows the differential diagnosis. Neuropathy and spasticity are seen in many spinocerebellar ataxias (SCAs). Spasticity is also a feature of Alexander disease and adult-onset leukodystrophy. Parkinsonism is seen in SCA2, SCA3, SCA9, SCA12, and SCA17, and in neuroferritonopathy. Epilepsy is often a component of SCA10 and dentatorubral-pallidoluysian atrophy (DRPLA). Myoclonus may be seen in SCA2, SCA14, DRPLA, and Gerstmann-Straussler-Scheinker syndrome, a rare familial prion disease caused by mutations in the *PRNP* gene. Chorea is a feature noted in SCA3, SCA17, and DRPLA. In cases with isolated ataxia, SCA5 and SCA6 are the most common entities. Of note, there can be considerable phenotypic heterogeneity between cases and even within families.

G. Episodic ataxias are characterized by attacks of ataxic symptoms. The two most common forms of episodic ataxia are EA1 and EA2. In EA1, episodes are brief, lasting seconds to minutes and classically provoked by startle or sudden movements. Interictal myokymia may be present. The attacks in EA2 are more prolonged, lasting from hours to days, and are often provoked by stress or exercise. Interictal extraocular movement abnormalities including downbeat nystagmus may be seen in EA2.

H. Associated neurologic signs can also help narrow the differential for autosomal recessive inherited cerebellar ataxias. Neuropathy is a prominent feature in Friedrich ataxia, ataxia with vitamin E deficiency (AVED), abetalipoproteinemia, ataxia telangiectasia, ARSACS, and ataxia with oculomotor apraxia types 1 and 2 (AOA1/2). Prominent spasticity is also seen in ARSACS, as well as in hereditary spastic paraplegia type 7 and cerebrotendinous xanthomatosis. Chorea can be a feature seen in ataxia telangiectasia and AOA1 or 2. Parkinsonism, psychiatric symptoms, and prominent dysarthria can be seen in Wilson disease. Dystonia is a feature of AOA2, ataxia telangiectasia, and Niemann Pick type C (NPC). Epilepsy may also be a feature of NPC, as well as autosomal recessive cerebellar ataxia 2 (ARCA2) and infantile onset spinocerebellar ataxia (IOSCA).

I. Ataxia is often present in mitochondrial encephalopathy, lactic acidosis, and stroke-like episodes (MELAS), myoclonic epilepsy with ragged red fibers (MERRF), neurogenic weakness with ataxia and retinitis pigmentosa (NARP), and *POLG*-related ataxia neuropathy spectrum diseases, which include sensory ataxia with neuropathy dysarthria and ophthalmoplegia (SANDO) and mitochondrial recessive ataxia syndrome (MIRAS). Given heteroplasmy and the relatively low number of mitochondria found in peripheral blood cells, muscle biopsy may be necessary to make a diagnosis.

J. FXTAS is the most common form of X-linked ataxia. A family history should include asking about children or grandchildren with intellectual disability and if women in subsequent generations suffered premature ovarian failure. FXTAS may present with a combination of action, postural, and rest tremor. Mild Parkinsonism and cognitive impairment may be present as well. Characteristic magnetic resonance imaging features are T2 hyperintensities in the middle cerebral peduncles and the splenium of the corpus callosum, but these features are neither sensitive nor specific for FXTAS.

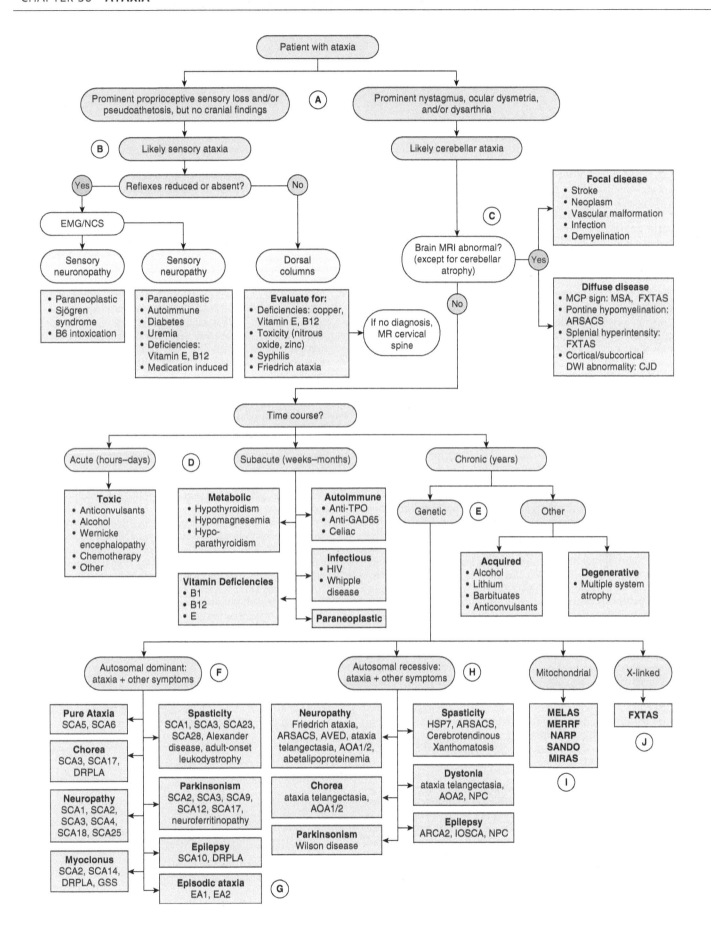

Difficulty Walking

Molly Cincotta and Raymond S. Price

Gait disorders can result from dysfunction of motor coordination systems, pyramidal or extrapyramidal motor pathways, or impairments in proprioceptive sensation. In addition, there are a number of nonneurologic causes of difficulty walking. Careful neurologic examination, including observation of the patient attempting to walk, can usually localize the lesion and focus the diagnostic evaluation.

A. Initial evaluation should focus on determining if significant leg weakness is present. If so, this is the likely cause of the gait disorder. If weakness is unilateral and acute, consider cerebral infarction or hemorrhage; rarely spinal cord infarction can cause acute unilateral leg weakness. If bilateral and acute, consider spinal cord infarction and cord compression. If weakness has been rapidly progressive over days, consider transverse myelitis, cauda equina syndrome, or Guillain-Barré syndrome. Patients with chronic unilateral leg weakness from a central nervous system (CNS) process such as stroke or spinal cord injury often have decreased flexion at the hip, knee and ankle when walking, which causes them to trip if they bring their leg directly forward. Instead, these patients move the affected leg in a circular direction ("circumduction gait") when walking. Patients with bilateral leg weakness from a CNS process may have spasticity, which causes their legs to cross when walking ("scissoring gait"). Patients with foot drop will trip over the dropped foot when walking and compensate with increased flexion of the legs at the hips ("steppage gait"). Lastly, patients with myopathy or neuromuscular junction disease may have proximal leg weakness causing excessive swaying of the trunk when walking ("waddling gait").

B. Acute onset of isolated gait ataxia can be seen with cerebellar lesions, particularly those affecting the cerebellar vermis; posterior circulation ischemic stroke or intracerebral hemorrhage must be considered. Acute gait imbalance can also be seen in conjunction with continuous vertigo, in which the main diagnostic distinction is between CNS lesions affecting the brainstem/cerebellum and peripheral lesions, such as vestibular neuritis, which affect the vestibulocochlear nerve.

C. Unlike patients with proprioceptive sensory loss, patients with cerebellar dysfunction are unable to stand with their feet together with their eyes open. Patients often compensate for this unsteadiness when their feet are close together by having a wide-based gait. With prominent involvement of the cerebellar vermis, patients may have truncal instability and not be able to sit up unassisted. Limb ataxia due to cerebellar lesions can be seen on finger-nose-finger or heel-knee-shin testing. Patients with weakness or proprioceptive loss will often also have difficulty with these tests, and thus one must be confident the difficulty is out of proportion to motor weakness or sensory impairment in order to attribute it to a cerebellar lesion. With cerebellar dysfunction, there may also be nystagmus and impaired saccadic eye movements.

D. Moderate to severe sensory loss in the legs, particularly proprioceptive loss, can cause difficulty walking. This is termed sensory ataxia. Impairment of proprioceptive sensation can be caused by injury to peripheral nerves or the dorsal column of the spinal cord; with the former, ankle reflexes are usually absent, whereas they are preserved in the latter. A patient with proprioceptive dysfunction typically will exhibit the Romberg sign, in which the ability to stand with the feet together is preserved with the eyes open but balance is lost when the eyes are closed.

E. Dystonia is characterized by sustained or intermittent muscle contraction causing stereotyped often twisting movements or postures, and is usually initiated or worsened by voluntary action including walking. A dystonic gait may appear bizarre and is often confused with a functional gait disorder, but can be differentiated by the stereotyped nature of the movements. Since gait dystonia is task-specific, the dystonia may disappear when the patient is asked to walk backwards.

F. Nonneurologic causes of gait dysfunction include visual loss, orthopedic or rheumatologic disorders, pain, drug or toxic effect, peripheral vascular disease, and cardiorespiratory problems.

G. Patients with unilateral vestibular dysfunction may have difficulty walking but additionally will describe symptoms of vertigo or a sensation of motion while standing still. Nausea and vomiting may also occur. Patients with bilateral vestibular dysfunction, as can be seen with gentamycin toxicity, will also have difficulty walking but not report vertigo. These patients typically have bilateral abnormal head impulse testing.

H. Frontal gait disorder, also described as a magnetic gait or gait apraxia, can be seen in syndromes that involve the subcortical white matter. The gait has a normal or wide base and may become more shuffling or magnetic when the patient is distracted. The difficulty with leg movements is often specific for walking; patients may be able to move their legs normally when asked to do alternative tasks such as pretending to ride a bike. Classically, magnetic gait has been associated with normal pressure hydrocephalus (NPH), a condition in which dementia and urinary incontinence may accompany the gait disorder. NPH should be considered when there is ventriculomegaly out of proportion to cortical atrophy on computed tomography or magnetic resonance imaging. To more quantitatively define this finding, the ratio of the maximum width of the frontal horns of the lateral ventricles is divided by the maximum internal diameter of the skull at the same level (Evans index). A ratio >0.3 is suggestive of NPH. If NPH is suspected, gait assessment should be performed before and after a large-volume lumbar puncture (~30 mL of cerebrospinal fluid is removed). More commonly, magnetic gait is due to chronic severe microvascular brain ischemic disease, in which case it does not improve with shunting.

I. Parkinsonism is the clinical constellation of tremor, bradykinesia, and rigidity. The most common cause is idiopathic Parkinson disease, although it can be caused by antidopaminergic medications, cerebrovascular disease, or other neurodegenerative processes.

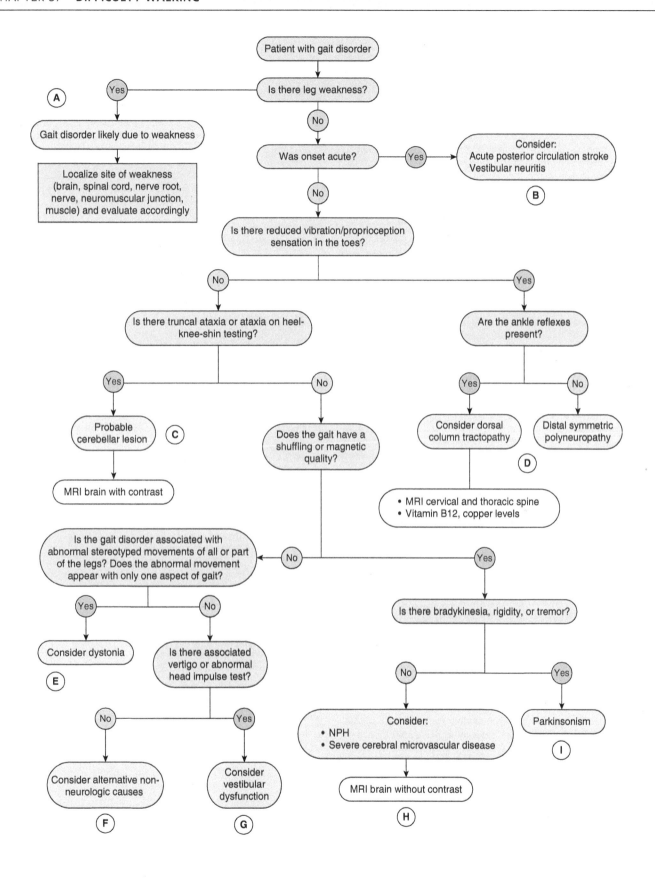

Bladder Dysfunction

Anne G. Douglas and Raymond S. Price

Urinary continence requires coordination of both the somatic and autonomic nervous systems, and also involves elements of volitional control and assessments of social appropriateness. Urinary storage is primarily mediated involuntarily by the sympathetic nervous system and volitionally by the somatic neurons to the external urethral sphincter. At low bladder volumes, contraction of the internal and external urethral sphincter is maintained via α-adrenergic receptors and detrusor muscle contraction in the bladder wall is inhibited via β-adrenergic receptors. Urinary voiding is primarily mediated by the parasympathetic nervous system in conjunction with the pontine micturition center. At higher bladder volumes, descending axons from the pontine micturition center activate the parasympathetic neurons in the sacral spinal cord, which cause both detrusor muscle contraction via muscarinic acetylcholine receptors and urethral relaxation. They also inhibit the sympathetic neurons to the bladder and the somatic neurons to the external urethral sphincter. The pontine micturition center is inhibited by cortical regions so that voiding occurs in the appropriate social context.

A. Bladder dysfunction may signal pathology at any level from the cortex and pons to spinal cord and sacral peripheral nerve roots. However, more often it is due to a primary urologic cause affecting the bladder or urethra, and thus urologic evaluation should be performed initially, including an evaluation for urinary tract infection, prostate disease in men, and gynecologic disease in women. Urinary incontinence or retention is a frequent medication side effect. Commonly implicated medications include anticholinergics, opiates, calcium channel blockers, and diuretics.

B. In patients with urinary hesitancy and/or urinary retention, there is dysfunction of detrusor muscle contraction indicating a loss of parasympathetic excitation. This can be seen in focal lesions of the sacral spinal cord (conus medullaris) or sacral nerve roots (cauda equina) or in diffuse processes affecting the autonomic nervous system. An acute cervical or thoracic spinal cord injury can result in acute urinary retention (spinal shock), but patients will develop detrusor overactivity in a few weeks or months.

C. Due to extensive autonomic innervation, bladder dysfunction may be seen in processes that preferentially involve the autonomic system, such as polyneuropathy from diabetes or amyloidosis, idiopathic small fiber polyneuropathy, and primary autonomic failure. Multiple system atrophy (MSA) may be a unifying diagnosis when an older patient presents with isolated, prominent autonomic dysfunction without other evidence of polyneuropathy. Accompanying evidence of Parkinsonism may not be seen in the early stages of MSA. In this context, patients with bladder dysfunction should be specifically asked about other symptoms of autonomic dysfunction, such as orthostasis, dry mouth, abnormal sweating, gastroparesis, and constipation. On examination, patients should be evaluated for distal loss of pain and temperature sensation and orthostatic hypotension.

D. Intermittent catheterization is the main treatment for urinary retention regardless of the etiology. Intermittent catheterization overrides the internal and external urethral sphincters, obviating the need for detrusor contraction, avoids damage to the upper urinary tract from chronic retention, and minimizes the infection risk relative to chronic catheterization. Scheduled voiding may also prevent overflow incontinence episodes and promotes patient independence.

E. Detrusor overactivity (detrusor muscle contraction at low filling volumes) often occurs after central nervous system injury and leads to urgency, frequency, and urge incontinence. When the lesion is in the spinal cord, there may also be a loss of upper motor neuron modulation of the external urethral sphincter resulting in detrusor-sphincter dyssynergia. Thus, in addition to frequent detrusor contractions at low filling volumes, the bladder and external sphincter often contract simultaneously, resulting in ineffective voiding.

F. The classic triad of normal pressure hydrocephalus (NPH) includes urinary incontinence (especially urgency), gait instability (magnetic gait), and dementia. Patients need not have all three features. Brain magnetic resonance imaging or computed tomography demonstrating ventriculomegaly out of proportion to cortical atrophy is present in NPH. To more quantitatively define this finding, the ratio of the maximum width of the frontal horns of the lateral ventricles is divided by the maximum internal diameter of the skull at the same level (Evans index). A ratio of greater than 0.3 is suggestive of NPH. Ventriculoperitoneal shunting may provide relief, largely depending on the stage of illness and comorbidities.

G. Cortical lesions, particularly in the frontal lobe, often result in urinary urgency. Frequently cited mechanisms include interruption of conscious control of voiding or mechanisms underlying the switch from storage to evacuation of urine.

H. Optimal treatment of bladder dysfunction with urgency often requires a multimodal approach. Anticholinergic or β-adrenergic medications promote detrusor relaxation by inhibiting parasympathetic and activating sympathetic pathways, respectively. In patients with detrusor-sphincter dyssynergia, intermittent catheterization is usually employed as well to combat incomplete emptying, which can exacerbate detrusor overactivity, cause symptoms of urgency and frequency, and lead to infection.

REFERENCE

1. Fowler CJ, Griffiths D, de Groat WC. The neural control of micturition. *Nat Rev Neurosci.* 2008;9(6):453–466.

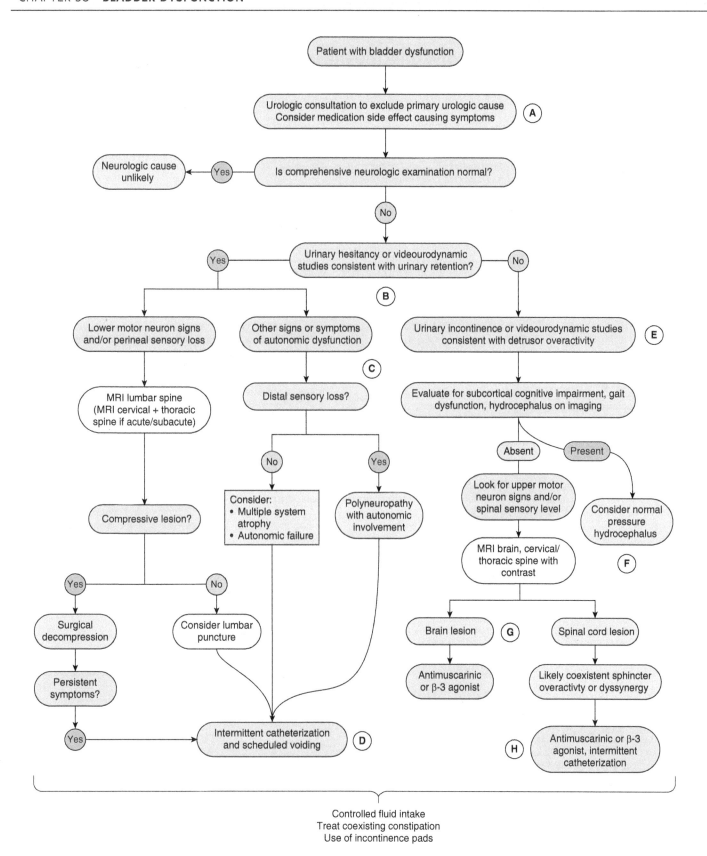

Transient Loss of Consciousness

Erin Conrad and Michael Gelfand

Dysfunction of either the brainstem or both cerebral hemispheres is necessary for loss of consciousness (LOC) to occur. Syncope, caused by global hypoperfusion of the brain due to a drop in blood pressure or cardiac output, is the most common cause of transient LOC. Seizures may also affect bilateral hemispheres of the brain leading to LOC. One of the challenges in transient LOC is that the underlying causes range from benign (e.g., vasovagal syncope) to extremely dangerous (cardiac arrhythmia). Misdiagnosis is common, particularly mistaking so-called "convulsive syncope," in which brief myoclonic jerks occur on losing consciousness in the setting of syncope, for seizure activity. Likewise, despite the perception that it is specific for seizure, urinary incontinence occurs frequently irrespective of underlying cause. Careful evaluation and testing guided by the clinical picture is thus important. As patients are by definition unconscious during the event itself, obtaining history from bystanders, family, and first responders is a priority. In rare cases where the patient is able to recall the event, consider mimics such as cataplexy.

A. Prodromal symptoms preceding LOC may be recalled by the patient or may have been mentioned to witnesses on the scene prior to losing consciousness. Syncope typically has a prodrome of lightheadedness, nausea, diaphoresis, tinnitus, and visual dimming. Chest pain, palpitations, or shortness of breath suggest a cardiac cause. In the rare cases where transient LOC is due to posterior circulation transient ischemic attack (TIA), there may be vertigo or focal neurologic symptoms (e.g., dysarthria, double vision, hemiparesis, or hemisensory loss) preceding the episode. Seizures with a focal onset and secondary generalization may begin with confusion associated with some preservation of consciousness, with focal motor activity, or with an aura.

B. Commonly described auras are a sense of déjà vu or fear, or visual, auditory, somatic, or olfactory (typically unpleasant) sensations. Seizure onset can also be accompanied by autonomic auras difficult to distinguish from symptoms seen in syncope, such as tachycardia, pallor, diaphoresis, or nausea. Seizures often occur without aura, or the patient may not recall the aura postictally. If convulsive activity is described, one must be careful to distinguish between focal convulsions (e.g., face twitching or arm shaking) *before* LOC, which strongly suggests seizure, and generalized myoclonic jerks *during* the period the patient is unconscious, which is nonspecific and, when brief, common in syncope.

C. The duration of LOC and postictal confusion helps distinguish between seizure and syncope. In syncope, LOC is usually brief (seconds), with rapid recovery once the cause is removed, such as returning to a recumbent position after orthostatic syncope. Seizures may lead to more prolonged LOC as well as a longer period of postictal dysfunction, such as confusion, which may last minutes to hours.

D. If posterior circulation TIA is suspected, vascular imaging of the head and neck with computed tomography or magnetic resonance angiography should be performed. Absence of high-grade stenosis or occlusion makes this diagnosis extremely unlikely.

E. Triggers and provoking factors may suggest a specific syncope etiology such as vasovagal, situational (e.g., tussive or micturition), or orthostatic syncope. Vasovagal syncope may be triggered by stress, fear, pain, physical exertion, or prolonged standing. Prior episodes of presyncope, most typically lightheadedness or vision dimming without LOC, provoked by the same triggers should be noted. Very rarely, LOC may be triggered by standing in patients with severe vertebrobasilar or bilateral carotid stenosis.

F. If seizure is suspected, perform electroencephalogram (EEG) and brain magnetic resonance imaging (MRI). Epileptiform abnormalities on EEG indicate a high probability that seizure is the cause; a normal EEG, however, does not rule out epilepsy and is common in patients with seizures. Brain MRI is performed to look for an obvious seizure focus, such as tumor. If initial testing is unrevealing, EEG should be repeated, and prolonged EEG monitoring considered, both of which increase the yield for finding epileptiform abnormalities.

G. Cardiogenic syncope is potentially life-threatening; it usually results from either arrhythmia (acquired or from genetic causes such as long QT or Brugada syndrome) or cardiac outflow obstruction (such as aortic stenosis or hypertrophic obstructive cardiomyopathy). Ask about known cardiac disease and family history of early sudden death. Evaluation for suspected cardiac causes of syncope includes electrocardiogram, echocardiography, and potentially long-term cardiac monitoring. When cardiac syncope is suspected, consult cardiology.

H. Consider psychogenic events in patients with recurrent unexplained episodes of LOC. Suggestive features include recurrent events with variable presentations, prolonged periods of unresponsiveness (often longer than several minutes) with a rapid return to baseline, and eye closure, particularly if forced, throughout the episode (with epileptic seizures the eyes are usually open). Testing to rule out other causes should generally be completed before considering this diagnosis. Continuous video-EEG monitoring in an epilepsy monitoring unit can confirm a diagnosis of psychogenic nonepileptic seizures.

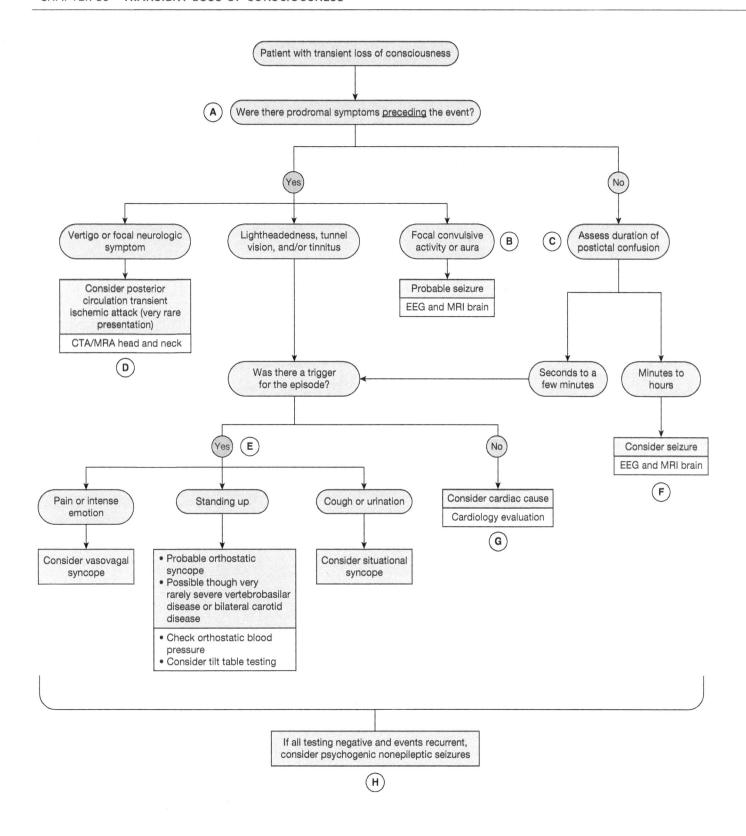

PART II

Specific Neurologic Conditions

Transient Ischemic Attack

Christopher Renner, Christopher G. Favilla, and Brett L. Cucchiara

A transient ischemic attack (TIA) represents focal brain ischemia that reverses before leaving a permanent neurologic deficit. Most TIAs present suddenly and last for minutes, though on occasion symptoms can persist or fluctuate for hours before recovery. Given the transient nature of the symptoms, initial suspicion for TIA often depends on the patient's description of the event. This may be imprecise depending on the patient's ability to accurately describe symptoms; a high level of suspicion for TIA is therefore always appropriate. TIA represents a warning sign of possible impending stroke, with the first 48 hours the highest risk period. Start antiplatelet therapy immediately and perform a diagnostic evaluation to determine the underlying mechanism that will guide long-term preventative therapy.

A. There are a number of nonvascular causes of transient neurologic symptoms. The most important are seizure with transient postictal deficits (usually apparent from the history), and migrainous phenomenon. Use care in making the latter diagnosis, as headache may also accompany TIA; a history of migraine with aura along with similar stereotyped events in the past argues for migraine as a cause. When the diagnosis is uncertain, it is generally advisable to pursue a TIA workup to ensure a vascular cause is not responsible for the episode.

B. Head computed tomography (CT) is commonly the initial imaging study. Rarely, patients with brain tumors or small subdural hematomas will present with transient focal neurologic symptoms, and these will generally be seen on CT. Magnetic resonance imaging (MRI) of the brain is a more sensitive test to identify acute ischemic changes (see section E), but in most centers is not easily and/or rapidly available.

C. If urgent vascular imaging is performed and shows large artery atherosclerotic disease, or if this is known to exist prior to the TIA, the short-term risk of stroke is substantially increased and aggressive therapy is appropriate (see section F).

D. The $ABCD_2$ score is a risk stratification tool that can be used to estimate the risk of stroke following TIA. It can be quickly calculated during the initial evaluation. A score of 0–3 suggests a 48-hour stroke risk of about 1%; higher scores are associated with higher risk of up to 10% in the first 48 hours.

E. MRI brain with diffusion-weighted imaging (DWI) sequences reveals acute infarction in about one-third of TIA patients. When present, the diagnosis of a vascular cause is confirmed and evaluation should proceed as for those with stroke; further, the risk of subsequent stroke is substantially greater. A negative MRI DWI study does not rule out TIA, but given the lower risk of future stroke and, in many cases, uncertainty about whether a vascular cause was responsible for symptoms, a more conservative evaluation for underlying etiology may be reasonable. MRI may also reveal an alternative diagnosis, such as tumor or demyelination. In patients with an obvious cause for TIA, such as atrial fibrillation or carotid stenosis, MRI may not be necessary.

F. In high-risk patients ($ABCD_2$ score ≥ 4 or large artery disease) who present within 24 hours, dual antiplatelet therapy with aspirin and clopidogrel lowers the risk of recurrent stroke and should be administered as soon as possible. A loading dose of both (aspirin 162–325 mg, clopidogrel 300–600 mg) should be given, followed by a 21-day course of treatment. After this, antiplatelet monotherapy should be continued indefinitely. If subsequent evaluation reveals a cardioembolic source warranting anticoagulation (e.g., atrial fibrillation), dual antiplatelet therapy should be discontinued and replaced with oral anticoagulation.

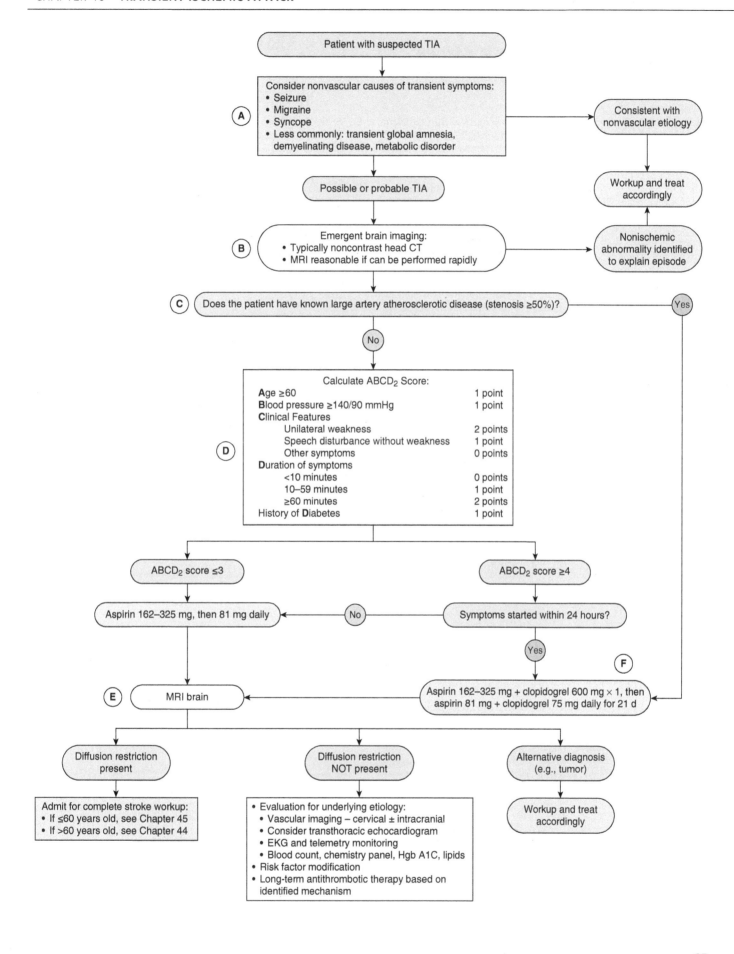

Acute Ischemic Stroke

Christopher G. Favilla

When a patient presents with acute focal neurologic deficits consistent with ischemic stroke, the immediate goal is to determine whether the patient is eligible for reperfusion therapies with intravenous thrombolysis (tissue plasminogen activator, tPA) and/or endovascular therapy with mechanical thrombectomy (MT). Assessment is based on clinical symptoms which are typically assessed with the National Institutes of Health Stroke Scale (NIHSS), timing, and neuroimaging. A detailed description of the NIHSS can be found in Appendix 2. Evaluation and treatment decisions must be made as quickly as possible, keeping in mind the mantra that "time is brain"—there is clear evidence that faster treatment results in a greater likelihood of neurologic recovery.

A. A focused history should establish the time of symptom onset. When the exact time of symptom onset is unclear, the time at which the patient was last known normal should be used. The NIHSS serves as a rapid neurologic exam to quantify the neurologic deficit. A fingerstick glucose should be checked to ensure hypo- or hyperglycemia is not causing a stroke mimic.

B. In patients with mild, non-disabling deficits, the risk of thrombolytic therapy likely outweighs the benefit, so withholding tPA is reasonable. No specific threshold value of the NIHSS can discriminate between disabling and non-disabling deficits, therefore clinical judgment in the individual patient is required.

C. Patients within 4.5 hours of the time last known normal may be eligible for intravenous (IV) thrombolysis. Noncontrast head computed tomography (CT) can exclude hemorrhage. IV tPA exclusion criteria should be quickly assessed (see Table 41.1), and tPA should be administered as rapidly as possible if the deficit is perceived to be disabling (see Table 41.1 in Appendix 1). If blood pressure elevation precludes tPA, administer IV antihypertensive medication such as labetalol or nicardipine to achieve an acceptable blood pressure. It is not necessary to wait for the results of laboratory testing other than fingerstick glucose unless the patient is on anticoagulation (if on warfarin, international normalized ratio [INR] >1.7 precludes tPA) or has a clinical history raising suspicion of thrombocytopenia (e.g., sepsis, malignancy).

D. A patient with a severe deficit and a contraindication to tPA may benefit from MT, so CT angiogram (CTA) should be obtained to evaluate for large vessel occlusion. Depending on workflow, CTA may also be obtained with the initial CT in order to speed evaluation.

E. When >4.5 hours from onset, tPA should not be given, but if significant neurologic deficit is present, then rapid CTA (MRA is also acceptable, though generally more time-consuming) should be used to assess for the presence of a large vessel occlusion, in which case MT should be considered. When <6 hours from onset, perfusion imaging is generally not necessary.

F. In the 6–24-hour time window, if large vessel occlusion is present, perfusion imaging should be performed to identify patients that are likely to benefit from MT (small infarct core and large territory at risk).

G. If occlusion of the internal carotid artery (ICA) or proximal middle cerebral artery (MCA) is identified, MT should be pursued in patients with significant deficits <6 hours from onset unless there is extensive ischemic injury on CT. In the 6-24-hour window, results of perfusion imaging should be considered in making an assessment of potential benefit of treatment. Thrombectomy for basilar artery occlusion has not been well studied, but given the severity of the disease, it is reasonable to treat based on similar principles. If no large vessel occlusion is present, the patient is not eligible for MT.

H. Beyond 24 hours, the benefit of MT is uncertain; urgent CTA is appropriate if there is symptom fluctuation or progression.

I. Patients that receive reperfusion therapy warrant intensive monitoring per a standard protocol, particularly during the first 24 hours, due the risk of intracranial bleeding. A blood pressure goal of <180/105 mmHg is appropriate. Antithrombotic therapy and deep vein thrombosis prophylaxis should be withheld for 24 hours following IV tPA, until head imaging confirms there is no hemorrhage. After MT, antithrombotic therapy can be started immediately if the risk of procedural bleeding complications is felt to be low; this is often assessed with a repeat head CT postprocedure to exclude intracranial bleeding.

J. In patients not treated with tPA or MT, early administration of aspirin is indicated to reduce the risk of recurrent stroke. Within the first 24 hours of symptom onset, patients with minor stroke should be treated with combination aspirin and clopidogrel, assuming no contraindication, for 21 days, then switched to antiplatelet monotherapy.

K. Aggressive intravenous hydration should be administered to all stroke patients unless there is concern for heart failure. Positioning the head of bed flat may improve cerebral blood flow in some patients. Formal dysphagia screening should be performed prior to allowing oral intake.

See Appendix 1 for Table 41.1: Criteria for selecting patients with acute ischemic stroke for thrombolysis.

See Appendix 2 for description of the National Institute of Health Stroke Scale (NIHSS).

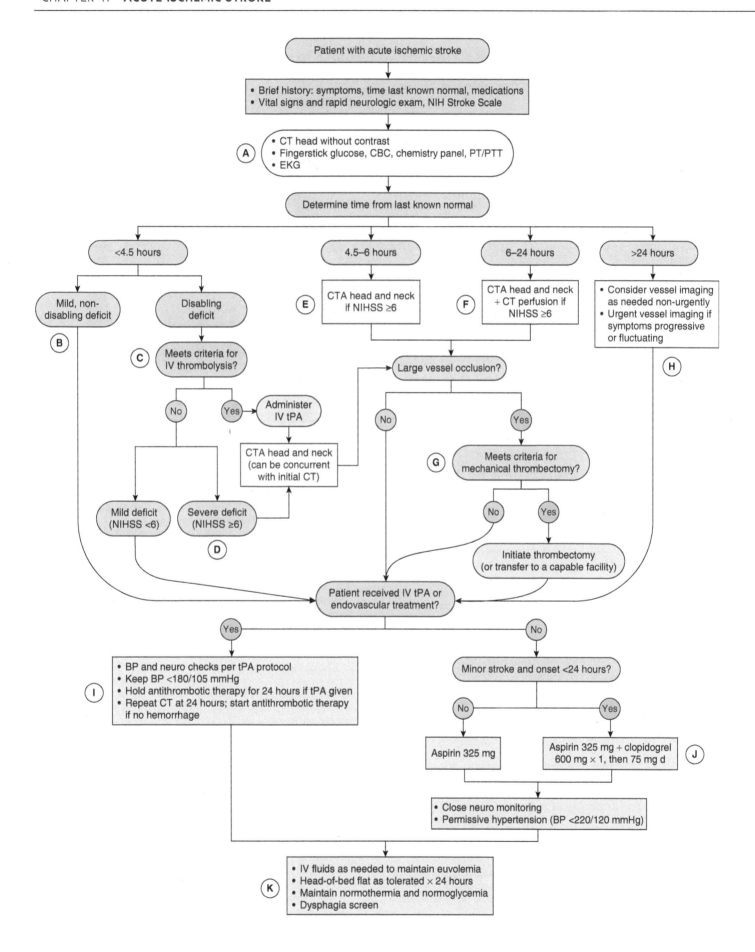

Patient with acute ischemic stroke

- Brief history: symptoms, time last known normal, medications
- Vital signs and rapid neurologic exam, NIH Stroke Scale

(A)
- CT head without contrast
- Fingerstick glucose, CBC, chemistry panel, PT/PTT
- EKG

Determine time from last known normal

<4.5 hours | 4.5–6 hours | 6–24 hours | >24 hours

Mild, non-disabling deficit

Disabling deficit

(B)

(C) Meets criteria for IV thrombolysis?

(E) CTA head and neck if NIHSS ≥6

(F) CTA head and neck + CT perfusion if NIHSS ≥6

- Consider vessel imaging as needed non-urgently
- Urgent vessel imaging if symptoms progressive or fluctuating

(H)

No   Yes → Administer IV tPA

Large vessel occlusion?

CTA head and neck (can be concurrent with initial CT)

No   Yes

(G) Meets criteria for mechanical thrombectomy?

Mild deficit (NIHSS <6)

Severe deficit (NIHSS ≥6)

(D)

No   Yes

Initiate thrombectomy (or transfer to a capable facility)

Patient received IV tPA or endovascular treatment?

Yes   No

(I)
- BP and neuro checks per tPA protocol
- Keep BP <180/105 mmHg
- Hold antithrombotic therapy for 24 hours if tPA given
- Repeat CT at 24 hours; start antithrombotic therapy if no hemorrhage

Minor stroke and onset <24 hours?

No   Yes

Aspirin 325 mg

Aspirin 325 mg + clopidogrel 600 mg × 1, then 75 mg d (J)

- Close neuro monitoring
- Permissive hypertension (BP <220/120 mmHg)

(K)
- IV fluids as needed to maintain euvolemia
- Head-of-bed flat as tolerated × 24 hours
- Maintain normothermia and normoglycemia
- Dysphagia screen

42 Malignant Middle Cerebral Artery Infarction

Izad-Yar D. Rasheed and Joshua M. Levine

"Malignant" infarction refers to a large hemispheric ischemic stroke characterized by severe cerebral edema; such infarction can lead to midline shift with resultant compression of contralateral hemispheric structures and downward herniation leading to death (Fig. 42.1). Edema following hemispheric stroke slowly evolves, generally peaking 3–5 days after stroke onset. The definitive therapeutic intervention is hemicraniectomy, in which a large segment of skull overlying the infarction is removed, allowing the brain to swell outward. Medical therapy with hyperosmolar agents such as mannitol and hypertonic saline also have roles as a bridge to hemicraniectomy or in those who are not surgical candidates.

A. Even with aggressive therapy, patients with malignant middle cerebral artery (MCA) infarction are uniformly left with long-term significant disability, with the vast majority (>80%) dependent on others for help with activities of daily living. The severity of brain injury should be clearly communicated to family. Discuss with family the patient's willingness to live with severe disability as expressed prior to the stroke. Rarely can the patient engage meaningfully in this discussion, as they typically are severely aphasic (dominant hemisphere involvement) or have dense neglect (nondominant hemisphere involvement), which precludes an accurate understanding of their condition. Many patients and families feel living with severe disability is a fate worse than death, and decline aggressive intervention.

B. Patient age has a major impact on outcome following malignant MCA infarction. In randomized trials of hemicraniectomy, younger patients (<60 years) treated surgically have both a dramatic reduction in mortality and a significantly greater likelihood of achieving mild-moderate disability. In contrast, mortality is reduced with surgery in older patients but almost all survivors are left with moderately severe disability or worse. Given this, in combination with the invasiveness of hemicraniectomy, it is generally avoided in older patients.

C. Clinical criteria for predicting which acute ischemic strokes become "malignant" are imperfect. Generally, those with involvement of two-thirds or more of the MCA territory, particularly if the basal ganglia is also affected, are likely to develop severe swelling and midline shift and benefit from decompressive surgery with hemicraniectomy. In many cases the degree of infarction is only apparent on early interval follow-up head computed tomography (CT); accordingly, patients without evidence of malignant infarction on initial scan should have an interval CT 12–24 hours after the initial scan. If radiographic evidence of likely malignant infarction is present in a patient otherwise eligible for surgery within the first 24–48 hours of stroke onset, proceed to hemicraniectomy even in the absence of neurologic decline.

D. In patients without clear radiographic evidence to suggest a high risk of malignant infarction (e.g., smaller MCA infarctions, lack of early edema and midline shift), close neurologic monitoring is indicated. Often the earliest sign of malignant infarction is increasing somnolence. Do not wait for symptoms of uncal (anisocoria or an unreactive pupil) or transtentorial (new field cut, bilateral small fixed pupils, impaired upgaze) herniation to develop prior to considering hemicraniectomy. Should deterioration occur, administration of osmotic agents and hyperventilation can be implemented. Perform immediate repeat head CT to exclude alternative causes of worsening, such as hemorrhagic conversion. Proceed to hemicraniectomy as soon as possible.

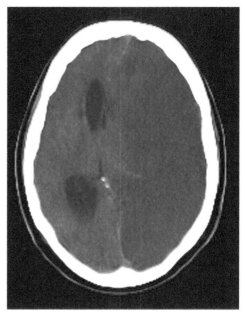

FIG. 42.1 Head computed tomography showing large left cerebral artery infarction with edema and midline shift.

E. Mannitol and hypertonic saline are osmotic therapies used to reduce cerebral edema. Mannitol is a reasonable initial choice, and is strongly preferred in volume-overloaded patients; hypertonic saline is preferred in patients with renal impairment. Administration through a central venous catheter is desirable but not essential. A bolus of 1 g/kg mannitol 20% can be given intravenously every 6 hours as needed. Determine the "osmolar gap" (calculated serum osmolarity subtracted from measured osmolarity) prior to redosing; if it exceeds 20 mOsm/L, do not give additional mannitol. Replete urine losses aggressively with normal saline to prevent hypovolemia. Hypertonic saline is an alternative to mannitol, given as a bolus (either 250 mL of 3%; 150 mL of 5%; or 30 mL of 23.4% solution) every 6 hours. Closely monitor serum sodium; if >160 mmol/L, hypertonic saline should be stopped. Osmotic therapy is best viewed as a bridge to decompressive surgery, as it is far less effective than hemicraniectomy. However, for patients who are not candidates for hemicraniectomy, osmotic therapy may be used in an attempt to minimize the impact of cerebral edema until swelling starts to resolve on its own, usually after day 3–5. It should not be used prophylactically.

REFERENCE

1. Vahedi K, Hofmeijer J, Juettler E, et al. Early decompressive surgery in malignant infarction of the middle cerebral artery: a pooled analysis of three randomized controlled trials. *Lancet Neurol.* 2007;6(3):215–222.

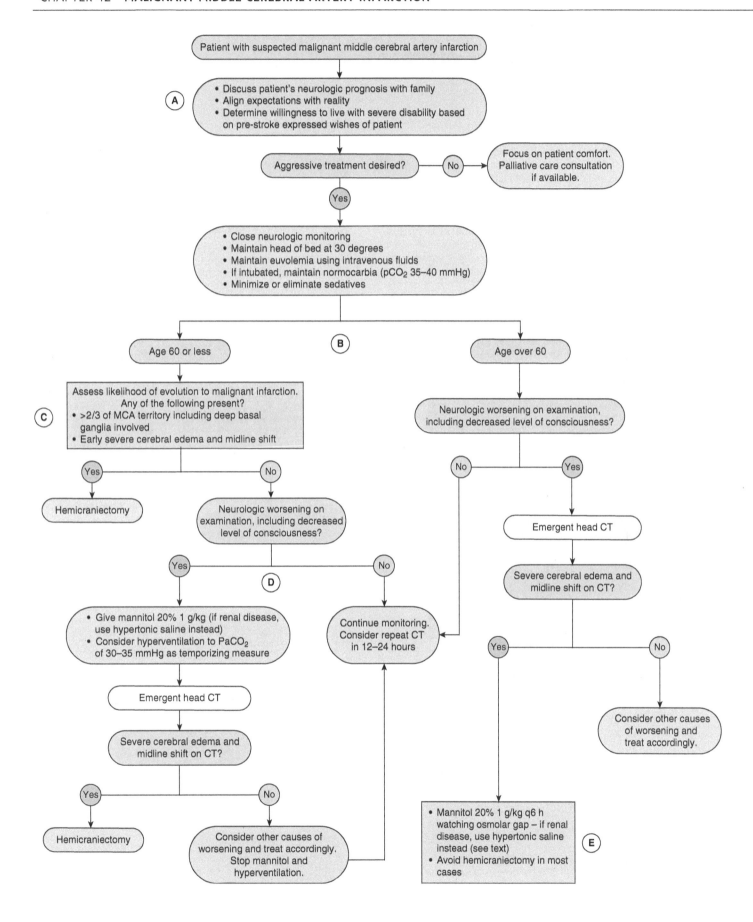

Large Cerebellar Infarction

Brett L. Cucchiara

Because of its unique position abutting the brainstem, infarction of the cerebellum can lead to a compression of the fourth ventricle with resulting hydrocephalus, direct compressive brainstem injury, and downward brainstem herniation, all with devastating neurologic consequences (Fig. 43.1). Vulnerable patients are those with large cerebellar infarctions associated with mass effect, typically caused by occlusion of the posterior inferior cerebellar artery or by occlusion of multiple cerebellar branch arteries. In the latter case, involvement of the vermis is associated with an increased risk of neurologic deterioration. Treatment is surgical decompression with suboccipital craniectomy, and placement of an external ventricular drain if there is hydrocephalus. Intervention must be performed urgently when signs of brainstem dysfunction are present to prevent progressive injury.

A. In patients at risk, close observation for signs of neurologic deterioration is mandatory. Serial brain computed tomography (CT) may be useful for monitoring the degree of mass effect and hydrocephalus. If neurologic signs or symptoms referable to brainstem dysfunction appear and are associated with a correlating change in the degree of compression on imaging, surgery should be pursued urgently. At times there may be uncertainty as to whether clinical signs of brainstem dysfunction are in fact due to brainstem compression, for instance when a significant change on serial imaging is not apparent. In these cases, osmotic therapy such as a bolus of mannitol can be given; if there is improvement in symptoms, this argues strongly to proceed with decompressive surgery.

B. In some patients, progressive swelling becomes apparent on serial scans without an obvious clinical change. Prophylactic decompressive surgery should be considered in these cases, as waiting until clinical symptoms appear carries some risk of irreversible brain injury.

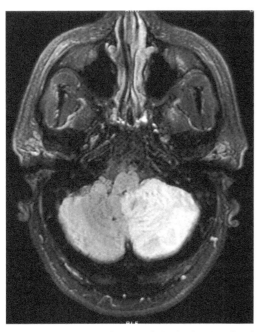

FIG. 43.1 Magnetic resonance image of the brain showing large left posterior inferior cerebellar artery infarction with early mild brainstem compression.

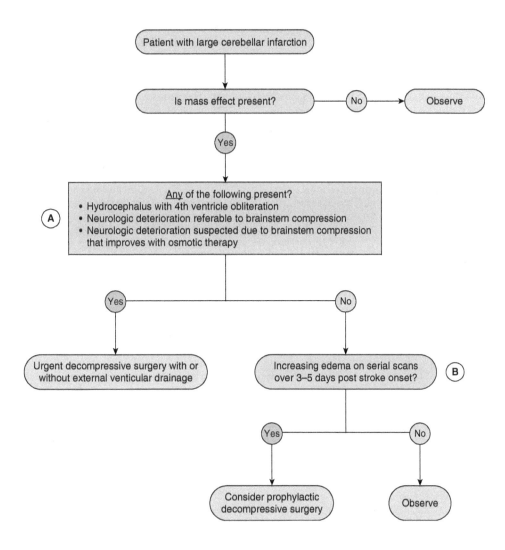

Prevention of Recurrent Ischemic Stroke

Saad Mir and Christopher G. Favilla

Mechanisms of ischemic stroke are heterogeneous, and therapies to prevent recurrent stroke vary based on underlying mechanism. Determining the specific cause of stroke in the individual patient is therefore critical. Major mechanistic categories in the typical patient with stroke (i.e., older or with traditional vascular risk factors) include large vessel atherosclerotic stenosis, cardioembolism, small-vessel (lacunar) disease, and a host of infrequent other specific causes. Occasionally, hypercoagulable states, unusual infectious causes of stroke, and other less common causes will need to be considered. Note that these less common causes of stroke are more likely to be present in younger patients (<60 years old), and thus evaluation is different in that group (see Chapter 45, Ischemic Stroke in the Young).

A. The location and pattern of infarction on brain imaging has mechanistic implications. Simultaneous acute infarctions in more than one vascular territory strongly implicates a proximal embolic source. When acute infarctions are present in all three vascular territories, consider hypercoagulability of malignancy. Carotid revascularization is an important intervention to prevent recurrent stroke, but it depends on the infarct being in the territory supplied by the carotid artery. For posterior circulation infarctions, there is little role for revascularization. Magnetic resonance imaging (MRI) of the brain is more sensitive than computed tomography (CT) at identifying and defining the infarction pattern; however, in a patient with an obvious mechanism (such as atrial fibrillation) it is not always necessary.

B. CT and MR angiography of the head and neck provide a comprehensive assessment of the cerebral vasculature and are highly sensitive for identifying significant stenosis. As an alternative in older patients (>60 years) with anterior circulation stroke, carotid ultrasound adequately evaluates the carotid bifurcation where the vast majority of carotid stenosis occurs, and transcranial Doppler can screen for intracranial stenosis. While less sensitive than CT or MR angiography, this strategy is also less expensive and resource intensive.

C. In the older patient, atrial fibrillation is a major cause of stroke; electrocardiography and cardiac monitoring should be performed in all patients. Unless an obvious cause of stroke is apparent, transthoracic echocardiography (TTE) should generally also be performed. This can identify important cardioembolic sources, such as dilated cardiomyopathy, severe heart failure, apical akinesis, valvular disease, and intracardiac thrombus. Transesophageal echocardiography (TEE) is more sensitive than TTE for some of these findings, but is invasive and relatively low yield. It should be reserved for those with multiple unexplained infarcts or concern for infective endocarditis. It can also be considered in those with embolic-appearing stroke in which a complete evaluation has been unrevealing. Basic laboratory testing is indicated for all patients to screen for hematologic or coagulation abnormalities, kidney disease, diabetes, and hyperlipidemia. D-dimer is a useful test in many patients, as extreme elevations are strongly associated with hypercoagulability of malignancy. Be aware, however, that D-dimer is not useful when measured after thrombolysis.

D. A number of uncommon causes of nonatherosclerotic vasculopathy exist. Arterial dissection should be treated with antiplatelet therapy; stenting or surgical revascularization should generally be avoided, as spontaneous healing of the vessel is common and early risk of recurrent stroke is low. Fibromuscular dysplasia (FMD), which can be associated with dissection, is also treated with antiplatelet therapy alone. In neither case is statin therapy necessary, as these conditions are not due to atherosclerosis. Syphilis, antiphospholipid antibody syndrome, Moyamoya disease, and vasculitis may also cause a nonatherosclerotic vasculopathy; all are quite rare.

E. Large artery atherosclerosis can involve the cervical or intracranial arteries. When stroke is in the territory of >50% cervical internal carotid artery stenosis, carotid endarterectomy (CEA) or carotid stenting (CAS) should be performed. Benefit is greatest when done within the first week after the stroke. CEA is preferred in most patients; CAS may be appropriate in younger patients and those with significant coronary disease. Vertebral artery and intracranial atherosclerosis are managed medically. With intracranial stenosis >50%, a 90-day course of aspirin and clopidogrel is appropriate, followed by monotherapy thereafter.

F. Long-term oral anticoagulation is imperative when atrial fibrillation is identified, reducing the risk of recurrent stroke by ~50%; it is also indicated if intracardiac thrombus is found. Severe cardiomyopathy with an ejection fraction <35% and an embolic-appearing stroke warrants long-term oral anticoagulation. If the ejection fraction subsequently improves, anticoagulation may be changed to antiplatelet therapy. Valvular vegetations may indicate infectious endocarditis, in which case antibiotic therapy and surgical consultation should be pursued, or nonbacterial thrombotic endocarditis, in which case evaluation for underlying hypercoagulability and rheumatologic disease is indicated and anticoagulation typically started. Surgical resection should be considered in patients with a cardiac mass (fibroelastoma, myxoma). Complex aortic atherosclerosis (>4 mm thickness or mobile) is generally treated with dual antiplatelet therapy for a period of at least 3–6 months.

G. Lacunar (small-vessel) infarctions, by definition <15 mm and located in deep, subcortical brain structures, are most often due to intrinsic disease in the small penetrating arteries, though embolism can mimic lacunar infarction. Classic lacunar syndromes include pure motor weakness, pure hemisensory loss, ataxia hemiparesis, and dysarthria–clumsy hand syndrome; the specificity of these clinical patterns for a small-vessel mechanism is poor, however.

H. Specific clinical scenarios should prompt consideration of less common causes of stroke. Fever, particularly if present on hospital arrival, should prompt suspicion for infectious endocarditis, as should bacteremia. Blood cultures and TEE should be performed. Always consider the possibility of cancer causing hypercoagulability in older patients with stroke, particularly those with multiple recurrent unexplained strokes, prior recent venous thromboembolism, or markedly elevated D-dimer. When suspected, CT of the chest/abdomen/pelvis is appropriate.

I. Vasculitis, either systemic or isolated to the central nervous system (CNS), is a rare cause of stroke. When suspected, a thorough diagnostic evaluation is critical, including serologic testing for systemic vasculitis, lumbar puncture to assess for cerebrospinal fluid inflammation and infectious processes, and catheter angiography to assess the smaller cerebral vessels. Brain/meningeal biopsy should be performed if isolated CNS vasculitis is strongly suspected, but a negative biopsy does not rule out the diagnosis. Treatment is usually steroids and cyclophosphamide. Rheumatology consultation is appropriate.

J. Paroxysmal atrial fibrillation is found on prolonged outpatient cardiac rhythm monitoring in 5%–10% of stroke patients with no identified mechanism on initial evaluation. Patients with cortical embolic appearing stroke and stroke in multiple vascular territories are particularly likely to have occult atrial fibrillation.

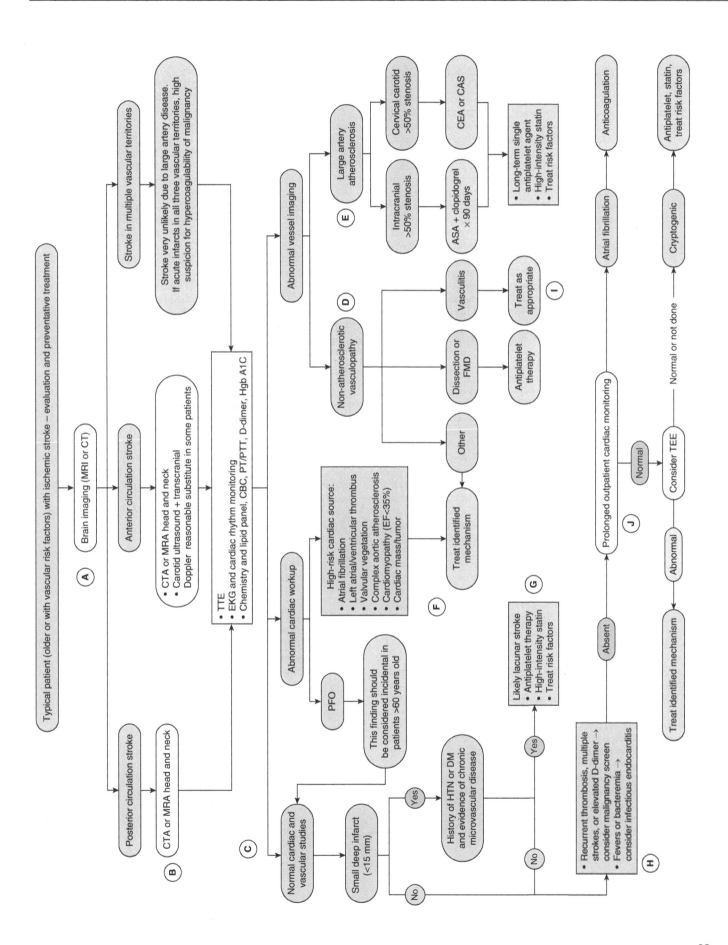

Ischemic Stroke in the Young

Christopher G. Favilla and Steven R. Messé

Ischemic stroke in a young adult (generally considered age <60 years), particularly when traditional vascular risk factors are absent, should raise suspicion for an unusual stroke mechanism.

A. Evaluate for traditional vascular risk factors, but note that arterial dissection, infective endocarditis, drugs of abuse, and thrombophilia are much more common stroke mechanisms in young compared to older patients. Careful inquiry into family history, preceding headache or neck pain, and illicit drug use are essential.

B. Brain magnetic resonance imaging (MRI) is useful to help determine the distribution and timing of stroke. Multifocal infarcts or infarcts of different ages suggest an embolic or hypercoagulable source. Carotid ultrasound is not adequate to evaluate for arterial dissection, a common stroke mechanism in the young, and thus computed tomography or MR angiography (CTA/MRA) of the head and neck should be performed. Initial laboratory testing should screen for hematologic abnormalities, renal dysfunction, risk for atherosclerosis, and syphilis. Depending on the context, more specific labs may be warranted (see sections F and H).

C. Carotid or vertebral arterial dissection is a common cause of stroke in the young. Dissection can occur spontaneously or as a consequence of trauma. A connective tissue disorder may predispose to dissection. Dissection carries a relatively low long-term risk of stroke recurrence. Short-term (1–3 months) aspirin plus clopidogrel is commonly used in those with minor stroke, followed by long-term aspirin monotherapy; the latter tends to be preferred in those with larger strokes to minimize the risk of hemorrhagic transformation. Anticoagulation can be considered if there is stroke recurrence despite antiplatelet therapy. Revascularization with stenting is rarely indicated and should be considered only in those with recurrent hemodynamic symptoms or stroke despite medical therapy.

D. Reversible cerebral vasoconstriction syndrome (RCVS) typically presents with recurrent thunderclap headaches. It is often associated with the use of sympathomimetic vasoconstrictive drugs such as stimulants and decongestants. A thorough history of prescription and over-the-counter medications as well as illicit drug use is essential. Potentially implicated drugs should be stopped. Verapamil may help mitigate vasoconstriction and treat headache.

E. Moyamoya disease is characterized by progressive bilateral narrowing of the internal carotid artery terminus extending into the anterior and middle cerebral artery accompanied by a network of small collateral vessels (so-called "puff of smoke"). Most often a primary process (moyamoya disease) likely to have a genetic basis, it can also occur secondary to a specific underlying disease (moyamoya syndrome) such as severe atherosclerosis, syphilis, or antiphospholipid antibody syndrome, amongst others. Moyamoya carries a risk of both ischemic and hemorrhagic stroke. In patients with an ischemic stroke, antiplatelet therapy is appropriate. Adequate hydration and avoidance of hypotension is crucial. Surgical procedures to facilitate collateral flow from the external carotid system to the intracranial circulation can be considered in patients with severe vascular compromise, progressive stenosis, and recurrent stroke.

F. Central nervous system (CNS) vasculitis may be a primary process or a component of a systemic vasculitis. Thorough evaluation of the kidneys, liver, eyes, and skin to identify a systemic process should be performed. Serum markers of inflammation, systemic autoimmune disease, and infection should be tested; erythrocyte sedimentation rate (ESR), C-reactive protein (CRP), anti-nuclear antibodies (ANA), anti-neutrophil cytoplasmic antibodies (ANCA), anti-double stranded DNA (Anti-dsDNA), anti-Sjögren's-syndrome-related antigen A and B (SSA/B), cryoglobulins, human immunodeficiency virus (HIV) and rapid plasma reagin (RPR) are commonly evaluated. Cerebrospinal fluid (CSF) should be evaluated for signs of inflammation with tests for specific infectious causes (such as varicella-zoster virus or fungal infections) based on the CSF profile. In the absence of an infectious or systemic process, primary CNS vasculitis should be considered. Brain/meningeal biopsy and rheumatology consultation are indicated in this scenario.

G. Transthoracic echocardiography (TTE) with bubble study is a reasonable starting point for cardiac imaging. If unrevealing, proceed to transesophageal echocardiography (TEE) with bubble study.

H. If no mechanism is found despite above evaluation, testing for high-risk thrombophilia should be performed. This may include testing for antiphospholipid antibodies and protein C and S and antithrombin III deficiency depending on the patient's age and clinical context. Notably, protein C, S, and antithrombin III measurements are unreliable in the setting of acute thrombosis, so should be measured at least 4–6 weeks after a thrombotic event. The factor V Leiden and prothrombin gene mutation tests are commonly performed, but only when the patient is homozygous or both are positive is anticoagulation generally warranted. In the appropriate clinical context, hypercoagulability of malignancy should also be considered.

I. Prolonged cardiac monitoring for atrial fibrillation is particularly low yield in patients <40 years old, but can be considered if older, if there is a family history of atrial fibrillation, or in the presence of cardiac disease by history or on echocardiography.

J. Cardiac thrombus, severe cardiomyopathy, and nonbacterial thrombotic endocarditis should be treated with long-term anticoagulation. Patients with a cardiac mass should be referred to cardiothoracic surgery. Aortic atherosclerosis >4 mm or with a significant mobile component is generally treated with dual antiplatelet therapy.

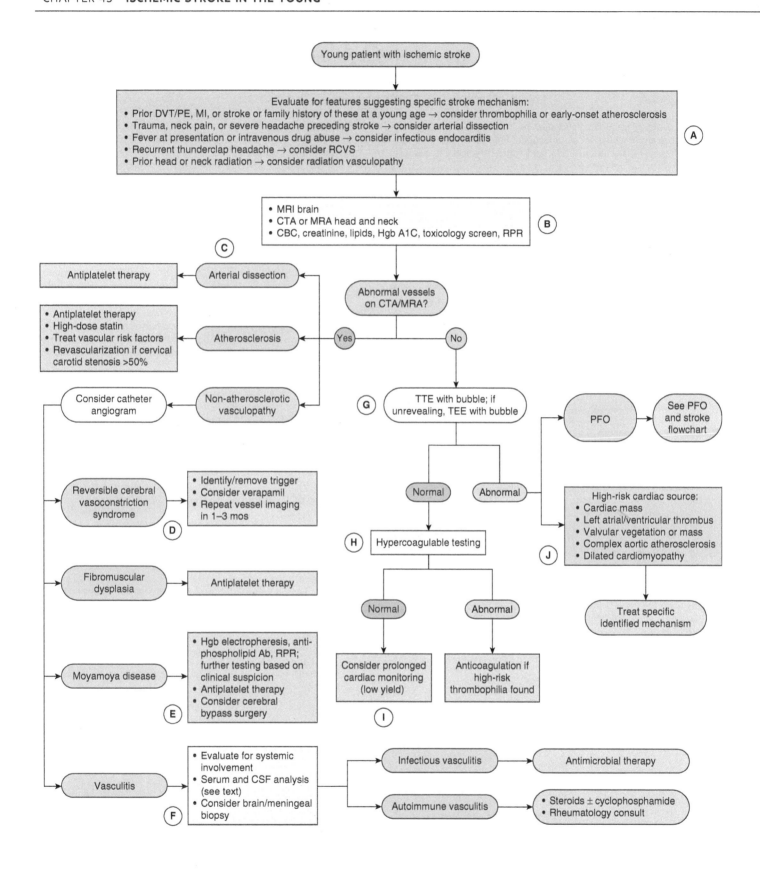

Patent Foramen Ovale and Ischemic Stroke

Christopher G. Favilla and Steven R. Messé

Patent foramen ovale (PFO) is a common congenital cardiac finding. The foramen ovale allows for unidirectional blood flow from the right atria to the left atria while in utero, and while it typically closes after birth, persistence of the foramen ovale is seen in ∼25% of healthy adults. It is, therefore, a very frequent incidental finding. PFO has been implicated as a potential source of ischemic stroke via paradoxical embolization, in which a clot from the systemic venous system travels to the right atrium and passes through the PFO in order to reach the left side of the heart and the systemic arterial circulation. The association between stroke and PFO is most robust for younger patients (≤60 years) with otherwise unexplained (cryptogenic) stroke; in this population, percutaneous PFO closure reduces the risk of recurrent stroke.[1-3] However, in cases where a specific alternative stroke etiology is identified, this is much more likely to be the cause of the stroke than the PFO, and closure is rarely indicated.

A. Trials of PFO closure in cryptogenic ischemic stroke included only patients 60 years old or younger. In older patients, the association of PFO and stroke is much weaker, likely due to the much higher prevalence of traditional stroke mechanisms in this population such that the PFO is most often an "innocent bystander." Given this, PFO closure in older patients is not recommended.

B. Confirmation of acute ischemic stroke on imaging is critical before considering PFO closure. In younger patients, symptoms suggestive of transient ischemic attack commonly are due to nonvascular mechanisms, such as migraine and seizure. Chronic infarctions are not infrequently found on imaging and are not an indication for PFO closure as the underlying stroke mechanisms in these cases are typically obscure, the risk of recurrence uncertain, and such patients are not eligible for inclusion in trials showing benefit for PFO closure.

C. A comprehensive evaluation to determine stroke mechanism is critical for all younger patients with ischemic stroke. This is outlined in Chapter 45. If an alternative mechanism is identified, PFO closure should not be pursued. The absolute risk of recurrent stroke associated with PFO is very low, so closure is not emergent, leaving time to complete a careful, thorough workup. The Risk of Paradoxical Embolization (ROPE) score is a simple scoring system that can be used to estimate the likelihood that stroke was related to PFO in the individual patient; it also can be used to predict the risk of recurrent stroke.[4]

D. The clinical trials that demonstrated the efficacy of PFO closure focused on patients with embolic appearing infarcts, typically excluding those with small deep infarcts thought to be due to lacunar disease.[3] Subgroup analysis of one trial that separately analyzed those with cortical compared with small deep infarcts (presumed to be nonlacunar by the enrolling investigator) suggested no benefit in the latter group.[2]

E. In the context of underlying thrombophilia that requires anticoagulation, it is unclear whether PFO closure conveys added benefit. Closure certainly does not preclude the need for anticoagulation, as it does not mitigate the risk of deep vein thrombosis or pulmonary embolism. While patients with thrombophilia were largely excluded from PFO closure trials, subgroup analysis of one trial revealed no additional benefit of closure in patients treated with anticoagulation.[2] In another trial that randomized patients between closure and anticoagulation, there was no significant difference in these treatments, raising the possibility that closure likely conveys little or no added benefit.[1]

F. A larger PFO or an associated atrial septal aneurysm may be associated with an increased risk of recurrent stroke, with the benefit of closure magnified in such patients.[2] In patients lacking any of these high-risk features, the benefit of closure is less clear, but may be considered.

G. Percutaneous PFO closure is performed with a small device deployed into the PFO via cardiac catheterization. Open surgical repair is generally only performed if cardiac surgery is required for a different issue.

REFERENCES

1. Mas JL, Derumeaux G, Guillon B, et al. Patent foramen ovale closure or anticoagulation vs. antiplatelets after stroke. *N Engl J Med*. 2017;377:1011–1021.
2. Saver JL, Carroll JD, Thaler DE, et al. Long-term outcomes of patent foramen ovale closure or medical therapy after stroke. *N Engl J Med*. 2017;377:1022–1032.
3. Søndergaard L, Kasner SE, Rhodes JF, et al. Patent foramen ovale closure or antiplatelet therapy for cryptogenic stroke. *N Engl J Med*. 2017;377:1033–1042.
4. Kent DM, Ruthazer R, Weimar C, et al. An index to identify stroke-related vs incidental patent foramen ovale in cryptogenic stroke. *Neurology*. 2013;81:619–625.

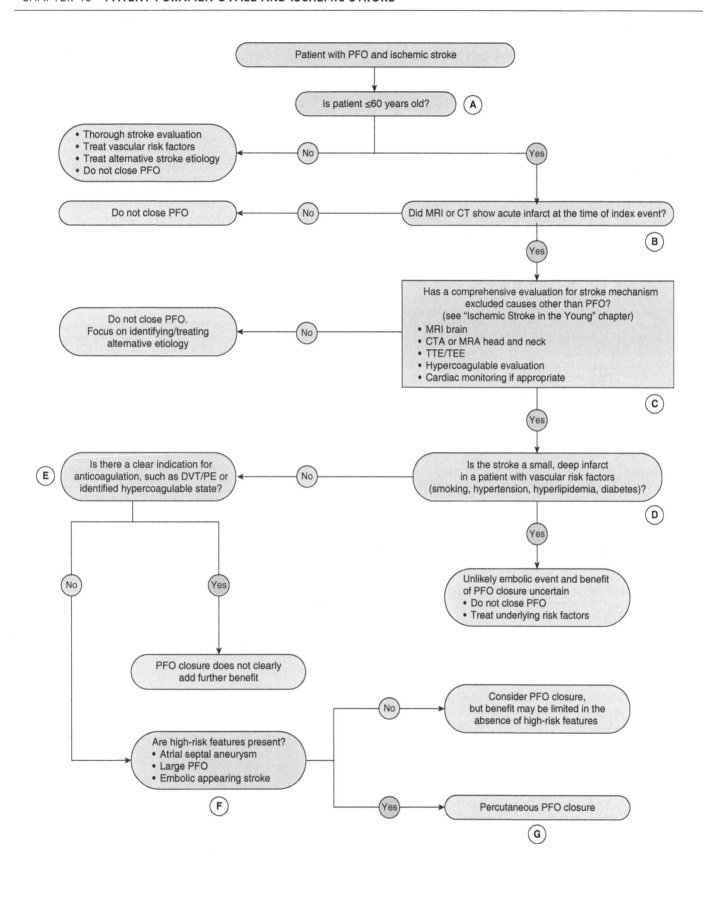

Spinal Cord Infarction

Michael McGarvey

Spinal cord infarction (SCI) is a rare but devastating disorder. A majority of infarctions involve anterior spinal cord and present with acute quadriparesis or paraparesis depending on the level of the spinal cord involved; rarely, weakness of a single limb may be seen, and even more rarely hemiparesis mimicking cerebral infarction. The diagnosis is made clinically and by excluding other potential explanations for the patient's symptoms. Spine magnetic resonance imaging (MRI) may confirm the diagnosis of infarction, although it can be normal in the acute period. Depending on the clinical scenario, urgent MRI may be needed to exclude compressive lesions of the cord which may cause similar symptoms but require a completely different therapeutic approach (e.g., decompressive surgery and/or steroids).

A. The etiology of SCI is critical to management. The most important distinction is whether SCI occurs in the perioperative or procedural setting or in a spontaneous outpatient setting. The vast majority of SCI occurs periprocedurally, typically complicating aortic surgery.

B. SCI is a major complication of spinal and descending aortic surgery that puts the spinal cord at risk due to loss or injury of critical intercostal arteries that collateralize the anterior spinal artery.[1] In an effort to reduce this complication, surgical techniques have been developed to identify and reduce this complication, including intraoperative neurophysiologic monitoring (IOM) and the use of lumbar cerebrospinal fluid drains to increase spinal cord perfusion.

C. If spinal cord ischemia is detected by IOM, spinal cord perfusion is enhanced by increasing systemic blood pressure. Blood pressure goals must be individualized due to the competing risk of hemorrhage or exacerbation of underlying aortic disease. It is reasonable to increase mean arterial pressure in increments of 10 mmHg until there is clinical improvement or it is felt unsafe to increase pressure further. Perfusion can also be augmented by placing a lumbar cerebrospinal fluid drain to reduce intracranial pressure to 8–12 cm H_2O. In some cases, a lumbar drain will already be present because it was prophylactically placed in the operating room. Additional considerations to augment cord perfusion include surgical vascular manipulations and optimizing oxygen delivery with transfusion.

D. Reversal of the ischemia in many cases occurs intraoperatively, but if a patient arouses from anesthesia with any degree of weakness, a similar protocol is followed.

E. SCI is associated with high morbidity and mortality, and patients require substantial supportive care. When there is neurologic improvement, aggressive support should be continued until stability has been present for at least 24 hours. These patients are at high risk for reoccurrence of ischemia, typically manifested as fluctuating or worsening weakness, particularly with even mild instances of hypotension and thus require vigilant observation as they are weaned from SCI treatment. After patients have stabilized, they may begin their typical postoperative care. If patients with complete paralysis do not improve despite aggressive management, the infarction can be considered complete after a 24-hour period and aggressive support can be discontinued.

F. The mechanisms of spontaneous spinal cord ischemia are diverse and include embolism and severe aortic atherosclerosis, but also unusual causes such as surfer's myelopathy and fibrocartilaginous emboli. Perhaps the most important and treatable cause is aortic dissection, resulting in loss of perfusion to critical spinal cord collateral blood flow. Computed tomography angiography of the chest should be performed to identify aortic dissection in patients with spontaneous SCI because management typically requires emergent surgical intervention.

G. While surgical repair of aortic dissection is critical, blood pressure should be supported to augment spinal cord perfusion. Extremity malperfusion syndromes should be excluded, as they often mimic or mask SCI in this setting.

H. Cervical cord infarction is more often embolic than perfusional. While reperfusion therapies such as thrombolysis are theoretically appealing, there is little data on such treatment and conservative management is generally pursued. Spontaneous thoracic SCI in the absence of aortic dissection is very uncommon, but can be due to atherosclerosis of perforating arteries, surfer's myelopathy, or fibrocartilaginous emboli. Thoracic ischemia is more likely to be perfusional, as compared to cervical ischemia, so blood pressure and volume support is more critical.

I. If a patient's SCI is persistent and greater than 24 hours in length, it is unlikely that aggressive management will change the outcome. If the onset of spontaneous SCI is less than 24 hours, in particular if symptoms are fluctuating or progressing, aggressive management should be pursued, very similar to that undertaken in the perioperative setting.

REFERENCE

1. McGarvey ML, Cheung AT, Szeto W, Mess SR. Management of neurologic complications of thoracic aortic surgery. *J Clin Neurophysiol.* 2007;24 (4):336–343.

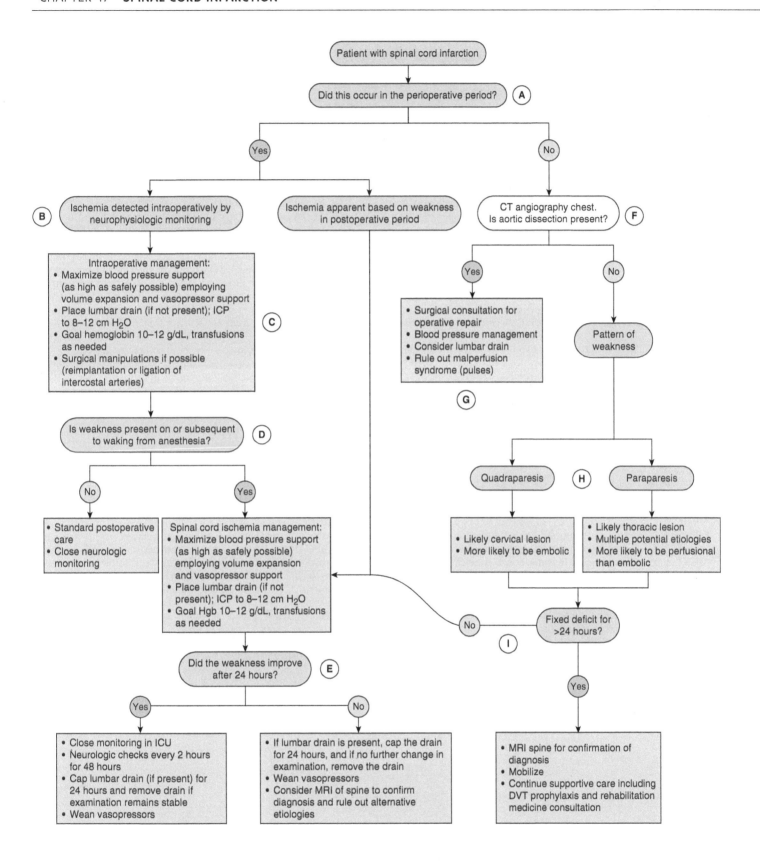

Asymptomatic Carotid Stenosis

Glenn Konsky and Michael Mullen

Asymptomatic carotid stenosis refers to atherosclerotic narrowing of the extracranial internal carotid artery, most commonly involving the proximal internal carotid artery at or just distal to the carotid bifurcation. To consider the stenosis asymptomatic, the patient must not have experienced ischemic stroke, transient ischemic attack (TIA), or retinal ischemia referable to the stenotic artery within the past 6 months. Randomized trials of carotid revascularization in asymptomatic patients have shown that revascularization is associated with approximately a 3% risk of perioperative stroke or death and a 1% per year absolute reduction in the risk of stroke (i.e., 2% per year with medical therapy vs. 1% per year after revascularization). Because the upfront procedural risk is substantial relative to the annual risk reduction, careful patient selection is critical. Further, recent evidence suggests that modern, more intensive medical therapy has reduced the risk of stroke attributable to asymptomatic carotid stenosis, possibly to as low as 0.5% per year. If true, this may limit the potential benefit from carotid revascularization.

A. Intensive medical therapy for all patients should include antithrombotic therapy, high-dose, high-intensity statin therapy, blood pressure control with a goal <130/80 mmHg, diabetes control with a goal HgbA1c <7.0% when applicable, and lifestyle modification including smoking cessation, healthy diet, exercise, and weight loss. Choice of antithrombotic therapy should be individualized. Low-dose aspirin monotherapy is reasonable for most patients; for those with significant carotid stenosis (>50%) and a low risk of systemic bleeding, the addition of low-dose rivaroxaban (2.5 mg bid.) to aspirin offers additional reduction in vascular risk and should be considered.

B. All patients with carotid stenosis ≥60% should be screened to confirm that they have not had a TIA, ischemic stroke, or retinal ischemia referable to the stenotic artery within the past 6 months. If any of these has occurred, the patient should be considered symptomatic and the risk of subsequent ischemic stroke is much higher; in this scenario, carotid revascularization is of substantial benefit and should be pursued.

C. Age, life expectancy, and medical comorbidities are important considerations. Patients with a life expectancy <5 years should generally avoid revascularization because the procedural risk is high relative to the short-term reduction in stroke. This is particularly true in the context of medical comorbidities that may increase the procedural risk. Current guidelines recommend carotid revascularization only be considered in asymptomatic patients if the surgical risk of stroke, death, or myocardial infarction is <3%.

D. Features which convey a greater likelihood of benefit from carotid revascularization include young age, male sex, and absence of significant medical comorbidities. Transcranial Doppler ultrasonography (TCD) can be used to evaluate for microembolic signals (MES) ipsilateral to the stenotic carotid artery. If present, MES suggest a high short-term risk of stroke. Additionally, progressive stenosis over time despite aggressive medical therapy is associated with a higher risk of stroke. Plaque morphology, including the presence of heterogeneous and/or ulcerated plaque, and impaired cerebral vasoreactivity on TCD may also be associated with an increased risk of stroke. Clinical decision making should be individualized, including shared decision making with the patient that incorporates their personal preferences, age, medical comorbidities, estimated life expectancy, and surgical risk. Notably, contrary to common belief, a higher degree of stenosis at initial presentation (i.e., 80% vs. 65%) has not been associated with an increased benefit from revascularization.

E. In carefully selected patients who have a life expectancy of ≥5 years and an estimated surgical risk of stroke, death, or myocardial infarction <3%, it is reasonable to proceed with carotid revascularization.

F. In the absence of high-risk features, it is reasonable to proceed with medical therapy alone. Given the equipoise between medical therapy and carotid revascularization, it is critical to engage the patient in a process of shared medical decision making. Consideration should be given to the patient's perceptions about immediate vs. long-term risk, as well as their level of anxiety about both the carotid disease and the risks of surgery.

G. When carotid revascularization is planned, both carotid endarterectomy (CEA) and carotid artery stenting (CAS) are options. CEA is typically preferred due to a lower perioperative risk of stroke and death. CAS can be considered in patients <70 years of age with high-risk cardiac disease and/or contralateral carotid occlusion. In some cases, carotid artery anatomy precludes CEA (e.g., high bifurcation), in which case CAS can be considered.

H. Patients treated with medical therapy alone should receive an annual carotid ultrasound. If there is progressive stenosis despite medical therapy, or the development of other high-risk features, it is reasonable to consider carotid revascularization.

REFERENCE

1. Moresoli P, Habib B, Reynier P, Secrest MH, Eisenberg MJ, Filion KB. Carotid stenting versus endarterectomy for asymptomatic carotid artery stenosis: a systematic review and meta-analysis. *Stroke.* 2017;48(8):2150–2157.

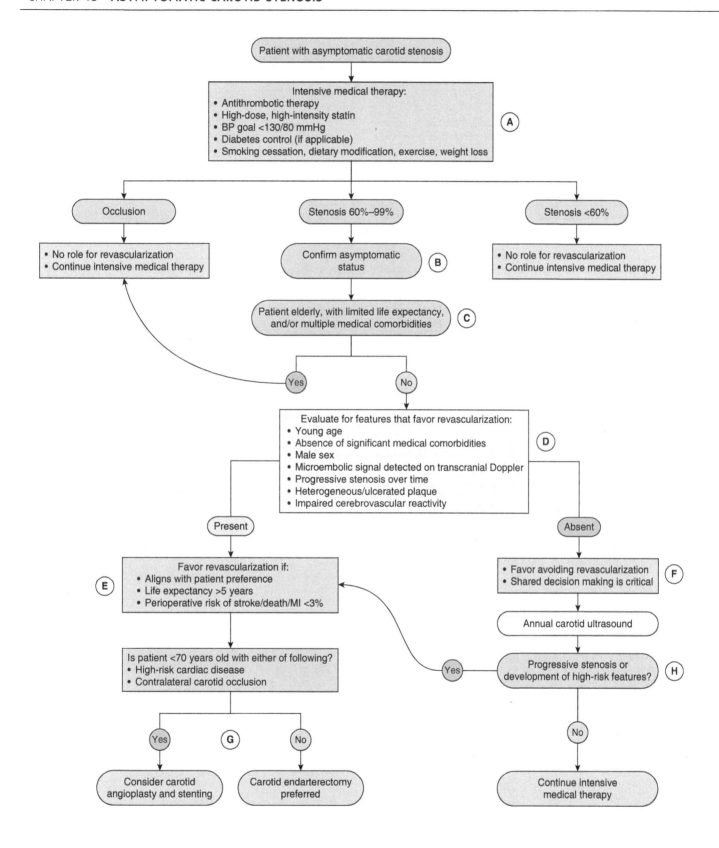

Preoperative Neurovascular (Carotid) Clearance

Michael Mullen

The risk of perioperative stroke varies dramatically based on the intervention being performed. Stroke risk is generally estimated to be <1% for cardiac catheterization, general surgery, and noncarotid vascular surgery. Carotid artery interventions, intracranial vascular procedures, and cardiac surgeries have higher rates of periprocedural stroke. Among cardiac surgeries, coronary artery bypass grafting (CABG) has been associated with a 1%–4% risk of stroke. Cardiac valve procedures and thoracic aortic surgeries have even higher risks, with estimates ranging from 2% to over 10% in some studies.

There are no existing guidelines for preoperative neurologic clearance. Studies, predominately conducted in cardiac surgery populations, have identified patient level risk factors for periprocedural stroke including age, a history of atherosclerotic risk factors and/or atherosclerotic disease, and a history of prior stroke. Additionally, there is evidence that the risk of periprocedural stroke is highest in the first 6 months after a prior stroke. Given the association between carotid stenosis and risk of stroke, a common and controversial clinical question is whether or not carotid artery imaging is necessary preoperatively.

A. Because symptomatic carotid artery stenosis is associated with a high short-term risk of stroke, patients should be screened to determine if they have a history of stroke, transient ischemic attack (TIA), or retinal ischemia within the past 6 months. If so, carotid imaging should be performed if not already done.

B. In patients with symptomatic carotid stenosis >50% the risk of stroke recurrence is substantial, and it is appropriate to pursue carotid revascularization with carotid endarterectomy (CEA) or carotid artery stenting (CAS) prior to planned surgery.

C. In patients with stroke within the past 6 months without carotid stenosis, there appears to be an elevated risk of perioperative stroke, regardless of the stroke mechanism. This is true even in otherwise low-risk, noncardiac surgeries. If the surgery is not urgent, it is reasonable to delay the planned surgery until at least 6 months poststroke.

D. Among asymptomatic patients (no stroke or TIA within the past 6 months), the utility of carotid imaging depends on the planned surgery. Noncardiac surgery is associated with a low risk of stroke even in the presence of carotid stenosis; this perioperative stroke risk is generally exceeded by the risk of stroke complicating CEA or CAS. Given this, there is no need for carotid imaging prior to the planned procedure in asymptomatic patients.

E. For patients undergoing nonurgent CABG or other cardiac surgery requiring cardiopulmonary bypass, it is reasonable to perform screening carotid ultrasound on high-risk patients. High-risk features include age ≥70 years, prior stroke, multivessel coronary artery disease, peripheral artery disease, and the presence of a carotid bruit.

F. The presence of no stenosis or unilateral stenosis, or bilateral moderate stenosis is not associated with a significantly increased risk of stroke after CABG. Carotid intervention is not necessary prior to the planned cardiac surgery in these patients.

G. When bilateral severe stenosis/occlusion is present, consider revascularization of the more severely stenotic vessel, or the dominant hemisphere if both hemispheres are equally stenotic. Revascularization should not be attempted on an occluded vessel. When carotid revascularization is pursued, treatment strategies could include staged CAS/CABG, staged CEA/CABG, or combined CEA/CABG. In patients who do not require urgent coronary revascularization, staged CAS/CABG is likely optimal, given increased cardiac risk associated with CEA, but typically requires a delay in CABG of 4–6 weeks due to the need for short-term dual antiplatelet therapy. Similar decision-making likely applies to non-CABG cardiac surgery, although this is less well studied.

REFERENCES

1. Aboyans V, Ricco JB, Bartelink MLE, et al. 2017 ESC Guidelines on the diagnosis and treatment of peripheral arterial diseases, in collaboration with the European Society for Vascular Surgery: Document covering atherosclerotic disease of extracranial carotid and vertebral, mesenteric, renal, upper, and lower extremity arteries. *Eur Heart J.* 2018;39(9):763–816.
2. Jørgensen ME, Torp-Pedersen C, Gislason GH, et al. Time elapsed after ischemic stroke and risk of adverse cardiovascular events and mortality following elective noncardiac surgery. *JAMA.* 2014;312(3):269–277.

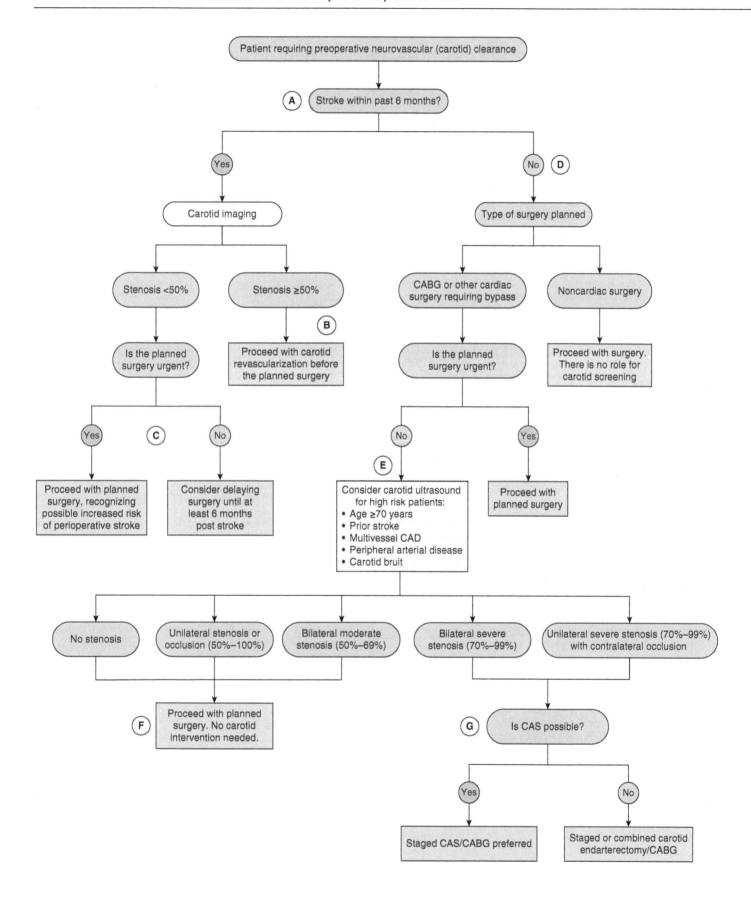

Acute Spontaneous Intracerebral Hemorrhage

Laura A. Stein and Christopher G. Favilla

A. Patients with intracerebral hemorrhage (ICH) have a high risk of neurologic deterioration, particularly early after presentation. Close neurologic monitoring is thus important. Intubation and mechanical ventilation are necessary in some patients due to obtundation or coma. Aggressive blood pressure control may reduce the risk of hemorrhage expansion in the acute period; an initial target of <160/90 mmHg is reasonable. Easily titratable intravenous antihypertensives with a short duration of action, such as labetalol or nicardipine, are preferred. Neurosurgical consultation is indicated for patients with mass effect or intraventricular hemorrhage potentially causing increased intracranial pressure as hemorrhage evacuation or external ventricular drainage may be needed. Head of bed should be positioned at 30 degrees or greater to reduce intracranial pressure. Patients with witnessed or suspected seizures should receive antiepileptic drugs, but prophylactic treatment is generally not indicated.

B. Urgent laboratory workup to evaluate for coagulopathy (complete blood count, prothrombin, and partial thromboplastin time) is important, and a urine toxicology screen should be sent to evaluate for potential sympathomimetic drugs (cocaine, amphetamines) that might contribute to ICH. Importantly, the presence of such drugs does not preclude another underlying ICH mechanism, so even if present a thorough evaluation should still be performed.

C. In addition to laboratory testing for coagulopathy, focused history to identify recent anticoagulant or thrombolytic use is essential. Reversal of any identified coagulopathy should be immediately undertaken (see Chapter 52). The presence of coagulopathy does not necessarily exclude another contributing cause of ICH (e.g., anticoagulant use may increase risk of bleeding into a brain metastasis), so additional evaluation may still be needed and should be based on clinical suspicion.

D. Common etiologies of hemorrhage vary based on the hemorrhage location. Deep, subcortical hemorrhages, for example in the thalamus or basal ganglia, are typically due to chronic hypertension. In contrast, superficial, lobar hemorrhages (i.e., cortical) are less commonly due to hypertension; in the elderly, amyloid angiopathy is a common cause. Look for finger-like projections of lobar ICH, which supports the diagnosis of amyloid angiopathy.

E. While most deep hemorrhages are hypertensive in etiology, in the absence of a history of hypertension or evidence of end-organ damage attributable to chronic hypertension, further diagnostic evaluation is warranted. Brain magnetic resonance imaging (MRI) showing severe microvascular disease or chronic deep microhemorrhages (see section G) strongly suggests a hypertensive etiology. The presence of elevated blood pressure in the acute period should not be considered to indicate chronic hypertension; this is a common physiologic response to the brain hemorrhage itself.

F. Simultaneous multifocal acute ICHs are rare and suggest an atypical hemorrhage etiology. Most of these specific causes will be identified with a contrast enhanced brain MRI. Venous sinus thrombosis sufficient to cause multifocal ICH is almost always visible on standard enhanced brain MRI; however, MR venography may be necessary to confirm the diagnosis and assess the degree of compromise to venous drainage. In some cases, it may be necessary to repeat imaging in 4–8 weeks after acute hemorrhage has cleared to better evaluate underlying lesions.

G. It is important to ensure brain MRI is performed with gradient echo (GRE) or susceptibility weighted imaging (SWI) sequences. These sequences identify chronic, often asymptomatic, areas of hemorrhage within the brain typically not visualized with standard MRI sequences. When multiple microhemorrhages are present in a cortical distribution in an elderly patient with lobar hemorrhage, amyloid angiopathy is usually the cause. Amyloid angiopathy is associated with a substantial risk of ICH recurrence, and thus antithrombotic therapy must be scrupulously avoided. While a superficial or lobar ICH location is atypical for hypertensive hemorrhages, long-term blood pressure control remains important and may reduce the risk of recurrent ICH. Other important causes of superficial or lobar hemorrhage include arteriovenous malformations, cavernomas, hemorrhagic metastasis, and venous sinus thrombosis. The latter diagnosis must always be carefully considered as management requires acute parenteral anticoagulation, completely different than that for all other causes of ICH. MR venography or computed tomography (CT) venography are used to confirm the diagnosis. Occasionally, hemorrhagic conversion of ischemic stroke may be confused with a primary ICH. A good rule of thumb is that if the initial CT scan is done within 6 hours of symptom onset and shows ICH, hemorrhagic conversion of ischemic stroke is highly unlikely.

H. A small subset of patients with arteriovenous malformation or dural arteriovenous fistulas will have normal CT or MR angiography. If there is high suspicion for vascular malformation and no other identified cause, catheter angiography should be pursued. Repeat MRI brain and vessel imaging should be considered 4–8 weeks after initial presentation if the etiology of ICH remains unknown. This allows time for resolution of the hematoma and surrounding edema that may mask underlying pathology.

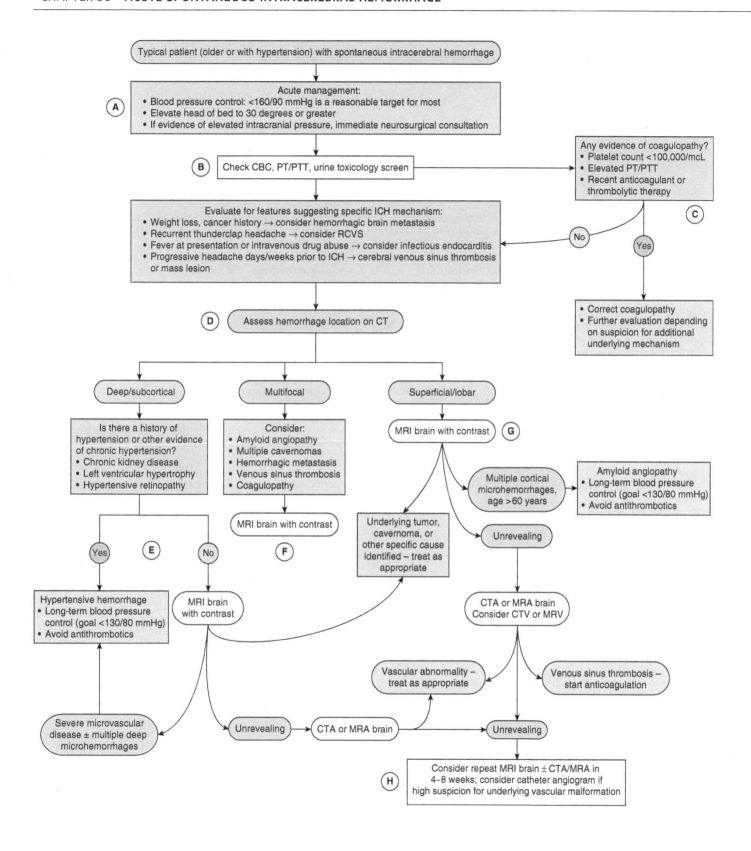

Intracerebral Hemorrhage in the Young

Ava Liberman and Christopher G. Favilla

Intracerebral hemorrhage (ICH) is uncommon in young adults (age <50 years) but is more likely to be associated with specific underlying vascular abnormalities than in older patients. Given this, diagnostic evaluation is often more involved and complex.

A. Acute medical management is broadly similar to that in older patients. Careful monitoring is critical due to the high risk of clinical deterioration. Aggressive blood pressure lowering may limit hemorrhage expansion. While there is very limited data for specific blood pressure targets in younger patients, considering premorbid blood pressure when determining the target is likely sensible, with more aggressive lowering in previously normotensive patients.

B. Given the higher prevalence of structural vascular abnormalities in younger patients, immediate vessel imaging is appropriate for almost all patients. Computed tomography angiography (CTA) can be obtained rapidly and is probably more sensitive than magnetic resonance angiography for identifying small vascular malformations. If the clinical scenario or hemorrhage pattern is concerning for cerebral venous sinus thrombosis, venous imaging should be obtained acutely. Lobar hemorrhage with associated edema or venous infarction should raise the suspicion for sagittal sinus or cortical vein thrombosis; bilateral thalamic hemorrhage should raise suspicion for straight sinus thrombosis. Testing for coagulopathy and a toxicology screen should be sent. While stimulants (e.g., cocaine, amphetamine) are associated with ICH in the young, a positive toxicology result should not prevent further diagnostic testing as vascular malformations often coexist in these patients.

C. Specific features of the medical history and clinical presentation may suggest an underlying mechanism for the ICH and help target diagnostic testing.

D. If vascular imaging does not reveal a clear etiology, perform brain magnetic resonance imaging (MRI) brain with contrast, being sure to include susceptibility-weighted or gradient-echo sequences to detect areas of chronic hemorrhage. Cerebral cavernous malformations are angiographically occult and thus best seen on MRI. While hypertension is a much less frequent cause of ICH in the young than in older patients, it still accounts for many cases. Severe microvascular disease with multiple microhemorrhages on MRI supports this as a cause. Evidence of contrast enhancement may suggest hemorrhage into tumor.

E. Noninvasive imaging studies such as CTA are less sensitive than catheter angiography for identifying some important causes of ICH in the young, including reversible cerebral vasoconstriction syndrome (RCVS), dural arteriovenous fistulas, and small arteriovenous malformations. If ICH is unexplained after noninvasive imaging, catheter angiography should be pursued.

F. Up to 25% of patients with RCVS will have a normal catheter angiogram early in their clinical course, with abnormalities becoming apparent on repeat angiogram several days to a week later. Therefore, if there is strong clinical suspicion for RCVS (i.e., recurrent thunderclap headaches, associated convexity subarachnoid hemorrhage), early repeat angiography should be done. Note also that concurrent arterial dissections can be seen with RCVS and may be an important clue to this diagnosis.

G. If initial evaluation is unrevealing, MRI brain with contrast should be repeated 4–8 weeks later. This time allows for resolution of the hematoma and associated edema, which may mask underlying pathology. If this study is unrevealing, consider repeat catheter angiography. Small arteriovenous malformations may initially be compressed by the acute hematoma and may only become apparent on follow-up angiography.

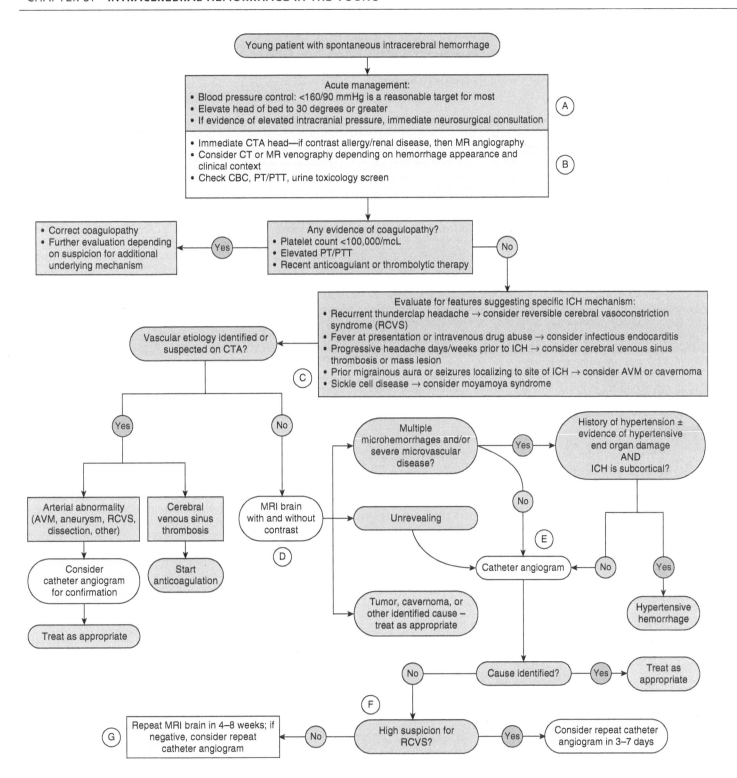

Intracerebral Hemorrhage Due to Anticoagulant Therapy

Paul J. Novello and Christopher G. Favilla

Patients taking anticoagulants have larger baseline intracerebral hemorrhage volume, greater early hemorrhage expansion, and increased morbidity and mortality compared to those not on anticoagulants. While there is little formal data proving that prompt reversal of anticoagulation improves outcome, most experts agree that aggressive, rapid reversal is an important intervention likely to limit brain injury in this scenario. Reversal protocols are largely based on expert opinion as opposed to clinical trial data, and institutions often have specific internal reversal protocols based on local expertise and resource availability. The recommendations presented here represent one of many reasonable approaches.

A. In the case of unfractionated heparin, protamine is the typical reversal agent. Protamine 1 mg neutralizes about 100 units of unfractionated heparin, with a maximal dose of 50 mg. Because intravenous heparin has a short plasma half-life, the amount administered within the preceding 2–3 hours may reasonably represent the total active dose that needs to be reversed. For example, if a heparin infusion has been running at 1000 units/hour for the past 3 hours, reversal of 3000 units would be appropriate, which requires 30 mg of protamine. A single dose of protamine is usually sufficient because of the short half-life of intravenous (IV) heparin, but activated partial thromboplastin time (aPTT) should be checked after protamine administration to ensure adequate reversal.

B. For patients receiving prophylactic doses of subcutaneous heparin, reversal is typically not warranted. aPTT levels should be checked, and if elevated, protamine can be dosed accordingly. If needed, the exact dose of protamine is unclear in the context of subcutaneous heparin, but the longer half-life warrants surveillance of aPTT and redosing of protamine as needed.

C. For low-molecular-weight heparin, protamine achieves partial reversal (about 60%–80% of anti-Xa activity). Protamine dosing depends on the timing and dose of low-molecular-weight heparin. Recombinant factor VIIa can be considered in patients with refractory life-threatening bleeding.

D. The need for reversal of direct oral anticoagulants (DOAC) depends on the time from last dose. Some conservative protocols advocate for reversal if the last dose was within 48 hours, but given the relatively short half-life of these medications, reversal for use within 24 hours is probably most reasonable. Betrixaban has a longer half-life, so late reversal might be considered with this agent. If the time of last DOAC dose in unknown, it is appropriate to proceed with reversal. If last dose was within 2 hours, activated charcoal can be considered to reduce absorption of any remaining unabsorbed drug.

E. Thrombin time is very sensitive to dabigatran, so if the thrombin time is normal, reversal is not needed. However, rapidly obtaining this measurement is difficult at many centers, and treatment should not be delayed to await thrombin time results. Idarucizumab is a humanized monoclonal antibody that uniquely binds dabigatran given as two separate 2.5 mg IV doses, separated by no more than 15 minutes. If idarucizimab is not available, prothrombin complex concentrate (PCC) can be considered (50 units/kg, maximum dose 5000 units). Alternatively, hemodialysis can also be considered to remove circulating dabigatran, particularly if there is renal insufficiency. Consultation with pharmacy and hematology is appropriate.

F. Andexanet alfa is a reversal agent specific to factor Xa inhibitors. Dosing depends on timing and dose of DOAC. If andexanet is not available, a dose of 50 units/kg of PCC should be administered, with a maximum of 5000 units. Factor Xa inhibitors are not readily dialyzable.

G. For warfarin related intracerebral hemorrhage, 10 mg of IV vitamin K should be administered immediately, but this does not rapidly correct the coagulopathy and normalize the international normalized ratio (INR). It is critical, then, to give 4-factor PCC for rapid warfarin reversal. The PCC dose should be selected based on INR. Typically, no reversal is needed if the INR is <1.4. In the case of mildly elevated INR (1.4–1.9), reversal can be considered depending on the severity of bleeding. If PCC is unavailable, fresh frozen plasma (FFP) can be considered, but slower administration time and the risk of volume overload make this less desirable. The preferred initial dose of FFP is 15mL/kg or 4 units. Rechecking the INR after reversal is important to ensure the coagulopathy has been corrected.

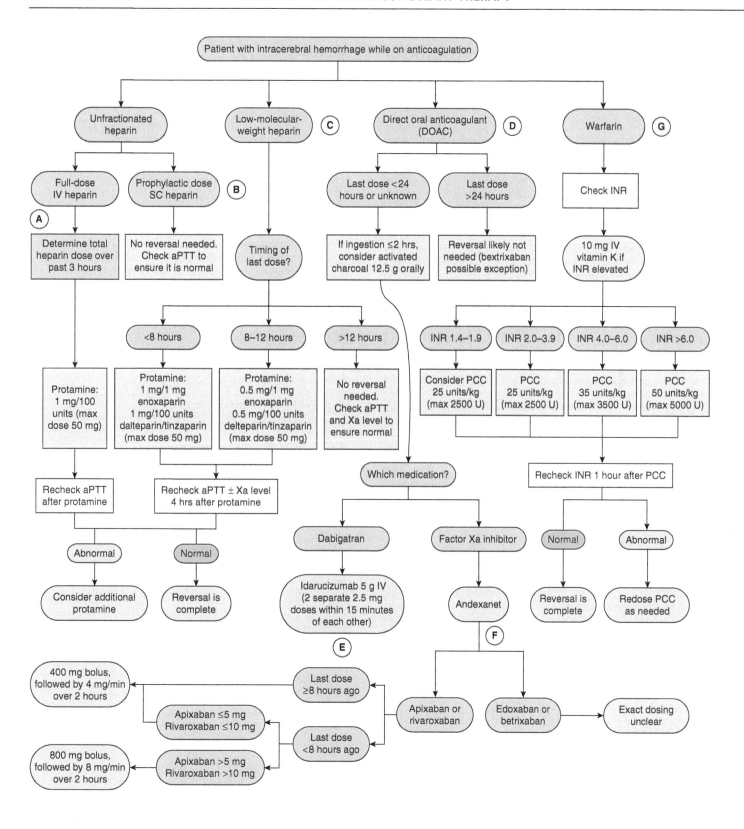

Restarting Antithrombotic Therapy After Intracerebral Hemorrhage

Donna George and Christopher G. Favilla

Patients with intracerebral hemorrhage often have concurrent ischemic vascular disease, venous thromboembolic disease, or atrial fibrillation for which antiplatelet (AP) or anticoagulant (AC) therapy would be indicated. Deciding if and when to start or restart antithrombotic therapy in these patients is a common challenge in clinical care. Determining the underlying cause of the intracerebral hemorrhage helps predict the risk of recurrent bleeding. Similarly, the risk of thromboembolism should be estimated based on the specific clinical scenario. This then allows one to weigh the risks and benefits of therapy. In general, those with a prior vascular event (secondary prevention) are at higher risk than those who are clinically asymptomatic (primary prevention), and those with a recent event more at risk than those with a remote event. Risk scores such as the CHA2DS2-VASc score can help stratify thrombotic risk in patients with atrial fibrillation; patients with mechanical heart valves are at high risk even without a history of prior ischemic events.

A. Hypertensive hemorrhage typically affects the deep, subcortical structures. The risk of recurrence is about 2% per year; this can be significantly reduced with aggressive blood pressure control.[1] Even so, the risk of recurrent hemorrhage often exceeds the risk of a future ischemic event in low-risk patients, such that antithrombotic agents are likely to cause more harm than benefit.

B. Amyloid angiopathy is a common cause of lobar or multicompartment hemorrhage in elderly patients. The risk of recurrent bleeding in patients with amyloid angiopathy is very high even in the absence of antithrombotic agents (~10% per year), and therefore it is generally recommended to avoid all antiplatelet and anticoagulant agents regardless of indication.[2]

C. Coagulopathic hemorrhages can occur in the setting of therapeutic or supratherapeutic anticoagulation, or when anticoagulation is combined with an antiplatelet agent. In general, if the hemorrhage occurred while on warfarin or in the setting of combination therapy with an anticoagulant and antiplatelet, transition to direct oral anticoagulant (DOAC) monotherapy should be considered given the lower risk of intracranial hemorrhage with these agents compared to warfarin.[3] When intracerebral hemorrhage occurs in the context of DOAC use, the cause of hemorrhage and the indication for therapy should guide decision-making.

D. Hemorrhagic transformation of an ischemic stroke is quite different from a primary intracerebral hemorrhage in that the underlying precipitating event is ischemia. Accordingly, the long-term risk of recurrent hemorrhage is low, and the risk of recurrent ischemia may be relatively high. Hemorrhagic conversion can be characterized on imaging as *petechial hemorrhage*, in which case antithrombotic therapy can usually be continued without cessation, or *parenchymal hematoma*, in which case antithrombotic therapy is typically held for at least 1 week and possibly as long as 4 weeks depending on the size of the infarction and the hemorrhage, and the short-term risk of recurrent ischemia (determined by stroke mechanism).

E. Cavernous malformations, or cavernomas, can be identified incidentally or in the context of acute hemorrhage. If identified incidentally, without prior clinical symptoms of hemorrhage, it is reasonable to start or continue antiplatelet agents or anticoagulation in most patients based on vascular indication; the exception is low-risk primary prevention in which the risk-benefit ratio is quite unclear. In the setting of prior clinical hemorrhage, antithrombotic therapy is reasonable for patients at high risk of recurrent vascular events. However, brainstem cavernomas often have higher risk of bleeding and the consequence of recurrent hemorrhage is more significant, so a patient-centered discussion of the risks versus benefits of therapy is warranted.

F. Once secured by either surgical or endovascular intervention, arteriovenous malformations (AVMs) and cerebral aneurysms have a low risk of recurrent hemorrhage and antiplatelet or anticoagulant therapy can be used as needed.

REFERENCES

1. Bailey RD, Hart RG, Benavente O, Pearce LA. Recurrent brain hemorrhage is more frequent than ischemic stroke after intracranial hemorrhage. *Neurology.* 2001;56:773–777.
2. Poon MT, Fonville AF, Al-Shahi Salman R. Long-term prognosis after ntracerebral haemorrhage: systematic review and meta-analysis. *J Neurol Neurosurg Psychiatry.* 2015;85:660–667.
3. López-López JA, Sterne JAC, Thom HHZ, et al. Oral anticoagulants for prevention of stroke in atrial fibrillation: systematic review, network meta-analysis, and cost effectiveness analysis. *BMJ.* 2017;359:j5058.

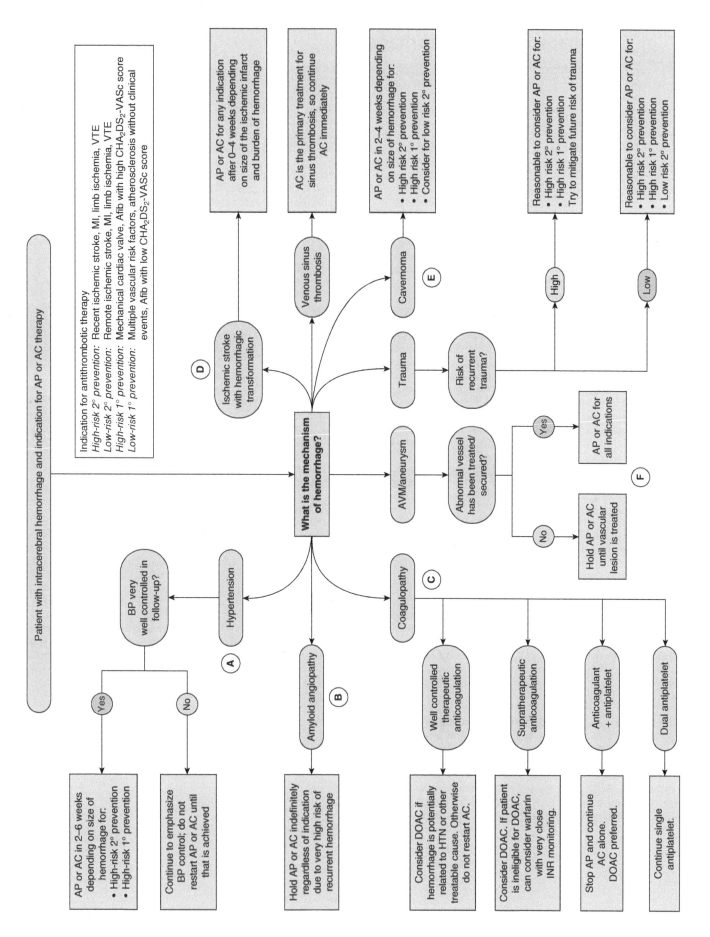

Subarachnoid Hemorrhage

Preethi Ramchand, Christopher G. Favilla, and David Kung

Subarachnoid hemorrhage (SAH) refers to bleeding within the cerebrospinal fluid (CSF)-filled subarachnoid space. The majority of spontaneous cases are due to ruptured cerebral aneurysms, but 15%–20% are due to another mechanism. SAH, particularly aneurysmal SAH, carries a high rate of morbidity and mortality. Prevention of recurrent SAH is paramount, and determining the mechanism of initial SAH is necessary to select the proper therapy to prevent recurrence.

A. Patients with SAH require intensive monitoring. Regardless of etiology, acute blood pressure management is critical. A goal of <160/90 mmHg is reasonable, though the optimal target is unclear. Elevated intracranial pressure is a common complication of SAH, so the head of bed should be maintained >30 degrees. If hydrocephalus is present, ventriculostomy should be placed to facilitate CSF drainage.

B. Cortical/convexity SAH in elderly patients is likely to represent amyloid angiopathy. Magnetic resonance imaging (MRI) of the brain demonstrating chronic lobar hemorrhage or cortical microhemorrhages supports this diagnosis, but must be performed with gradient echo/susceptibility weighted images which are sequences sensitive to chronic hemorrhage. There is no specific treatment for SAH due to amyloid angiopathy, but all antithrombotic therapy should be stopped as there is a high risk of recurrent bleeding.

C. Vascular imaging, starting with brain computed tomography angiography (CTA), is indicated in young patients with cortical/convexity SAH and in older patients without evidence of amyloid angiopathy on MRI. CTA is highly sensitive for identifying arteriovenous malformations and larger aneurysms, but less sensitive for dural arteriovenous fistulas, reversible segmental vasoconstriction syndrome, and smaller, particularly distal, aneurysms.

D. Reversible cerebral vasoconstriction syndrome (RCVS) is a vasospastic condition associated with multifocal segmental narrowing of cerebral vessels. It is often visible only on catheter angiography; further, segmental narrowing seen on CTA is not infrequently artifactual. Consider catheter angiography to confirm the diagnosis. RCVS can be associated with conditions such as pregnancy and migraine, and may be triggered by use of vasoconstrictive drugs, including sympathomimetics, triptans, and decongestants. A thorough history of prescription, over-the-counter, and illicit drug use is essential. Potentially implicated drugs should be stopped. Calcium channel blockers such as verapamil are commonly used to mitigate vasoconstriction. Repeat vessel imaging in 1–3 months should confirm normalization of the vessels.

E. If CTA is unrevealing, brain MRI with contrast should be performed; MR venography should also be considered if there is suspicion for cerebral venous thrombosis (i.e., prodromal progressive headache, known hypercoagulable state, or significant parenchymal edema, venous infarction, or adjacent parenchymal hemorrhage on imaging). Isolated cortical vein thrombosis and superficial cavernomas may also cause focal convexity SAH and are best visualized on brain MRI. If negative, catheter angiography should be pursued.

F. When SAH is isolated to the perimesencephalic region, an underlying etiology is rarely identified; aneurysms are found in only about 5% of cases. Initial evaluation with CT and catheter angiography is appropriate, but if negative, repeat vascular imaging is not necessary.

G. Hemorrhage in the basal cisterns typically represents aneurysm rupture. CTA is the preferred initial study, but MRA can also be considered. Both are very sensitive to aneurysms >3 mm, but can miss smaller aneurysms. Catheter angiography is indicated regardless of the results of CTA (to ensure an aneurysm has not been missed if CTA is negative, and to better define aneurysm anatomy if previously identified), but CTA is useful to help target the catheter-based study to areas of concern. Also, occasionally a thrombosed aneurysm may be better seen on CTA.

H. A ruptured aneurysm should be secured within 24 hours in order to reduce the risk of rebleeding. An unsecured aneurysm carries ~15% risk of early rebleeding; if this occurs, the mortality rate approaches 50%. An aneurysm can be secured via endovascular coiling or surgical clipping, a determination that is based on specific anatomic and clinical features of the patient.

I. Medical management after aneurysmal SAH focuses on reducing the risk of secondary complications, specifically seizures, hydrocephalus, and vasospasm. Prophylactic levetiracetam is administered for 1 week; clinical seizures will require a longer course of antiepileptic drug therapy. Aside from rebleeding, vasospasm causing delayed cerebral ischemia is one of the most devastating consequences of SAH. Monitoring for vasospasm and ischemia is done with frequent neurological exams and daily transcranial Doppler ultrasonography. Elevations in blood flow velocities indicate evolving vasospasm. When present and severe, treatment options include induced hypertension and aggressive volume expansion, angioplasty of affected vessels, and direct intraarterial administration of vasodilators. Oral nimodipine (60 mg every 4 hours) for 21 days has been shown to improve outcome after SAH; the putative mechanism is reduction of vasospasm induced delayed cerebral ischemia.

J. Small aneurysms may initially be obscured by hemorrhage, vasospasm, or thrombosis within the aneurysm, so if an underlying vascular abnormality is not identified catheter angiography should be repeated between 4 and 10 days.

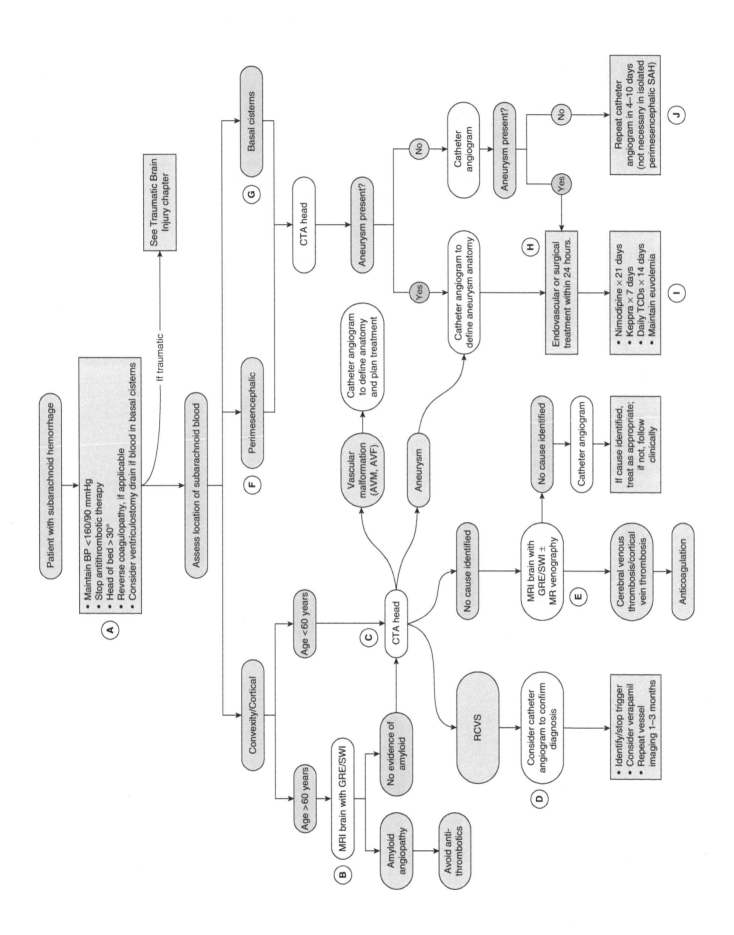

Unruptured Intracranial Aneurysm

Michael E. Kritikos, Preethi Ramchand, and David Kung

Management of unruptured intracranial aneurysms (UIAs) poses a conundrum to physicians. The prevalence of UIAs is approximately 3%, the majority of which are discovered incidentally. Rupture of an aneurysm can have devastating effects with high morbidity and mortality, but the vast majority of aneurysms do not rupture. Aneurysm repair, which can be performed with either open surgical or endovascular approaches, effectively eliminates the risk of rupture, but carries a risk of procedural complications. Shared decision-making, taking into account age, general health status, personal preferences, and the patient-specific risk of rupture and procedural complications is advisable.

A. Modifiable risk factors for aneurysm rupture include smoking, hypertension, and alcohol abuse; these should be addressed in all patients with UIA.

B. If an aneurysm is causing a cranial neuropathy, a classic example being a third nerve palsy from a posterior communicating artery aneurysm, repair should be pursued as this indicates an expanding aneurysm.

C. Aneurysms in the cavernous carotid artery do not cause subarachnoid hemorrhage, as the blood is contained within the cavernous sinus; they should only be repaired if causing a cranial neuropathy or rarely if very large in size.

D. Risk of rupture increases with aneurysm size, with 7 mm often considered a threshold of increased risk warranting intervention. However, other risk factors such as anatomical configuration of the aneurysm, location, and personal or family history (two or more first-degree relatives) of prior rupture also influence risk (see box in algorithm). Patient age is important. Younger patients are exposed to greater risk of rupture given their longer life span; they are also at lower risk of procedural complication. Scores to predict the risk of rupture may assist with decision making.[1,2]

E. For patients with smaller aneurysms (<7 mm), decision-making is complex and there is not consensus on which patients to treat. Most of those with very small aneurysms (<4 mm) should be observed unless multiple high-risk features are present. Neurovascular consultation is indicated when the optimal treatment strategy is in question.

F. Both open surgical clipping and endovascular treatment of aneurysms are effective. A meta-analysis of surgical treatment showed a 1.7% mortality rate and an overall morbidity rate of 6.7%.[3] Patient age ≥50 years, aneurysm size ≥12 mm, and aneurysms located in the posterior circulation were predictors of poor surgical outcome. Endovascular treatment options include coiling, stent-assisted coiling, and endoluminal flow diversion. A meta-analysis showed a 4.8% total unfavorable outcome rate for endovascular treatment, but also a 9.1 % retreatment rate.[4] Aneurysm morphology (e.g., wide neck) and size should be considered when choosing which strategy to use for repair. In general, endovascular coiling is associated with lower treatment morbidity and mortality, but clipping offers a lower recurrence rate.

G. Aneurysm growth is significantly associated with rupture, but the likelihood of growth is generally low, particularly for small aneurysms. A typical recommendation is to perform follow-up vascular imaging at 1 year. Magnetic resonance angiography is the preferred noninvasive imaging method, since it does not expose patients to radiation and an exogenous contrast agent is not needed. If stability is demonstrated on follow-up imaging, the ideal long-term surveillance plan is controversial, but interval imaging can be decreased or even stopped for many patients.

REFERENCES

1. Greving JP, Wermer MJ, Brown Jr RD, et al. Development of the PHASES score for prediction of risk of rupture of intracranial aneurysms: a pooled analysis of six prospective cohort studies. *Lancet Neurol.* 2014;13:59–66.
2. Etminan N, Brown Jr RD, Beseoglu K, et al. The unruptured intracranial aneurysm treatment score: a multidisciplinary consensus. *Neurology.* 2015;10:881–889.
3. Kotowski M, Naggara O, Darsaut TE, et al. Safety and occlusion rates of surgical treatment of unruptured intracranial aneurysms: a systematic review and meta-analysis of the literature from 1990 to 2011. *J Neurol Neurosurg Psychiatry.* 2013;84(1):42–48.
4. Naggara ON, White PM, Guilbert F, Roy D, Weill A, Raymond J. Endovascular treatment of intracranial unruptured aneurysms: systematic review and meta-analysis of the literature on safety and efficacy. *Radiology.* 2010;256:887–897.

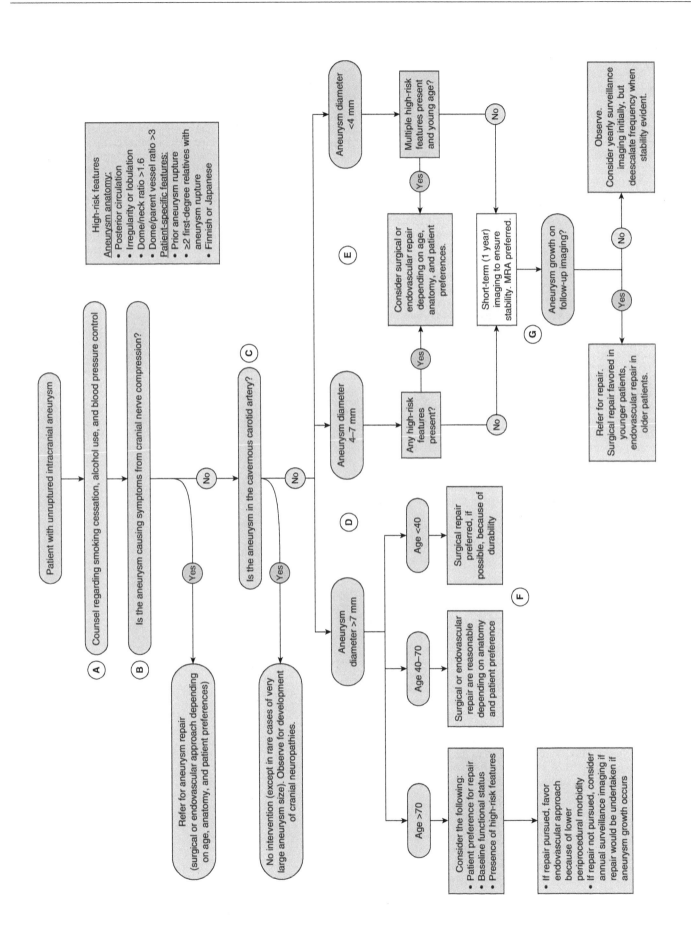

High-risk features
Aneurysm anatomy:
• Posterior circulation
• Irregularity or lobulation
• Dome/neck ratio >1.6
• Dome/parent vessel ratio >3
Patient-specific features:
• Prior aneurysm rupture
• ≥2 first-degree relatives with
  aneurysm rupture
• Finnish or Japanese

Patient with unruptured intracranial aneurysm

(A) Counsel regarding smoking cessation, alcohol use, and blood pressure control

(B) Is the aneurysm causing symptoms from cranial nerve compression?

Yes → Refer for aneurysm repair (surgical or endovascular approach depending on age, anatomy, and patient preferences)

No

(C) Is the aneurysm in the cavernous carotid artery?

Yes → No intervention (except in rare cases of very large aneurysm size). Observe for development of cranial neuropathies.

No

(D) Aneurysm diameter >7 mm

Age <40 → Surgical repair preferred, if possible, because of durability

Age 40–70 → Surgical or endovascular repair are reasonable depending on anatomy and patient preference

Age >70 → Consider the following:
• Patient preference for repair
• Baseline functional status
• Presence of high-risk features

(F)

• If repair pursued, favor endovascular approach because of lower periprocedural morbidity
• If repair not pursued, consider annual surveillance imaging if repair would be undertaken if aneurysm growth occurs

Aneurysm diameter 4–7 mm

Any high-risk features present?

Yes → (E) Consider surgical or endovascular repair depending on age, anatomy, and patient preferences.

No → Short-term (1 year) imaging to ensure stability. MRA preferred.

(G) Aneurysm growth on follow-up imaging?

Yes → Refer for repair. Surgical repair favored in younger patients, endovascular repair in older patients.

No → Observe. Consider yearly surveillance imaging initially, but deescalate frequency when stability evident.

Aneurysm diameter <4 mm

Multiple high-risk features present and young age?

Yes → Consider surgical or endovascular repair depending on age, anatomy, and patient preferences.

No → Short-term (1 year) imaging to ensure stability. MRA preferred.

Vascular Malformations

Charles Esenwa and Bryan Pukenas

Vascular malformations of the brain can be organized into five subtypes: (1) cavernous malformations, (2) capillary telangiectasias, (3) arteriovenous malformations (AVMs), (4) developmental venous anomalies, and (5) dural arteriovenous fistulas (dAVFs). Vascular malformations most often come to clinical attention when they cause intracerebral hemorrhage. Occasionally, they may be found in patients with epilepsy as a seizure focus. Increasingly, vascular malformations are discovered incidentally on brain imaging performed to evaluate an unrelated neurologic complaint. In patients with vascular malformations, the most important driver of treatment decisions is whether or not the lesion is symptomatic.

A. Cavernous malformations, or cavernomas, are thin-walled venous cavities that can be found in the cortex, white matter, basal ganglia, brainstem, and spinal cord. They are usually sporadic, but familial syndromes associated with multiple cavernomas exist and are important to recognize. Cavernomas are angiographically occult, and vascular imaging is not indicated. Bleeding risk is increased in patients with prior hemorrhage or focal neurologic deficits attributed to cavernoma and in those with brainstem cavernoma location. For example, in patients with asymptomatic, incidentally discovered non-brainstem cavernomas, the risk of bleeding is <1% per year, increasing to 3%–4% per year in patients with prior hemorrhage and non-brainstem cavernomas, and as high as 5%–6% per year in those with brainstem cavernoma with prior hemorrhage. Surgical resection of a cavernoma should be considered in patients with recurrent hemorrhage or intractable epilepsy, particularly if easily accessible surgically. Resection is generally not performed after a single hemorrhage in isolation.

B. Capillary telangiectasias are small clustered capillary-like anomalies usually found in the brainstem and cerebellum. They are most often incidental imaging findings and do not require monitoring or further investigation except when part of a genetic disorder such as hereditary hemorrhagic telangiectasia. Symptomatic hemorrhage is extremely unusual.

C. AVMs are tortuous collections of histologically abnormal vessels that are supplied by feeding arteries and drain into deep or superficial veins. Their lack of an organized capillary network can cause high-flow arteriovenous shunting of blood. The most feared complication is intracranial hemorrhage, which can be subarachnoid, from an associated feeding artery aneurysm, or intraparenchymal, from intranidal rupture. Bleeding risk is increased with prior hemorrhage, deep location, deep venous drainage pattern, and if an associated aneurysm is present. In patients with prior hemorrhage, annual risk of recurrent bleeding is ~5%. Seizures and headache can also occur with AVMs. Catheter angiography is necessary to define AVM anatomy to guide treatment decisions. Given their complexity, evaluation and management of a ruptured AVM should be done by an experienced multidisciplinary team. Treatment options include endovascular embolization, radiosurgery, and surgical resection. Staged intervention is sometimes necessary.

D. Developmental venous anomalies are normal venous channels that have an anomalous location or radiographic appearance. While they can be very rarely associated with hemorrhage, especially when associated with a cavernoma, surgical intervention is almost always contraindicated because of their physiologic role in venous drainage of functional brain tissue; disturbance can lead to venous infarction and further hemorrhage.

E. A dAVF is a dural-based arteriovenous shunt, typically supplied by extracranial arterial branches that anastomose with an intracranial dural vein and sinus. A dAVF is typically acquired through trauma or aberrant revascularization after cerebral vein thrombosis. Cerebral dAVF may present with symptomatic intracranial hemorrhage, cerebral edema, seizure, or pulsatile tinnitus. One commonly encountered form of dAVF is cavernous-carotid fistula, which can present with local eye abnormalities such as scleral injection, proptosis, double vision, and visual blurring or loss of vision. Spinal dAVF may also occur, typically manifesting with progressive myelopathy. Catheter angiography is necessary for adequate diagnostic evaluation; note that dAVFs are often not well seen on noninvasive vascular imaging studies (computed tomography or magnetic resonance angiography). In general, symptomatic dAVFs should be treated, often requiring a multidisciplinary approach (endovascular embolization, open surgical resection, less commonly stereotactic radiosurgery). Lesions are classified based on location and involvement of cortical veins. The presence of cortical venous drainage carries an increased risk of hemorrhage, which typically justifies referral for intervention.

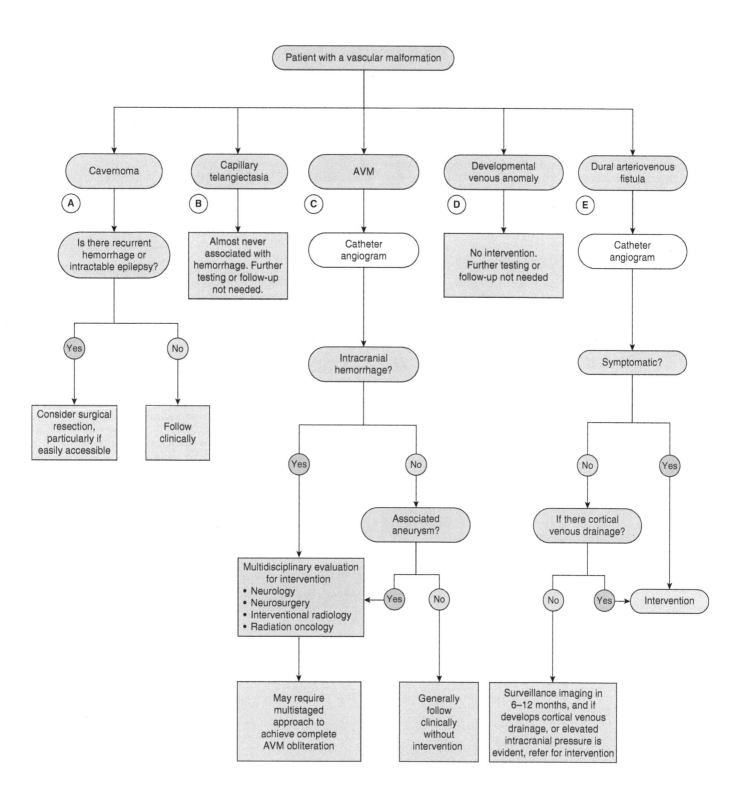

Cerebral Venous Sinus Thrombosis

Kelley Humbert and Christopher G. Favilla

Cerebral venous sinus thrombosis (CVST) presents with progressive headache, papilledema, changes in mental status, focal neurologic deficits, and/or seizures. Obstructed venous drainage causes venous congestion, resulting in cerebral edema, hemorrhage, or ischemia if the arterial pressure cannot overcome the venous pressure (venous infarction). CVST is often overlooked in patients with progressively worsening unexplained headache and young patients with lobar hemorrhage. Early identification is critical, as when unrecognized, progression and neurologic deterioration are common. Note that intracerebral hemorrhage due to CVST is the rare hemorrhagic condition in which anticoagulation is indicated. This reflects the fact that hemorrhage is due to venous outflow obstruction, not arterial bleeding. Hyperdensity in the sinuses on non-contrast computed tomography (CT) may suggest the diagnosis, but brain magnetic resonance imaging (MRI) with contrast and/or MR venography is usually necessary; CT venography is an alternative.

A. Anticoagulation is necessary regardless of the presence or absence of hemorrhage. If hemorrhage is present, it is reasonable to start therapeutic intravenous heparin because of its rapid reversibility and the ability to closely monitor anticoagulant levels. In the absence of hemorrhage, low-molecular-weight heparin (LMWH) may be more convenient and is likely of similar efficacy. Direct oral anticoagulants (DOACs) can also be considered once clinical stability is apparent.

B. With clinical deterioration and progressive edema despite therapeutic anticoagulation, consider endovascular therapy to mechanically remove venous sinus clot. Hyperosmolar therapy should also be considered when edema is severe, particularly as a bridge to endovascular therapy. Because of the high risk of seizures, continuous electroencephalogram monitoring is reasonable in patients with progressive symptoms or depressed mental status.

C. With clinical deterioration and worsening hemorrhage despite therapeutic anticoagulation, consider endovascular therapy as mentioned above. In rare cases of focal hematoma expansion causing herniation (i.e., temporal lobe hemorrhage), decompressive surgery can be considered. However, surgery necessitates temporary cessation of anticoagulation, which may result in worsening venous congestion and infarction.

D. Determine the underlying etiology of CVST to guide choice of optimal treatment, including duration and type of anticoagulant therapy. If intravenous heparin or LMWH was initially administered, this can be transitioned to an oral agent (DOAC or warfarin), assuming that medication is appropriate for the particular patient and underlying etiology.

E. During pregnancy and the postpartum period, there is an elevated risk of venous thrombosis. LMWH is the treatment of choice in pregnancy, although initial heparin use is also reasonable. Warfarin should be avoided in pregnancy due to teratogenicity. Hypercoagulability typically persists several weeks after delivery, so treatment is recommended to continue at least 6 weeks postpartum.

F. Both LMWH and DOACs are reasonable for hypercoagulability of malignancy. If cancer treatment is curative, consider discontinuing anticoagulation eventually.

G. When CVST is unprovoked and without clear cause, life-long anticoagulation is generally recommended although there is little data specific to CVST.

H. Oral contraceptive pills increase the risk of venous thrombosis, a risk that is compounded with age and smoking. A nonhormonal intrauterine device is the ideal alternative birth control plan, although some second-generation progesterone OCPs may not carry a risk of venous thrombosis. Similarly, estrogen supplementation contributes to venous thrombosis, in which case it should be stopped immediately. Some chemotherapeutic agents may also cause venous thrombosis and should be avoided.

I. If CVST occurs in the context of a high-risk thrombophilia, life-long oral anticoagulation is warranted. Choice of optimal anticoagulant agent (i.e., warfarin vs. DOAC) should be made in discussion with an expert in disorders of coagulation. With antiphospholipid syndrome, warfarin is preferred; DOACs may be appropriate in other scenarios.

J. Repeat venous imaging, typically with MR venography, should be repeated in 3–6 months to evaluate for recanalization of the venous sinuses and to establish a baseline study for comparison in the future should new or recurrent symptoms develop. Incomplete recanalization is not uncommon and generally well tolerated.

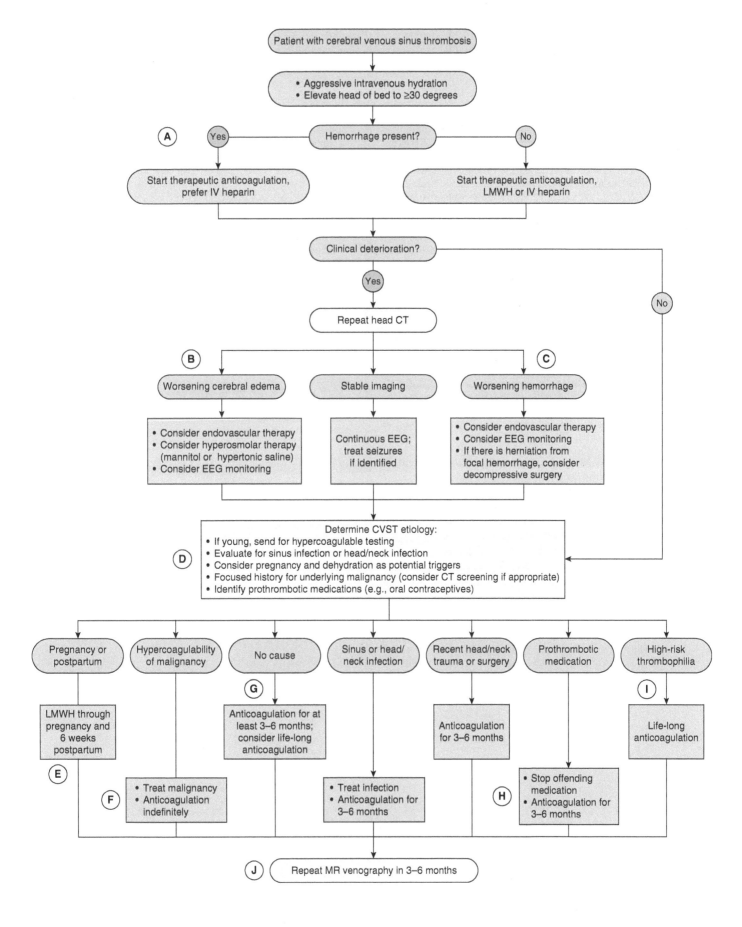

Brain Death

Joshua M. Levine

A. Brain death is defined, in the United States and many other countries, as permanent and irreversible cessation of whole brain function. Some countries, such as the United Kingdom, consider loss of all brainstem function sufficient to meet criteria for brain death. Brain death is a clinical diagnosis and, in localities that recognize the determination, is legally equivalent to death from permanent cessation of cardiac function. While various guidelines exist for determination of brain death, practice is determined by local law and by institutional policy. It is therefore incumbent upon the physician to know and to follow these.

B. Examples of etiologies sufficient to account for loss of whole brain function include global hypoxic-ischemic injury and herniation from severe cerebral edema or hydrocephalus.

C. The concept of brain death is frequently confusing to both physicians and the lay public. While permission to determine brain death is generally not required, it is good practice to educate families about the concept of brain death and to describe the process of brain-death determination.

D. Some institutions require two clinical examinations separated by a waiting period, while others require only a single examination. An examination that is consistent with brain death establishes that the patient is comatose and lacks all brainstem reflexes, including spontaneous breathing. The following examination elements should be assessed and documented:

- Coma – there should be no motor responses to pain except for reflexes mediated by the spinal cord.
- Pupillary light reflex – the pupils should be nonreactive to bright light.
- Corneal reflexes – there should be no reflex eye closure when the corneas are touched with a gauze.
- Oculocephalic reflexes – there should be no reflex movement of the eyes when the head is turned. This test should be deferred in patients with known or suspected instability of the cervical spine.
- Oculovestibular reflexes – there should be no movement of the eyes after instillation of cold water into each external auditory canal.
- Cough – there should be no cough when the carina is stimulated with a deep suction catheter.
- Gag – there should be no gag when the posterior pharynx is stimulated with a tongue depressor or firm plastic suction tip.
- Spontaneous breathing – there should be no patient-initiated breaths on the mechanical ventilator. Spontaneous breathing is also tested more rigorously by a formal apnea test.

E. In general, confirmatory studies are not required to determine brain death. However, under certain circumstances and in some areas, confirmatory testing may be mandated. When portions of the clinical examination cannot be completed (e.g., due to severe facial trauma), confirmatory testing is indicated. Confirmatory tests might include a nuclear blood flow scan or a catheter cerebral angiogram showing no cerebral blood flow, or a brain-death protocol electroencephalogram showing no cerebral electrical activity.

F. Formal apnea testing should be performed and aims to demonstrate absent function of medullary breathing centers. Typically, after a brief period of preoxygenation, the patient is removed from the ventilator and observed for 10–15 minutes. An apnea test is considered consistent with brain death if the patient makes no respiratory effort and the patient's arterial partial pressure of carbon dioxide rises from a normal baseline to >60 mmHg or to 20 mmHg above baseline.

REFERENCES

1. EFM Wijdicks. Current concepts: the diagnosis of brain death. *NEJM.* 2001;344:1215–1221.
2. Wijdicks EFM, Varelas PN, Gronseth GS, Greer DM. Evidence-based guideline update: determining brain death in adults. Report of the Quality Standards Subcommittee of the American Academy of Neurology. *Neurology.* 2010;74:1911–1918.

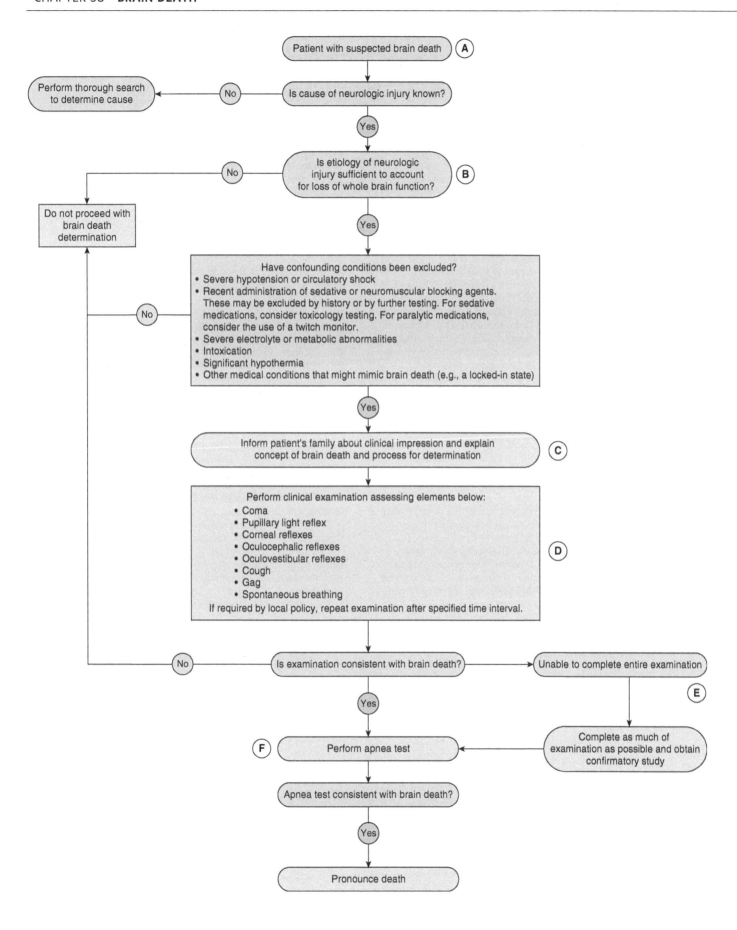

Patient with suspected brain death (A)

Is cause of neurologic injury known?

No → Perform thorough search to determine cause

Yes

Is etiology of neurologic injury sufficient to account for loss of whole brain function? (B)

No → Do not proceed with brain death determination

Yes

Have confounding conditions been excluded?
- Severe hypotension or circulatory shock
- Recent administration of sedative or neuromuscular blocking agents. These may be excluded by history or by further testing. For sedative medications, consider toxicology testing. For paralytic medications, consider the use of a twitch monitor.
- Severe electrolyte or metabolic abnormalities
- Intoxication
- Significant hypothermia
- Other medical conditions that might mimic brain death (e.g., a locked-in state)

No

Yes

Inform patient's family about clinical impression and explain concept of brain death and process for determination (C)

Perform clinical examination assessing elements below:
- Coma
- Pupillary light reflex
- Corneal reflexes
- Oculocephalic reflexes
- Oculovestibular reflexes
- Cough
- Gag
- Spontaneous breathing
If required by local policy, repeat examination after specified time interval. (D)

Is examination consistent with brain death?

No

Unable to complete entire examination (E)

Yes

Complete as much of examination as possible and obtain confirmatory study

(F) Perform apnea test

Apnea test consistent with brain death?

Yes

Pronounce death

Management of Increased Intracranial Pressure

Jessy Walia and Monisha A. Kumar

Brain tissue, cerebrospinal fluid (CSF), and blood are contained within the confined space of the skull. An increase in volume of one of these components necessarily results in a compensatory reduction in another. Normal physiologic compensatory mechanisms include egress of CSF or venous blood into the lumbar cistern or extracranial blood compartment. However, with a sufficiently large intracranial mass lesion, such as intracranial hemorrhage, or diffuse brain swelling, such as with traumatic brain injury, these compensatory mechanisms are overwhelmed, leading to decreased intracranial blood flow and/or direct compression of brain tissue, both of which may cause brain injury and potentially brain death. As a general rule, the patient with increased intracranial pressure (ICP) should be intubated and mechanically ventilated to facilitate management. Measures to lower ICP aim to prevent this injury and can be broadly divided into therapies that (1) reduce brain tissue volume, typically osmotic agents (e.g., mannitol, hypertonic saline) or surgical procedures to remove mass lesions; (2) reduce intracranial blood volume, typically through hyperventilation, which causes vasoconstriction; and (3) reduce the volume of CSF, typically through an external ventricular drain. An ICP greater than 20–25 mmHg that is sustained for a period of greater than 5 minutes generally warrants treatment.

A. Simply raising the head of the bed may reduce ICP. Likewise, the head should be maintained in the midline position to avoid compression of the jugular veins. Hypoosmotic fluids should be avoided. Seizure activity may increase cerebral metabolic demand and result in ICP elevation, so if present, it should be aggressively treated.

B. Mild hyperventilation (PaCO$_2$ 30–35 mm Hg) will rapidly reduce ICP by causing vasoconstriction, but the effect is not durable. It should therefore generally be used only in the setting of impending herniation as a bridge to more definitive ICP-lowering therapy.

C. If ICP is elevated due to a focal mass lesion, such as hemorrhage or tumor, surgical evacuation of the mass or decompressive craniectomy should be pursued if appropriate. CSF diversion with an external ventricular drain (EVD) may also be considered. If there is hydrocephalus, placement of an EVD is essential, and allows both direct monitoring of ICP and treatment by draining CSF. Steroids may be used when a tumor is present. For other conditions, such as intracerebral hemorrhage, traumatic brain injury, and ischemic stroke, steroids are ineffective and should be avoided.

D. Administration of an intravenous (IV) bolus of 20% mannitol (1 g/kg) rapidly reduces ICP. It may be repeatedly administered every 6 hours. The osmolar gap (measured serum osmolarity minus calculated serum osmolarity) should be calculated prior to each dose to assess for accumulation; if >20 mOsm/L, additional mannitol should not be given. Given the osmotic diuresis induced by mannitol, urinary losses should be carefully repleted to avoid hypovolemia. If hypovolemia is present initially, a bolus of hypertonic saline (150 mL of 5%; or 30 mL of 23.4% solution every 6 hours) may be used instead of mannitol. If serum sodium is ≥160, hypertonic saline (HTS) should be stopped; it should also be avoided in the setting of severe acidosis. In the setting of renal failure, mannitol should be avoided and HTS used instead.

E. HTS is available in various concentrations and for bolus or continuous administration. It is preferable to administer higher-concentration formulations via a central venous catheter to minimize infusion site reactions. Serial assessment of serum sodium is recommended for patients receiving repeated doses or continuous infusion of HTS. HTS induces a hyperchloremic metabolic acidosis and may cause volume overload or pulmonary edema.

F. Neuromuscular paralysis may reduce ICP in patients with refractory persistently elevated ICP. A test bolus should be given first, and a continuous infusion may be instituted if the patient responds.

G. Barbiturate (e.g., pentobarbital) coma can be considered for those who fail to respond to all other aggressive interventions to control ICP. Hypotension is a side effect, so patients should be carefully volume resuscitated, and vasopressors may be used as needed. Pentobarbital has potent immunosuppressive effects, and prolonged use should therefore be with caution. Continuous electroencephalogram should be used to target the infusion to burst suppression or ICP within target range (whichever occurs sooner). Therapeutic hypothermia may also be considered. If there is felt to be increased intraabdominal pressure, for instance in cases of major abdominal or thoracic injuries, laparotomy to reduce intraabdominal pressure may in some cases lower ICP by increasing venous drainage.

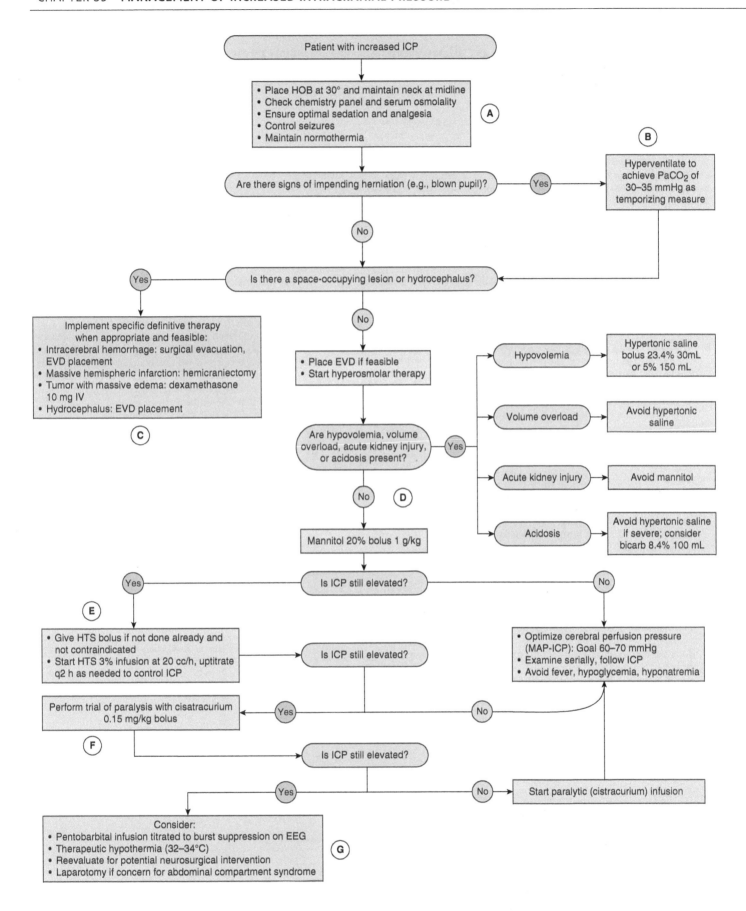

Management of Neuromuscular Respiratory Failure

Elizabeth Mahanna-Gabrielli

Patients with neuromuscular disease presenting with severe weakness require close monitoring of their respiratory status, as progression to respiratory failure can occur relatively suddenly. As the fundamental problem is one of ventilation as opposed to oxygenation, patients may continue to have normal oxygen saturation despite progressively worsening respiratory function. Similarly, hypercarbia represents a late manifestation of neuromuscular respiratory insufficiency and indicates impending respiratory failure; ventilatory support should start before hypercarbia is present. It is therefore critical to monitor ventilatory capacity frequently in these patients, typically with bedside measures of vital capacity and negative inspiratory force (NIF).

A. For patients with myasthenia gravis or Guillain-Barré syndrome, preparation and planning for starting plasmapheresis or intravenous immunoglobulin therapy should begin as soon as respiratory concerns are identified.

B. Respiratory status should be assessed a minimum of every 4 hours. The goal is to gauge whether the patient requires ventilatory support. Forced vital capacity (FVC) and NIF are both measurements of a patient's respiratory muscle strength and also correlate with the ability to cough and clear secretions. A simple bedside maneuver to roughly estimate FVC is to have the patient count as high as they can in a single breath; each number counted is equivalent to approximately 100 mL of FVC. For example, if a patient is able to count to 25, her FVC is about 2500 mL. The "20/30" rule is a good rule of thumb—if the FVC drops below 20 mL/kg, the NIF below 30 cm H_2O, or the patient is more than mildly dyspneic, ventilatory support should be started. A drop of 30% or more in either FVC or NIF should also prompt consideration of elective ventilatory support. The presence of facial weakness can sometimes confound measurement of FVC and NIF in the nonintubated patient, due to an inability to maintain a tight seal on the measurement device. This should be taken into consideration when these parameters are interpreted.

C. If the cause of weakness is Guillain-Barré syndrome, intubation and invasive mechanical ventilator support should be started, as these patients typically have progressive worsening over days before improvement starts to occur, even with immunotherapy.

D. If the patient is oxygenating well on room air, one can assume the patient is not markedly hypercapnic and does not have significant consolidation; noninvasive positive pressure ventilation in the biphasic positive airway pressure (BiPAP) mode can be started.

E. If supplemental oxygen is required, arterial blood gas (ABG) and chest radiograph (CXR) should be checked. If hypercapnia is present or CXR shows consolidation concerning for aspiration pneumonia or pneumonitis, BiPAP is not appropriate and intubation should be undertaken.

F. If inspiratory pressures (IPAP) greater than 20 cm H_2O are required, there is a risk of overcoming the lower esophageal sphincter tone and insufflating the stomach, and intubation should be pursued.

G. An increasing oxygen requirement or increasing IPAP are signs the patient may be failing BiPAP. An ABG should check for hypercapnia and CXR for signs of consolidation and aspiration. If present, intubation should be pursued.

H. When intubating a patient with neuromuscular disease, special attention should be paid to the choice of paralytic agent. If possible, intubation of patients with myasthenia gravis or Guillain-Barré syndrome should be performed without a neuromuscular blocking agent; when necessary, one-third to one-half the usual intubating dose of a nondepolarizing agent should be used. Depolarizing agents such as succinylcholine should be avoided given the unpredictable response in myasthenia and the risk of hyperkalemia in Guillain-Barré syndrome. Be prepared for a prolonged effect, and sedate and monitor the patient appropriately.

I. As muscle weakness begins to improve, daily spontaneous breathing trials (SBTs) with FVC and NIF measurements should occur. When the patient passes the SBT, FVC is >10 cc/kg, and NIF >20 cm H_2O, a trial of extubation should be considered. BiPAP ventilation can be used as a bridge immediately following extubation as needed.

REFERENCES

1. Lizarraga AA, Lizarraga KJ, Benatar M. Getting rid of weakness in the ICU: an updated approach to the acute management of myasthenia gravis and Guillain-Barré syndrome. *Semin Neurol.* 2016;35(6):615–624. https://doi.org/10.1055/s-0036-1592106.
2. Rabinstein AA. Noninvasive ventilation for neuromuscular respiratory failure: when to use and when to avoid. *Curr Opin Crit Care.* 2016;22 (2):94–99. https://doi.org/10.1097/MCC.0000000000000284.

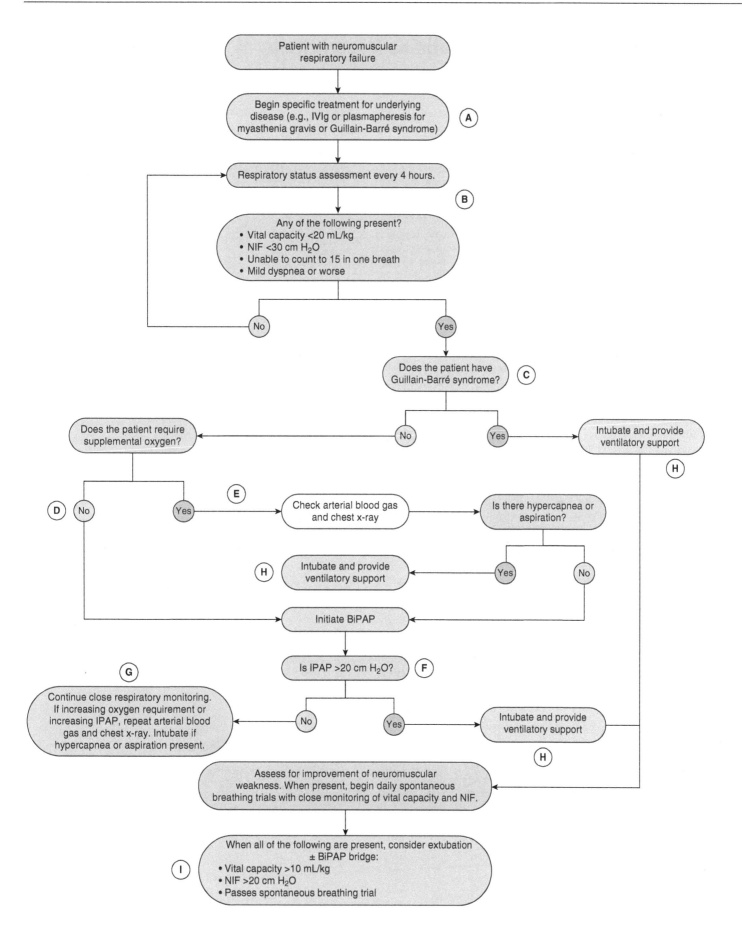

Paroxysmal Sympathetic Hyperactivity

Meghan M. Caylor and Arun K. Sherma

A. Paroxysmal sympathetic hyperactivity (PSH) is a syndrome encountered in patients with severe acute neurologic injury. Patients with PSH may have episodic tachycardia, hypertension, tachypnea, fever, diaphoresis, and posturing. Episodes may last minutes to hours and recur several times per day. Features supporting the diagnosis include multiple autonomic symptoms occurring simultaneously, multiple recurrent episodes over several days, and response to specific abortive therapy. The triggering of paroxysms by both noxious and nonnoxious stimuli is also an important defining feature of PSH. The pathophysiology of the condition is poorly understood, but impaired descending inhibitory control of excitatory spinal circuits, permitting unregulated sympathetic outflow, is a commonly proposed mechanism. PSH is often seen in severe traumatic brain injury, but may occur with any type of acute brain injury. Historically, terms used to describe this condition include "dysautonomia," "diencephalic seizures," "sympathetic storming," and "paroxysmal autonomic instability with dystonia."[1] Numerous medications are used to treat PSH, but there is little strong evidence to guide therapy. The most common agents employed in clinical practice are listed in Table 61.1. Often a combination of agents is necessary to achieve control of PSH episodes.[2,3]

B. Abortive therapy encompasses the initial intervention phase, utilizing rapid-acting intravenous (IV) agents to terminate acute episodes. Morphine is the prototypical IV opiate used in PSH and is particularly effective to abort multiple symptoms due to the additive effect of histamine release (lowers blood pressure, normally regarded as an adverse effect of IV morphine); other opiates may also be useful. Propranolol is considered the β-blocker of choice in PSH, as its lipophilicity allows it to cross the blood-brain barrier; labetalol is an alternative nonselective agent used frequently. Abortive agents can also be used to pretreat known triggers to prevent/minimize severity of paroxysms early in the course, as maintenance therapies are being uptitrated.

C. Preventative/maintenance therapies (oral agents) should be instituted after excluding alternative diagnoses and establishing a pattern of symptoms. Treatment may be optimized by using drugs with varied mechanisms of action. If no contraindications, oral opiates (such as oxycodone) and oral propranolol are recommended first-line maintenance agents. Additional agents may be selected based on the patient's predominant symptoms and comorbidities. Reevaluate every 24 hours and consider escalating current agents (every 1–3 days) or adding additional agents based on patient symptoms or occurrence of dose-limiting side effects.

D. Deescalation can be considered once acceptable control is achieved (episode-free or infrequent abortive therapies required). Therapeutic doses may be maintained for a period of time (several days or 1–2 weeks or longer) depending on the severity of symptoms, or immediately titrated down if mild PSH. The rate of downtitration should depend on duration of therapy and pharmacologic class with attention to minimize the risk of withdrawal.

TABLE 61.1 DOSING AND TITRATION OF MEDICATIONS FOR PAROXYSMAL SYMPATHETIC HYPERACTIVITY

ACUTE ABORTIVE THERAPIES			
	Starting dose	Titration	Maximum dose
Morphine IV	2–4 mg IV q1–2 h prn	2-mg increments	Doses up to 10 mg IV may be needed
Propranolol IV	1–3 mg IV q1–2 h prn	1–2-mg increments	5 mg IV per dose
Labetalol IV	10–20 mg IV q1–2 h prn	10-mg increments	80 mg IV per dose
Midazolam IV	1–2 mg IV q2–4 h prn	1–2-mg increments	10 mg IV per dose
MAINTENANCE/PREVENTATIVE THERAPIES			
Oxycodone PO	5–10 mg q4–6 h	5-mg increments	–
β-blockers			
Propranolol PO	10–20 mg q8–12 h	10–20-mg increments	320 mg/day[a]
Labetalol PO	100–200 mg q8–12 h	100–200-mg increments	2400 mg/day[a]
Clonidine PO	0.1 mg q8–12 h	0.1–0.2-mg increments	2.4 mg/day[a]
Gabapentin PO	100–300 mg q8 h	200–300-mg increments	3600 mg/day[a]
Benzodiazepines			
Clonazepam PO	0.25–1 mg q12 h	0.5-mg increments	–
Diazepam PO	2.5–10 mg q8–12 h	5 mg increments	–
Bromocriptine PO	1.25–2.5 mg q8–12h	2.5-mg increments	40 mg/day (divided q8–12 h)
Baclofen PO	5 mg q8 h	5 mg/dose every 2–3 days	80 mg/day[a]
Dantrolene PO	25 mg daily	After 7 days increase to 25 mg tid. Titrate dose by 25–50 mg increments weekly.	400 mg/day (divided q6 h)

IV, Intravenous; *PO*, per os;
[a]Total maximum daily doses should be divided q6–q8 h

REFERENCES

1. Baguley IJ, Perkes IE, Fernandez-Ortega JF, Rabinstein AA, Dolce G, Hendricks HT. For the Consensus Working Group. Paroxysmal sympathetic hyperactivity after acquired brain injury: consensus on conceptual definition, nomenclature, and diagnostic criteria. *J Neurotrauma.* 2014;31:1515–1520.
2. Perkes I, Baguley IJ, Nott MT, Menon DK. A review of paroxysmal sympathetic hyperactivity after acquired brain injury. *Ann Neurol.* 2010;68:126–135.
3. Rabinstein AA, Benarroch EE. Treatment of paroxysmal sympathetic hyperactivity. *Curr Treat Options Neurol.* 2008;10:151–157.

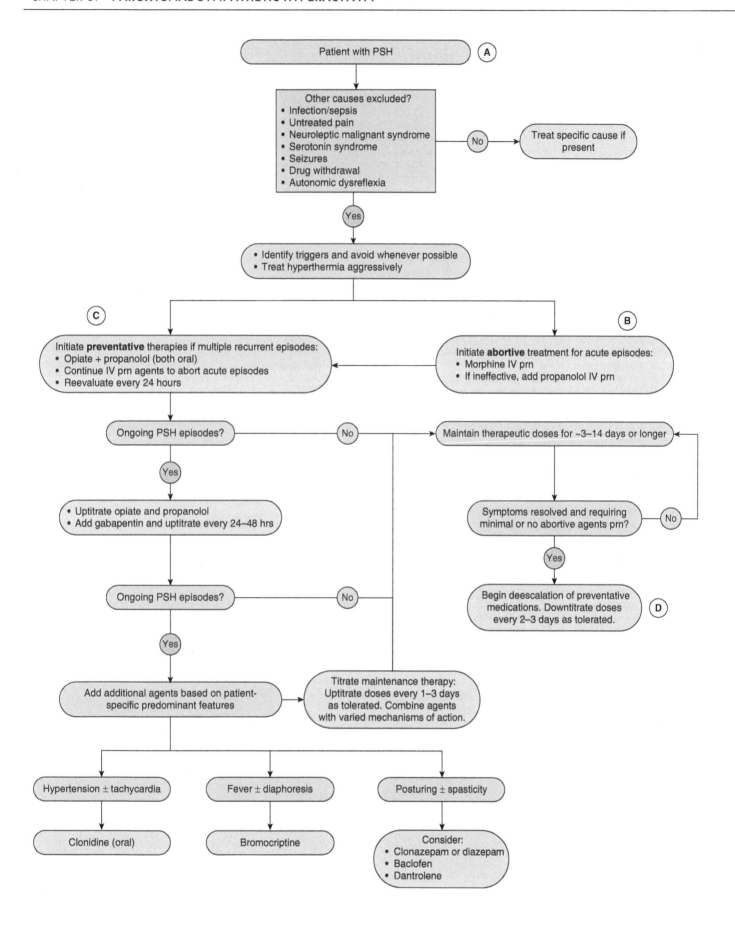

Traumatic Brain Injury

Lindsay Raab and Danielle K. Sandsmark

Initial primary brain injury following trauma occurs immediately at the time of head impact and is largely irreversible. Public health measures such as airbags, seat belts, bike helmets, and fall prevention measures are therefore essential to limit traumatic brain injury (TBI). Pathology at this initial stage includes diffuse axonal injury, intraparenchymal hemorrhage and contusion, and extraaxial hemorrhages including epidural and subdural hematoma, subarachnoid hemorrhage, and intraventricular hemorrhage. Secondary insults, including a variety of ischemic, metabolic, and inflammatory disturbances, develop over hours to days after injury and exacerbate the now injured, vulnerable brain tissue. Monitoring for secondary brain injury is the focus of hospital-based care following TBI. Main targets for intervention include limiting cerebral edema and brain compression, optimizing tissue perfusion, and minimizing metabolic distress.

A. Neurologic status on hospital arrival, commonly measured with the Glasgow Coma Scale (GCS), is an important predictor of prognosis. Other factors indicative of the degree of brain injury include duration of loss of consciousness (LOC) and duration of posttraumatic amnesia. These factors are most helpful in predicting outcomes in severe injuries but are less reliable for mild injuries. Severity of TBI is often classified as mild (GCS 13–15, LOC <30 minutes, posttraumatic amnesia <24 hours), moderate (GCS 9–12, LOC 30 minutes–24 hours, posttraumatic amnesia 24 hours–7 days), and severe (GCS <8, LOC >24 hours, posttraumatic amnesia >7 days).

B. Patients with TBI frequently have additional traumatic injuries; a complete trauma survey must be conducted. Securing the airway, stabilization of the spine, and treatment of immediately life-threatening issues such as pneumothoraces, cardiac tamponade, or shock should be undertaken. Serial examinations and assessments should be performed to avoid missed injuries.

C. Coagulopathy may be present in TBI and lead to additional secondary injury from ongoing bleeding. Prior antiplatelet and anticoagulant use should be identified, and prothrombin and partial thromboplastic times as well as platelet count measured. When present, coagulopathy should be corrected as appropriate.

D. Urgent surgical intervention is usually required for epidural hematoma, large or acute subdural hematomas, or any hemorrhage leading to mass effect with midline shift and impending herniation.

E. Following TBI, intracranial pressure (ICP) may be increased due to diffuse cerebral injury, focal intracranial hemorrhage, or contusions. Seizure activity may exacerbate elevations in ICP. Simple bedside measures to increase venous drainage should be implemented to lower ICP; more aggressive measures are often necessary, particularly in severe TBI. These are outlined in Chapter 59.

F. Monitoring of cerebral metabolism is available in some neurointensive care units and may include measurements of cerebral perfusion pressure, brain oxygen, cerebral blood flow, and cerebral microdialysis. In general, cerebral perfusion pressure (CPP) should be kept >60 mmHg and brain oxygen should be maintained >20 mmHg, but treatment must be individualized with the goal of matching glucose and oxygen delivery to meet cerebral metabolic demands based on the available monitoring data. In the absence of advanced neuromonitoring devices, the focus should be on minimizing systemic metabolic derangements through optimizing hemodynamics and pulmonary mechanics. A reasonable target for $PaCO_2$ is 35–40 mmHg; targeting lower values with prolonged hyperventilation is not advised. Oxygen saturation should be kept >88%, and hemoglobin >7 g/dL.

G. TBI patients are at high risk of both clinical and subclinical seizures, which if present should be treated with antiepileptic drug therapy. Continuous electroencephalogram (EEG) monitoring may detect subclinical seizures. Prophylactic antiepileptic drug therapy is for the first 7 days after injury is reasonable, but longer treatment has not been shown to prevent posttraumatic epilepsy.

H. Fever is common after severe TBI and is associated with poor neurological outcomes. Temperature >38°C should be aggressively treated with acetaminophen and/or induced normothermia using surface or intravascular cooling devices. Hypothermia has been shown to have no benefit, and may even cause harm, so should be avoided. Nonsteroidal antiinflammatory drugs should be avoided in most patients given the concomitant presence or risk of intracranial hemorrhage.

I. Hyperglycemia is associated with worse neurologic outcomes in TBI, and it is thus reasonable to treat with insulin to maintain glucose <200mg/dL. Overly stringent glycemic control (glucose levels maintained at 70–140mg/dL) does not improve mortality and results in more hypoglycemic episodes.

REFERENCES

1. Citerio G, Oddo M, Taccone FS. Recommendations for the use of multimodal monitoring in the neurointensive care unit. *Curr Opin Crit Care.* 2015;21:113–119.
2. Maas AIR, Menon DK, Adelson PD, et al. Traumatic brain injury: integrated approaches to improve prevention, clinical care, and research. *Lancet Neurol.* 2017;16:987–1048.

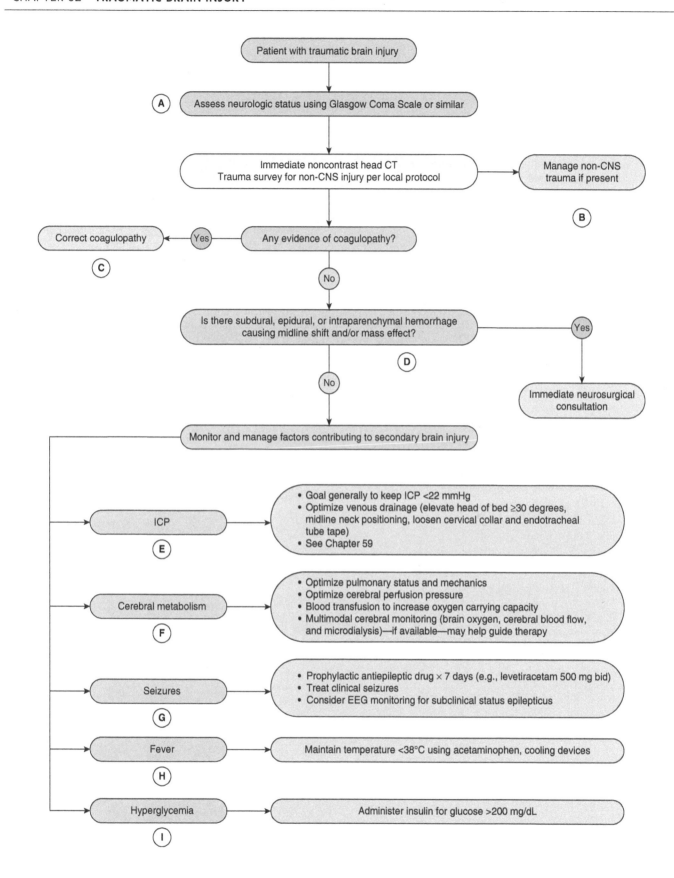

Patient with traumatic brain injury

A Assess neurologic status using Glasgow Coma Scale or similar

Immediate noncontrast head CT
Trauma survey for non-CNS injury per local protocol

Manage non-CNS trauma if present

B

Any evidence of coagulopathy?

Yes → Correct coagulopathy

C

No

Is there subdural, epidural, or intraparenchymal hemorrhage causing midline shift and/or mass effect?

D

Yes → Immediate neurosurgical consultation

No

Monitor and manage factors contributing to secondary brain injury

ICP

E
- Goal generally to keep ICP <22 mmHg
- Optimize venous drainage (elevate head of bed ≥30 degrees, midline neck positioning, loosen cervical collar and endotracheal tube tape)
- See Chapter 59

Cerebral metabolism

F
- Optimize pulmonary status and mechanics
- Optimize cerebral perfusion pressure
- Blood transfusion to increase oxygen carrying capacity
- Multimodal cerebral monitoring (brain oxygen, cerebral blood flow, and microdialysis)—if available—may help guide therapy

Seizures

G
- Prophylactic antiepileptic drug × 7 days (e.g., levetiracetam 500 mg bid)
- Treat clinical seizures
- Consider EEG monitoring for subclinical status epilepticus

Fever

H

Maintain temperature <38°C using acetaminophen, cooling devices

Hyperglycemia

I

Administer insulin for glucose >200 mg/dL

Concussion

Danielle K. Sandsmark

A. Concussion, more appropriately called mild traumatic brain injury, refers to any trauma-induced alteration in brain function. An obvious corollary of this is that patients must have head trauma causing some neurologic symptoms (though these may be very brief) in order to be diagnosed as having had a concussion. Common symptoms are confusion and amnesia, imbalance, dizziness, and headache. The injury may or may not involve loss of consciousness, but when present, the period of alteration of mental status is generally brief (less than 30 minutes).

B. Initial assessment of the patient with concussion should be focused on determining whether urgent neuroimaging is required. When indicated, computed tomography (CT) is the preferred modality to rule out intracranial hemorrhage, which might require close monitoring and/or urgent neurosurgical intervention. Clinical decision tools, such as the Canadian CT Head Rule, are useful in this assessment.[1] Basic information on the mechanism of injury and specific high-risk patient features should be obtained first, as this information may lead to a rapid decision to proceed directly to imaging. For example, imaging is recommended for all patients over age 60 years with concussion, regardless of specific neurologic symptoms or findings.

C. If no high-risk patient features are present, then a thorough assessment of neurologic symptoms and function should be performed to guide the decision on whether imaging is necessary. Milder neurologic symptoms, such as headache, dizziness, balance difficulties, and confusion, are common after head impacts but do not necessarily warrant head imaging unless one of these more concerning features is present.

D. If brain CT is abnormal and demonstrates acute hemorrhage, hospital admission with close neurologic monitoring should be undertaken given the risk of hemorrhage expansion, particularly in the first 24 hours after injury.

E. The vast majority of individuals with concussion will have normal head CT scans and do not require hospital admission. Providing anticipatory guidance to these patients has been associated with improved outcomes. Patients should receive a description of their injury and its severity, education regarding common symptoms and those that warrant emergency room reevaluation, details of the recovery process and return to activity, and contact information for appropriate community resources.[2] Symptom management beyond over-the-counter analgesics and antiemetics is generally not required, as the vast majority of patients will experience a slow recovery over the next 1–4 weeks without pharmacologic intervention. In the past, patients had been counseled to undertake complete cognitive and physical rest until their symptoms resolve. However, more recent evidence demonstrates that this approach is associated with increased symptoms and prolonged recovery. Therefore, a graduated return to normal daily activities is recommended after a brief period of rest (24–72 hours).

REFERENCES

1. Stiell IG, Wells GA, Vandemheen K, et al. The Canadian CT Head Rule for patients with minor head injury. *Lancet.* 2001;357:1391–1396.
2. Levin HS, Diaz-Arrastia RR. Diagnosis, prognosis, and clinical management of mild traumatic brain injury. *Lancet Neurol.* 2015;14:506–517.

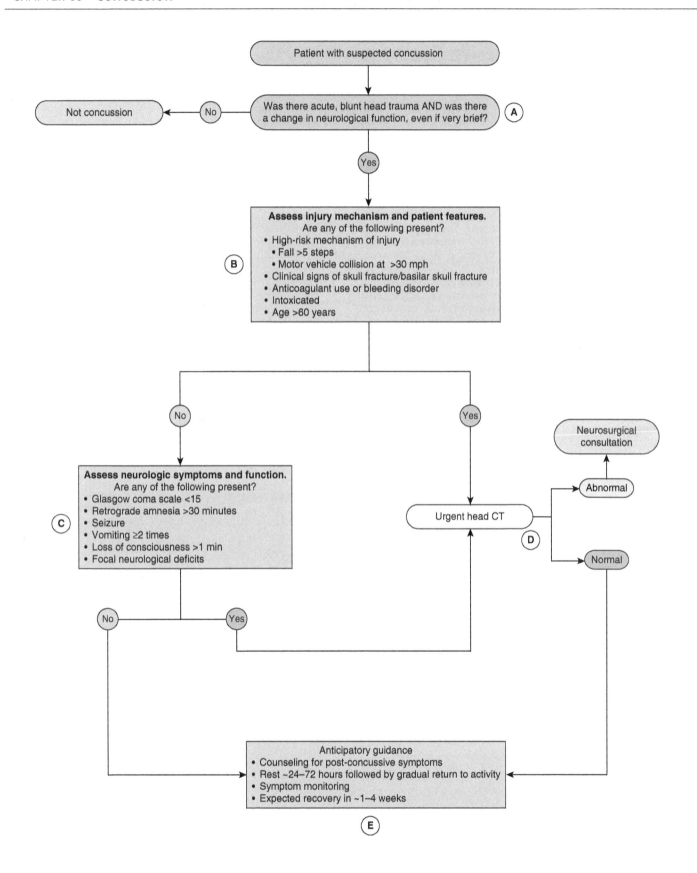

Patient with suspected concussion

A — Was there acute, blunt head trauma AND was there a change in neurological function, even if very brief?

No → Not concussion

Yes

B — **Assess injury mechanism and patient features.**
Are any of the following present?
- High-risk mechanism of injury
  - Fall >5 steps
  - Motor vehicle collision at >30 mph
- Clinical signs of skull fracture/basilar skull fracture
- Anticoagulant use or bleeding disorder
- Intoxicated
- Age >60 years

No

Yes

C — **Assess neurologic symptoms and function.**
Are any of the following present?
- Glasgow coma scale <15
- Retrograde amnesia >30 minutes
- Seizure
- Vomiting ≥2 times
- Loss of consciousness >1 min
- Focal neurological deficits

No

Yes

D — Urgent head CT

Abnormal → Neurosurgical consultation

Normal

E — Anticipatory guidance
- Counseling for post-concussive symptoms
- Rest ~24–72 hours followed by gradual return to activity
- Symptom monitoring
- Expected recovery in ~1–4 weeks

Postconcussive Syndrome

Megan T. Moyer and Danielle K. Sandsmark

While the initial neurologic symptoms following concussion typically resolve quickly, many will have symptoms that evolve over the ensuing 1–3 days. The majority of patients experience a complete recovery in 2–4 weeks. However, about 20% of patients experience persistent symptoms lasting months to years.[1] Postconcussive symptoms vary significantly between individuals but include headache, neck pain, sleep disturbances and fatigue, vestibular dysfunction, mood disturbances, and cognitive changes. Identifying the specific symptoms helps individualize treatment.[2] Women, those with prior traumatic brain injury, and those with preexisting anxiety and depression are at higher risk of developing persistent symptoms.

A. Precise definitions vary, but generally postconcussive syndrome can be considered when persistent symptoms are experienced for greater than 1–3 months after injury. If symptoms persist at 1 month postinjury, it is reasonable to start treatment to facilitate recovery.

B. Headaches are common in the acute period after head impact but can become persistent. Many of these have migrainous features, though other headache types can also develop. Pharmacologic therapy is identical to that used for abortive and preventative management in headache not related to concussion (see Chapters 65 and 66).

C. Neck pain is a frequent complaint, particularly after hyperextension injuries. Muscular tension in the neck may cause cervicogenic headaches. Occipital neuralgia may be present. Physical therapy is the mainstay of treatment. Occipital nerve blocks may be considered for those with symptoms consistent with occipital neuralgia. Pharmacologic therapy with muscle relaxants and/or benzodiazepines, particularly diazepam, may be helpful but should be limited to short-term use of not more than 1 week.

D. Sleep disturbances after concussion are common. While the immediate postinjury period is typically characterized by hypersomnolence, chronic sleep disturbances include insomnia, excessive daytime sleepiness, and sleep fragmentation. Obstructive sleep apnea can develop or become symptomatic. As poor sleep can aggravate other symptoms, screening for and treating sleep disturbances early is particularly important. A variety of pharmacologic and nonpharmacologic approaches can be used (see Chapter 78), though they have not been studied specifically in postconcussive syndrome.

E. Vestibular dysfunction, characterized by dizziness and imbalance, and tinnitus can be particularly disabling after concussion. These disturbances are closely related to oculomotor dysfunction, which may manifest as abnormalities of near-point convergence, saccades, and smooth pursuits. Patients often describe worsening symptoms with visual scanning, such as when reading, using phone or computer screens, being in crowds, or driving, or with rapid head and eye movement, such as bending over or turning around quickly. Vestibular physical therapy is the primary treatment. Pharmacologic agents like meclizine or benzodiazepines are of little benefit and should not be routinely used.

F. Mood disturbances are both a risk factor for persistent postconcussive symptoms and a consequence of concussion. Depressive symptoms, including fatigue, irritability, difficulty sleeping, impaired concentration, and anxiety, are associated with poorer recovery after concussion. Posttraumatic stress and anxiety disorders are also commonly associated with these injuries. Treatment should incorporate a multimodal approach that includes pharmacologic management and psychological support. Serotonin selective reuptake inhibitors (SSRIs) are generally favored over other antidepressants, although tricyclic antidepressants can be considered in those with concurrent chronic headache or neck pain.

G. Cognitive complaints can include trouble concentrating, irritability, and short-term memory impairment. Other symptoms that can exacerbate cognitive deficits, such as headaches, poor sleep, and depressive symptoms, must be treated. Neuropsychological testing can identify areas of difficulty and help to guide cognitive therapy. There are limited data regarding the use of stimulants and agents like amantadine to improve cognitive functioning after concussion.

REFERENCES

1. van der Naalt J, Timmerman ME, de Koning ME, et al. Early predictors of outcome after mild traumatic brain injury (UPFRONT): an observational cohort study. *Lancet Neurol.* 2017;16:532–540.
2. Levin HS, Diaz-Arrastia RR. Diagnosis, prognosis, and clinical management of mild traumatic brain injury. *Lancet Neurol.* 2015;14:506–517.

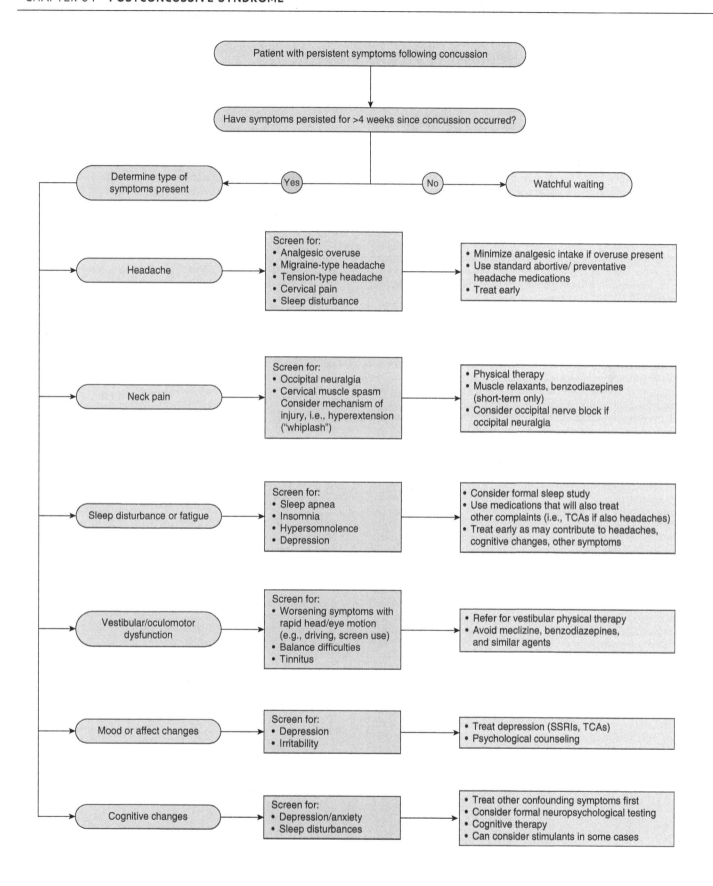

Migraine Headache: Acute Treatment

Carlyn Patterson-Gentile and Ana Recober

Acute treatment of migraine should target both head pain and, if present, associated symptoms such as nausea and vomiting. The latter may limit absorption of oral medications; in these cases, intranasal or subcutaneous formulations may be useful in the outpatient setting, and intravenous formulations in the hospital setting. Abortive medications are most effective when taken early in the migraine attack. Supportive measures should include aggressive hydration and rest or sleep when feasible. Caffeine may potentiate the effects of abortive medications and often helps relieve migraine. In general, use of abortive medications should be limited to 2–3 days per week to avoid medication overuse headache. Emerging alternatives to abortive medications include neurostimulation and occipital or other cranial nerve blocks with anesthetics; these may be particularly useful in patient for whom specific medications are ineffective or contraindicated.

A. In the hospital setting, the range of options for migraine treatment is broad due to the ability to give parenteral agents. Selection of therapy depends on which agents may have already been used in an attempt to abort headache, prior history of response or lack of response to particular agents, and potential contraindications to specific medications. In patients who have not already tried a triptan, subcutaneous sumatriptan and metoclopramide are a reasonable choice for initial therapy. Prochlorperazine or chlorpromazine can be used as alternatives to metoclopramide. When given parenterally, all three of these antiemetics have efficacy for relieving headache as well as associated nausea/vomiting. Pretreatment with diphenhydramine helps to prevent extrapyramidal side effects from these drugs. Ondansetron may be a more efficacious antiemetic but does not seem to have antimigraine effects. For patients previously unresponsive to triptans or who have not been able to abort their current migraine with a triptan, intravenous dihydroergotamine (DHE) can be an effective treatment strategy, but should not be used if a triptan has been administered within the previous 24 hours. DHE is contraindicated in patients with hemiplegic migraine, basilar migraine, cardiovascular disease, and severe renal or hepatic impairment. DHE should not be used within 2 weeks of monoaminoxidase inhibitors due to risk of serotonin syndrome. Finally, monotherapy with parenteral metoclopramide (prochlorperazine or chlorpromazine are alternatives) can be used if a patient has taken a triptan within 24 hours of presenting to the emergency department (ED) or has contraindications to triptans or DHE (Table 65.1).

B. When severe nausea or vomiting are present, subcutaneous sumatriptan should be used. It can be easily self-administered by patients at home. This is often effective at treating both the headache and nausea. If not, an antiemetic such as metoclopramide may be given as adjunctive therapy. Intranasal sumatriptan or zolmitriptan can also be considered in this situation, but nasal sprays can be difficult to tolerate in the presence of nausea.

C. Triptans should be used as a first-line abortive therapy for severe migraine headache, and can also be used when pain is moderate but does not respond to simple or combination analgesics. Subcutaneous and intranasal formulations have faster onset of action (10–20 min) and are preferred for headaches that are severe at the beginning of the attack or are present in the morning upon awakening. Eletriptan and rizatriptan appear to be the most effective oral triptans, but also may have more side effects. Almotriptan is often better tolerated with reasonable efficacy. Naratriptan has a slower onset of action and tends to have the least side effects. Frovatriptan has a longer half-life and should be considered if the pain usually returns within 24 hours. Importantly, response to individual triptans varies across patients, and it is reasonable to switch to a different triptan before trying other classes of medications. Triptans are contraindicated in patients with hemiplegic migraine, basilar migraine, or cardiovascular disease. Common side effects are dizziness, fatigue, flushing, tingling, and chest pain.

D. Combining a triptan with a nonsteroidal antiinflammatory drug (NSAID) has been shown to be more effective than either used as a monotherapy, and should be considered if triptans alone are ineffective.

E. Not infrequently, migraine headache will initially respond to intravenous therapy in the ED, but subsequently recur within 24 hours. Administration of a single dose of intravenous dexamethasone reduces the risk of headache recurrence and should be considered for most patients treated for headache in the ED.

F. In patients for whom triptans and DHE are contraindicated, simple analgesics, combination analgesics, occipital and other cranial nerve blocks with anesthetics, and neurostimulation devices are alternatives available in the outpatient setting. Neurostimulation devices for acute migraine treatment include transcutaneous trigeminal nerve stimulation, noninvasive vagus nerve stimulation, and transcranial magnetic stimulation. The use of butalbital-containing analgesic combinations (Fioricet and Fiorinal) is discouraged due to concerns of medication overuse headache. However, they may be considered when all other options are contraindicated or ineffective as long as they are used sparingly.

See Appendix 1 for Table 65.1: Medications for treating migraine headaches.

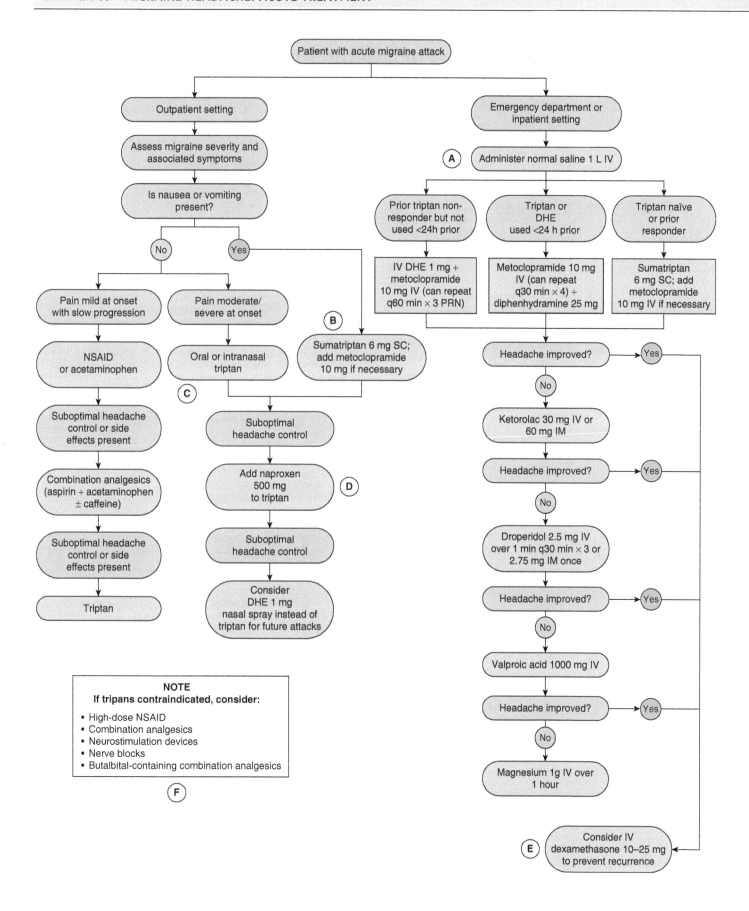

Patient with acute migraine attack

Outpatient setting

Assess migraine severity and associated symptoms

Is nausea or vomiting present?

No / Yes

Pain mild at onset with slow progression

Pain moderate/severe at onset

NSAID or acetaminophen

Oral or intranasal triptan

(C)

Suboptimal headache control or side effects present

Combination analgesics (aspirin + acetaminophen ± caffeine)

Suboptimal headache control or side effects present

Triptan

Sumatriptan 6 mg SC; add metoclopramide 10 mg if necessary

(B)

Suboptimal headache control

Add naproxen 500 mg to triptan

(D)

Suboptimal headache control

Consider DHE 1 mg nasal spray instead of triptan for future attacks

Emergency department or inpatient setting

(A) Administer normal saline 1 L IV

Prior triptan non-responder but not used <24h prior

Triptan or DHE used <24 h prior

Triptan naïve or prior responder

IV DHE 1 mg + metoclopramide 10 mg IV (can repeat q60 min × 3 PRN)

Metoclopramide 10 mg IV (can repeat q30 min × 4) + diphenhydramine 25 mg

Sumatriptan 6 mg SC; add metoclopramide 10 mg IV if necessary

Headache improved? — Yes

No

Ketorolac 30 mg IV or 60 mg IM

Headache improved? — Yes

No

Droperidol 2.5 mg IV over 1 min q30 min × 3 or 2.75 mg IM once

Headache improved? — Yes

No

Valproic acid 1000 mg IV

Headache improved? — Yes

No

Magnesium 1g IV over 1 hour

(E) Consider IV dexamethasone 10–25 mg to prevent recurrence

NOTE
If tripans contraindicated, consider:

- High-dose NSAID
- Combination analgesics
- Neurostimulation devices
- Nerve blocks
- Butalbital-containing combination analgesics

(F)

66 Migraine Headache: Prophylactic Treatment

Carlyn Patterson-Gentile and Ana Recober

Prophylactic therapy for migraine is aimed at reducing the frequency, and possibly severity, of recurrent migraine headaches. To maximize tolerability, it is important to start with low doses and titrate slowly (Table 66.1). Patients should be given realistic expectations of the benefit likely to be achieved (about 50% improvement in general) and the time to achieve benefit (often 1–3 months). Keeping a headache diary helps evaluate therapeutic response more objectively.

TABLE 66.1 PROPHYLACTIC TREATMENT FOR MIGRAINE		
Medication	**Dosing**	**Special considerations**
Nutraceuticals:		
Riboflavin	400 mg/day	Well tolerated
Magnesium	400–800 mg/day	May cause diarrhea
Coenzyme Q10	100 mg tid	Well tolerated
Melatonin	1–9 mg qhs	May help with insomnia
Tricyclic Antidepressants		
Amitriptyline	25–100 mg qhs	Consider if sedation is desired.
Nortriptyline	25–100 mg qhs	Better tolerated than amitriptyline.
β-Blockers		
Metoprolol	50–200 mg/day	Avoid in athletes, asthma, and diabetes
Propranolol	120–240 mg/day	
Timolol	10–15 mg/day	
Antiepileptics:		
Topiramate	50–200 mg/day	Teratogenic. Monitor for cognitive side effects and weight loss.
Valproic acid	500–1000 mg/day	Teratogenic. Monitor for weight gain.
Other Antihypertensives		
Candesartan	8–32 mg/day	Teratogenic. Well tolerated.
Lisinopril	10–20 mg/day	Can cause dizziness
Other Agents:		
Onabotulinumtoxin A	155–195 U IM every 12 weeks	Well tolerated
Monoclonal Antibodies		
Erenumab	70–140 mg SC monthly	Blocks CGRP receptor. Well tolerated. Can cause constipation and injection site reactions
Fremanezumab	225 mg SC monthly or 675 mg SC quarterly	Blocks CGRP ligand. Well tolerated. Can cause injection site reactions.
Galcanezumab	120–240 mg SC monthly	

CGRP, Calcitonin-gene-related peptide; *IM,* Intramuscular; *SC,* subcutaneous.

A. Keeping a regular schedule for meals and sleep hours (including weekends), exercising regularly, and reducing stress are central aspects of migraine prevention. Careful attention to the frequency with which acute medications are used, including over-the-counter medications, is important to avoid medication overuse headache. If migraine headache frequency is greater than 1 day per week, consider starting a prophylactic medication.

B. Choice of preventive therapy depends on migraine frequency and severity, as well as patient preference and comorbidities. For patients who do not have significant migraine-related disability or functional impairment such as missed school, work, family or social activities, choosing a treatment with few side effects but potentially lesser efficacy is reasonable (e.g., magnesium or riboflavin). For those with significant migraine-related disability, preventive therapy is often selected based on comorbidities and patient preference (Table 66.1). For example, some medications have additional effects that may be desirable in certain cases, such as weight loss in patients with obesity or sedation in patients with insomnia. Reduction in heart rate with β-blockers may be desired in a patient with anxiety but undesired in an athlete. While it is appealing to use a single medication to address multiple conditions, avoid compromising optimal disease management by choosing a less effective medication purely for this reason.

C. Chronic migraine, defined as 15 or more days with headache per month for 3 months or longer, is usually more difficult to treat than episodic migraine. Most standard prophylactic treatments for episodic migraine can also be tried in chronic migraine, but only botulinum toxin, topiramate, and calcitonin-gene-related peptide (CGRP) inhibitors have demonstrated efficacy in chronic migraine in randomized control trials. Route and frequency of administration of each of these treatments, as well as cost, play an important role in choosing therapy.

D. Neuromodulation has emerged as an alternative or complement to other established preventive treatments. Multiple neuromodulation therapies have been tested and may have a role in migraine prophylaxis, acute migraine treatment, or both (transcutaneous trigeminal nerve stimulation, noninvasive vagus nerve stimulation, minimally invasive sphenopalatine ganglion stimulation, subcutaneous occipital nerve stimulation). However, some of these devices are still undergoing clinical trials and/or are of uncertain long-term benefit in migraine prevention. Peripheral cranial nerve blockade and trigger point injections with lidocaine and/or bupivacaine are also used for migraine prophylaxis. The most common targets are the greater and lesser occipital nerves. The trigeminal branches (auriculotemporal, supraorbital, and supratrochlear nerves) can also be blocked.

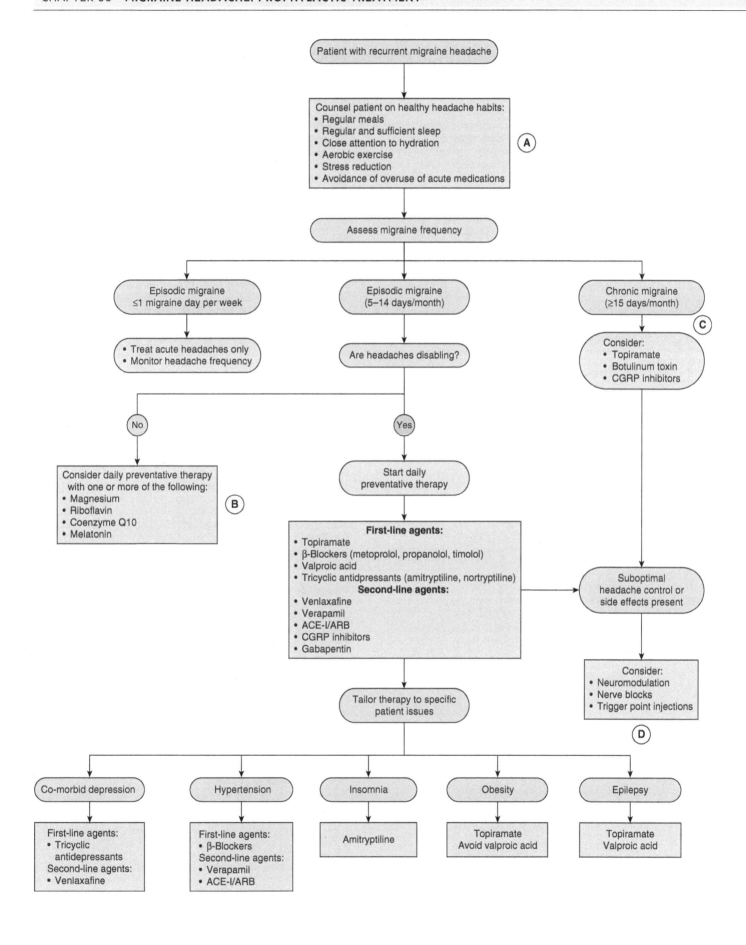

Trigeminal Autonomic Cephalalgias: Treatment

Adys Mendizabal and Ana Recober

Trigeminal autonomic cephalalgias (TACs) encompass a group of primary headache disorders characterized by unilateral headache with ipsilateral cranial autonomic symptoms such as conjunctival injection, lacrimation, nasal congestion, rhinorrhea, facial sweating, miosis, ptosis, and eyelid edema. A sense of restlessness or agitation is often associated with the pain.

A. In some cases, it may be difficult to differentiate between TACs, particularly when the duration or frequency of the attacks is not clear. Therefore, it is reasonable to consider a 3-week trial of indomethacin (Table 67.1) in patients with unilateral headache associated with ipsilateral cranial autonomic symptoms. Paroxysmal hemicrania and hemicrania continua are by definition prevented absolutely by therapeutic doses of indomethacin, in contrast to cluster headache and short-lasting unilateral neuralgiform headache attacks with conjunctival injection and tearing (SUNCT) or short-lasting unilateral neuralgiform headache attacks with cranial autonomic symptoms (SUNA).

TABLE 67.1 DOSING AND TITRATION OF MEDICATIONS FOR TRIGEMINAL AUTONOMIC CEPHALALGIAS

Drug	Starting dose	Titration	Maximum dose
Indomethacin	25 mg tid	Increase by 25 mg tid every 7 days (discontinue if not effective at maximum dose for 7 days)	225 mg daily
Sumatriptan	4–6 mg SC	Repeat dose if no response in 1 hour	12 mg in 24 hour
Zolmitriptan	5 mg intranasal	Repeat dose if no response in 1 hour	Two doses in 24 hour
Sumatriptan	20 mg intranasal	Repeat dose if no response in 1 hour	Two doses in 24 hour
Dihydroergotamine (DHE)	1 mg IM, SC or intranasal	Repeat dose if no response in 1 hour	3 mg in 24 hour
Intranasal lidocaine	4–10% 1 mL	Repeat once after 15 minutes	
Prednisone	60–80 mg	80 mg × 5 days, then decrease by 10 mg every 2 days	Two to three courses/year
Verapamil	80 mg tid (short-acting preferred)	Increase by 80 mg every 10–14 days	960 mg daily
Lithium carbonate	200 mg tid	May increase to 300 mg tid after 7 days	300 mg tid
Topiramate	25 mg qhs	Increase by 25 mg daily every 7 days	200 mg daily
Melatonin	5 mg qhs	Increase by 3–5 mg every week	20 mg daily
Lamotrigine	25 mg daily	Increase by 25 mg q2 week	200 mg bid
Gabapentin	100 mg tid	Increase by 100–300 mg every 4–5 days	1200 mg tid
Sodium valproate	250 mg daily	Increase by 250 mg every 7 days	2000 mg daily
Methylergonovine	0.2 mg tid		0.6 mg daily
Ergotamine	2 mg bid		

IM, Intramuscular; *SC*, subcutaneous.

B. Patients that do not respond to indomethacin or cannot tolerate it may try melatonin, typically needed at high doses (9–20 mg nightly), celecoxib, topiramate, verapamil, or gabapentin. These agents are usually selected based on comorbidities and patient preference. Greater occipital nerve blockade is an alternative to preventive oral drugs. The level of evidence supporting effectiveness for any of these second-line therapies is low. For greater occipital nerve blocks, a mixture of 2–4 mL of an anesthetic (2% lidocaine or 0.5% bupivacaine) and 80 mg of methylprednisolone is injected unilaterally or bilaterally 1–2 cm below the midpoint between the inion and mastoid process.

C. Lamotrigine may be useful for prevention of SUNCT or SUNA. Topiramate, gabapentin, intravenous lidocaine, and greater occipital nerve blockade can also be used for these typically refractory headache syndromes. Because the headache pain with these conditions is so brief, abortive therapy is not practical.

D. First-line abortive treatment for cluster headache is 100% oxygen inhaled via a nonrebreather face mask at a rate of 7–15 L/min for 15–20 min in the sitting position. Injectable and intranasal triptans are alternative abortive treatments for cluster attacks. Dihydroergotamine (DHE) given intranasally (IN), subcutaneously (SC), or intramuscularly (IM) can be used as an alternative to triptans if these are not effective or tolerated. Triptans and DHE are contraindicated in patients with coronary artery disease or stroke due to concerns about vasoconstriction.

E. Transitional therapy is often needed while waiting for long-term cluster headache preventive treatments to begin to work, which typically takes several weeks. Prednisone 60–80 mg daily for 5 days followed by a 14-day taper is a common strategy. Other options include greater occipital nerve blockade, DHE 1 mg SC, IM, or IN daily for 1 week, or ergotamine 2 mg PO twice daily for 1 week.

F. Verapamil is the preferred preventive drug for cluster headache. Lithium is considered a second-line agent due to potential toxicity (renal, thyroid, and liver) and a narrow therapeutic window (target level of 0.4–0.8 mEq/L). Melatonin, topiramate, sodium valproate, gabapentin, or methylergonovine can be used based on patient preference and comorbidities. Calcitonin-gene-related peptide (CGRP) monoclonal antibodies are being investigated for preventive treatment of cluster. Neuromodulation can be used for acute and/or preventive treatment (noninvasive vagal nerve stimulation, sphenopalatine ganglion stimulation, and occipital nerve stimulation). Deep brain hypothalamic stimulation is not recommended. Invasive destructive surgical procedures (radiofrequency ablation of the trigeminal ganglion, trigeminal rhizotomy, gamma knife surgery, and microvascular trigeminal nerve decompression) are reserved as a last-resort therapy for refractory cases.

REFERENCES

1. International Headache Society. *Trigeminal Autonomic Cephalalgias. IHS Classification ICHD-3.* 2018. Available at https://www.ichd-3.org/3-trigeminal-autonomic-cephalalgias/. Accessed May 10, 2018.
2. Robbins MS, Starling AJ, Pringsheim TM, Becker WJ, Schwedt TJ. Treatment of cluster headache: the American Headache Society Evidence-Based Guidelines. *Headache.* 2016;56(7):1093–1106.

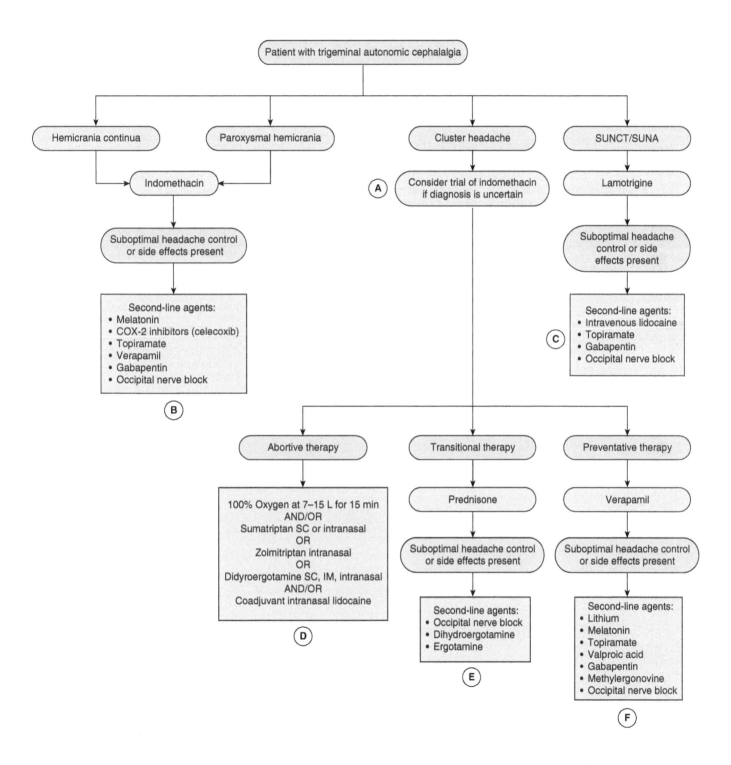

Trigeminal Neuralgia

Adys Mendizabal and Ana Recober

Trigeminal neuralgia, also known as tic douloreux, manifests as recurrent attacks of abrupt, unilateral, severe stabbing (or electric-like) pain in the distribution of the trigeminal nerve. Typically, the mandibular or maxillary region is involved, with the ophthalmic region only rarely affected. Pain persists for seconds to 2 minutes, then resolves. Episodes may recur multiple times per day. Symptoms are often triggered by chewing, brushing teeth, touching the face, or eating or drinking. Detailed neurological examination should demonstrate no abnormalities, specifically including no sensory loss in the distribution of the trigeminal nerve between attacks, and normal trigeminal nerve motor function (e.g., muscles of mastication). If abnormalities are present on examination, an alternative diagnosis should be considered. Trigeminal neuralgia may be idiopathic or due to a compressive or demyelinating lesion; brain magnetic resonance imaging with contrast can be performed to exclude secondary causes. Symptomatic treatment is generally similar regardless of the presence of an underlying identifiable cause.

A. The mainstay of treatment is carbamazepine, which is effective at controlling pain in about 75% of patients. A low dose should be started, with upward titration until good symptomatic relief is achieved. Oxcarbazepine is an alternative, and appears to have similar efficacy.

B. Other agents that can be used in addition to or instead of carbamazepine include gabapentin, baclofen, and lamotrigine, though evidence for efficacy of these drugs is weaker.

C. For refractory cases unresponsive to medical therapy or in cases where medications result in severe side effects, surgical procedures can be considered to relieve pain. These include microvascular decompression, percutaneous rhizotomy, and stereotactic radiosurgery (gamma knife radiosurgery). Of these, microvascular decompression is the only one that is not an intentionally destructive procedure. Through an incision behind the ear, the surgeon explores the cerebellopontine angle to identify sites of physical compression of the trigeminal nerve, typically caused by an adjacent vessel, and relieves the compression. Microvascular decompression appears to produce the most durable response of the surgical procedures for trigeminal neuralgia, but is also the most invasive procedure. Percutaneous rhizotomy is an intentionally destructive procedure with direct injury (heat, chemical, or mechanical) targeted to the trigeminal nerve via a needle placed through the face into the gasserian ganglion. Pain relief is often accompanied by numbness, but it produces near immediate results. It is recommended for patients who are deemed poor surgical candidates or who experience recurrent pain despite microvascular decompression. Stereotactic radiosurgery is also a destructive procedure; in this case utilizing high doses of focused radiation to damage the trigeminal nerve root. It is the least invasive procedure, but pain relief takes weeks to months to fully develop.

REFERENCES

1. Bick SKB, Eskandar EN. Surgical treatment of trigeminal neuralgia. *Neurosurg Clin N Am.* 2017;28:429–438.
2. Gronseth G, Cruccu G, Alksne J, et al. Practice Parameter: the diagnostic evaluation and treatment of trigeminal neuralgia (an evidence-based review): report of the Quality Standards Subcommittee of the American Academy of Neurology and the European Federation of Neurological Societies. *Neurology.* 2008;71:1183–1190.

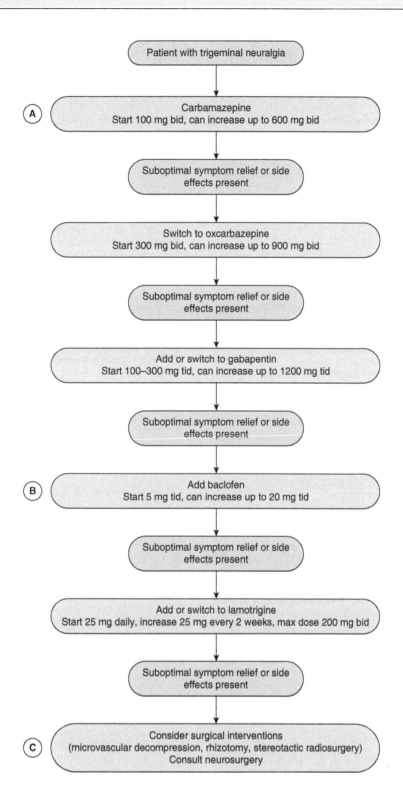

Intracranial Hypotension

Whitley Aamodt and Raymond S. Price

Intracranial hypotension, or low cerebrospinal fluid (CSF) pressure, should be suspected in a patient with a positional headache that worsens within 15 minutes of standing and improves with recumbency. The positional component of the headache may become less prominent or absent over time if the intracranial hypotension is untreated. Patients can also experience nonspecific symptoms such as dizziness, photophobia, blurred vision, nausea, vomiting, and neck pain and stiffness. Uncommonly, spinal manifestations of intracranial hypotension may appear, including radiculopathies, myelopathy secondary to compression by an extradural fluid collection or enlarged venous plexus, or bibrachial amyotrophy from a ventral extradural fluid collection. Some patients with intracranial hypotension have nonpositional headaches or present without headache. In these patients, intracranial hypotension is suggested by findings on magnetic resonance imaging (MRI). Classic MRI findings in intracranial hypotension include diffuse dural enhancement, subdural fluid collections, pituitary enlargement, brainstem sagging (such as descent of the mammillary bodies and narrowing of the interpeduncular fossa), and tonsillar descent through the foramen magnum (pseudo-Chiari malformation). The presence of any of these findings on brain MRI should raise the possibility of intracranial hypotension; no one finding is consistently present in all cases. Diffuse dural enhancement is the most common MRI finding, but this may disappear with prolonged intracranial hypotension.

A. Intracranial hypotension is a common complication of lumbar puncture (LP) and can also complicate more invasive procedures that disrupt the dura, such as the administration of spinal anesthesia or spinal or sinus surgery. In cases of iatrogenic intracranial hypotension, further brain imaging is not necessarily required depending on the context.

B. Intracranial hypotension can occur spontaneously secondary to a dural tear or fistula between the cerebrospinal fluid and the venous system. In a patient with clinical symptoms, an MRI brain with gadolinium is the preferred imaging modality to confirm the diagnosis. However, this can be normal in up to 20% of patients with low CSF pressure. If there remains high clinical suspicion, an LP can be performed to assess the opening pressure taking care not to exacerbate symptoms. Low CSF pressure is defined as less than 6 cm H_2O; note that opening pressure must be measured in the lateral decubitus position. A normal opening pressure does not exclude a diagnosis of intracranial hypotension.

C. Regardless of etiology, mild to moderate symptoms associated with intracranial hypotension should be treated with conservative measures that aim to restore CSF volume, including strict bed rest, oral or intravenous hydration, and high-dose caffeine intake.

D. If symptoms persist despite conservative management, a blind epidural blood patch should be performed. An epidural blood patch involves the injection of 5–10 cc of autologous blood into the epidural space. While an epidural blood patch can result in immediate clinical improvement, up to 50% of patients require more than one.

E. If symptoms persist despite epidural blood patches, spinal imaging should be performed to attempt to identify the site of CSF leakage. Common findings on MRI spine with gadolinium include an extradural fluid collection or engorgement of the epidural veins.

F. If MRI spine is normal or nondiagnostic, computed tomography (CT) or MR myelogram or radioisotope cisternography should be pursued. CT and MR myelogram are preferred as they provide better spatial resolution.

G. If the site of CSF leakage is known, a targeted epidural blood patch or epidural patching with fibrin glue may be performed at the corresponding level. If nonsurgical therapies are unsuccessful, surgical repair can be considered, which involves the placement of sutures or metallic clips around dural tears or leaking meningeal diverticula.

REFERENCE

1. Schievink WI. Spontaneous spinal cerebrospinal fluid leaks and intracranial hypotension. *JAMA.* 2006;295(19):2286–2296.

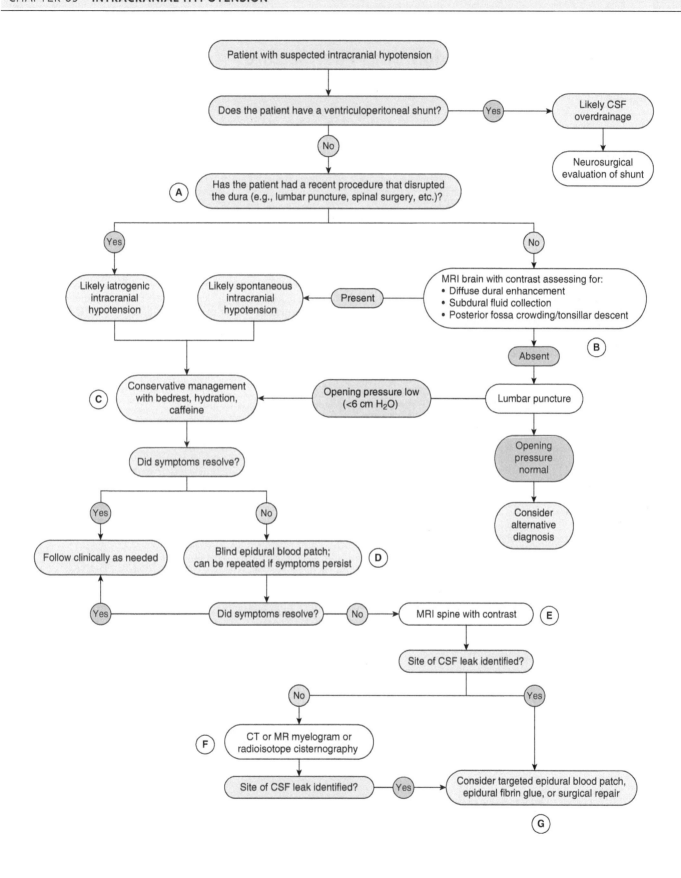

Evaluation of Adult With First Seizure

Michael Gelfand

Evaluation of the patient with a first seizure is focused on determining (1) the risk of recurrence and whether antiepileptic drug (AED) therapy is warranted to reduce this risk, and (2) whether there is sufficient concern for an underlying cause to warrant further specific diagnostic testing. About 8%–10% of the population will experience a seizure in their lifetime. On average, patients with a single seizure have a risk of recurrence of 32% in the first year, reaching 46% over 5 years. This risk is substantially lower in patients with provoked seizures (e.g., following acute infection or metabolic derangement) and substantially higher in patients with structural brain injury or an abnormal electroencephalogram (EEG). Further, if there have been two unprovoked seizures occurring on different days (meeting the criteria for a diagnosis of epilepsy), the chance of recurrent seizures is at least 60%. In general, those with a risk of seizure recurrence of 60% of greater should be treated with an AED.

A. Patients should be asked about prior known seizures and about possible previously unidentified subtle seizure activity, such as auras, that may immediately suggest a diagnosis of epilepsy. If prior seizures are confirmed or seem likely, an AED should be started, and magnetic resonance imaging (MRI) of the brain with contrast to identify structural lesions that might serve as a seizure focus and EEG should be done. The latter is important for estimating risk of recurrence, but also to help determine whether generalized or focal epilepsy is present, which affects AED choice.

B. If there is an identified reversible provoking factor, the risk of seizure recurrence is likely to be substantially lower than otherwise, and AED therapy is generally not indicated. Brain imaging and EEG can be considered in select cases to help better estimate this risk, but are not uniformly necessary.

C. Nocturnal seizure (occurring from sleep), history of prior brain injury including stroke, severe traumatic brain injury, or central nervous system infection, and neurologic examination findings consistent with focal cortical injury (e.g., as seen in cerebral palsy or prior stroke) are all associated with an increased risk of seizure recurrence. Epileptiform activity is seen on EEG in approximately 30% of patients with epilepsy and approximately doubles the chance of seizure recurrence. Note that a normal EEG does *not* exclude the diagnosis of epilepsy. Brain MRI has a higher yield than computed tomography (CT) and should be obtained, most often as an outpatient. A structural abnormality felt to constitute a seizure focus is found in ~10% of patients with an unprovoked first seizure, and increases recurrence risk by ~2.5-fold. Other testing, such as toxicology screen, and analysis of electrolytes and cerebrospinal fluid may be useful in the appropriate setting, although these are not universally needed. In cases where the diagnosis of seizure is uncertain, an elevated lactic acid level and anion gap may help to distinguish seizures from syncopal or psychogenic events, but has not been shown to predict the chance of seizure recurrence.

D. Patients with an increased risk of recurrence are typically treated with an AED. However, the decision to treat or not should be based on an individual assessment. Patients with a prolonged aura, or without loss of consciousness, may opt not to treat even in the setting of a high probability of recurrence; other patients may have experienced multiple events of uncertain etiology, where seizure is not clearly proven, and may prefer to confirm the diagnosis prior to treatment. Conversely, patients with high-stress jobs, a need to resume driving as soon as possible, or whose single seizure episode included a cluster of generalized convulsions may opt to treat even in the absence of a clear epilepsy diagnosis.

E. The benefits of starting AED treatment presumptively after a first seizure in a potentially lower-risk patient include decreasing the chance of recurrence within the first two years by ~35%, possible earlier return of driving privileges, possible decreased severity of future seizures, and peace of mind. However, early AED treatment, as compared to waiting, does not affect quality of life, and is *not* believed to affect the long-term prognosis for seizure recurrence. Any benefits should be weighed against medication side effects, pregnancy concerns, convenience, and cost. In general, AED therapy is not started in this scenario.

REFERENCES

1. Krumholz A, Wiebe S, Gronseth G, et al. Practice parameter: evaluating an apparent unprovoked first seizure in adults (an evidence-based review)—Report of the Quality Standards Subcommittee of the American Academy of Neurology and the American Epilepsy Society. *Neurology.* 2007;69 (21):1996–2007.
2. Krumholz A, Wiebe S, Gronseth GS, et al. Evidence-based guideline: management of an unprovoked first seizure in adults: Report of the Guideline Development Subcommittee of the American Academy of Neurology and the American Epilepsy Society. *Neurology.* 2015;84:1705–1713.

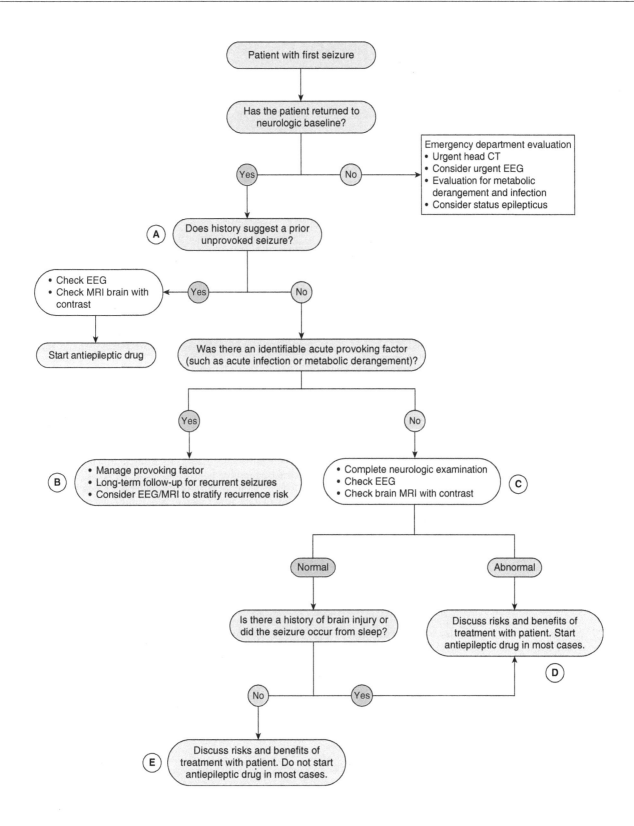

Initial Treatment of Epilepsy

Michael Gelfand

A. When choosing initial antiepileptic drug (AED) therapy for a patient with epilepsy, assess whether the suspected diagnosis is a focal or generalized epilepsy. In focal epilepsies, there is felt to be a discrete seizure focus within a local network, typically in a single hemisphere. Progression to a bilateral tonic-clonic seizure may ensue. The majority of AEDs are effective for focal epilepsy. In contrast, generalized epilepsies are characterized by seizures that rapidly engage diffuse bilateral networks; in addition to generalized-onset tonic-clonic seizures, common examples include absence and generalized myoclonic seizures. A smaller group of AEDs are considered effective for generalized epilepsy, and some commonly used drugs, such as carbamazepine, oxcarbazepine, and gabapentin, may actually worsen the condition. These drugs should be avoided in generalized epilepsy or in cases where the diagnosis is uncertain. In some situations, there may be a need for an AED to treat another condition in addition to epilepsy. Common examples include comorbid migraine headaches or neuropathic pain. This should be considered when choosing initial therapy (see Chapter 73).

B. In generalized epilepsies, commonly used drugs including levetiracetam, lamotrigine, valproate, zonisamide, and topiramate. Clobazam and perampanel are also reasonable choices, and ethosuximide is appropriate if absence seizures are the only seizure type (not shown). Of these, levetiracetam is frequently chosen first due to its rapid titration, absence of drug interactions, and excellent safety profile. However, it does have the potential to worsen mood or cause irritability. In fact, most so-called "broad spectrum" AEDs appropriate for generalized epilepsy have frequent adverse psychiatric effects, the main exceptions being lamotrigine and valproate. Lamotrigine is very well tolerated but requires a several-week titration and is often ineffective against myoclonus, and is therefore a poor choice if rapid seizure control is needed or if myoclonus is common. Initial treatment with levetiracetam with early consideration of transition to lamotrigine is a reasonable approach in the common situation where mood is a concern *and* rapid treatment is needed. Valproic acid has adverse effects including weight gain, hair loss, tremor, and decreased bone density, but is considered the most effective drug for generalized epilepsy. However, it must be avoided if pregnancy is a possibility, as it has a high risk of teratogenesis (Table 71.1).

C. Commonly used drugs in focal epilepsies include levetiracetam, lamotrigine, carbamazepine, and oxcarbazepine. Zonisamide, topiramate, lacosamide, and several others are also reasonable choices. Levetiracetam is again the most commonly chosen initial agent, particularly if rapid seizure control is needed and mood is not an immediate concern. Lamotrigine is an excellent alternative in outpatients who do not require rapid seizure control, particularly in young female patients or in patients with known mood disorder. In the common situation where rapid seizure control is needed—typically frequent tonic-clonic seizures—and where levetiracetam is either poorly tolerated or not appropriate due to known severe mood disorder, oxcarbazepine is an appropriate initial therapy, with carbamazepine and lacosamide as reasonable alternatives.

Drug	Starting dose	Titration	Usual maintenance dose
Lamotrigine	25 mg daily[a]	To 100 mg twice daily over 6+ week titration[a]	100–200 mg twice daily,[a] adjusted to clinical response
Levetiracetam	500 mg twice daily	By 500 mg/day each week if needed	500–1500 mg twice daily, adjusted to clinical response
Oxcarbazepine	300 mg twice daily	By 300 mg/day each week if needed	300–1200 twice daily, adjusted to clinical response
Valproic acid (extended release formulation)	500–1000 mg daily at bedtime, or 250–500 mg twice daily	By 500 mg/day each week if needed	500–1000 mg twice daily, adjusted to level and clinical response

TABLE 71.1 **ANTIEPILEPTIC DRUGS COMMONLY USED AS INITIAL THERAPY**

[a]Lamotrigine starting dose, titration and maintenance dose should all be slowed (approximately halved) in the presence of valproic acid due to inhibition of lamotrigine metabolism.

D. If the initial drug fails to control seizures, a second agent should be tried. The second agent can either replace the first or be added for combination therapy. A reasonable approach is to initiate combination therapy with a plan to later withdraw the initial failed drug if the second drug is effective. Ideally, the chosen second agent should have a different mechanism of action than the first. For example, with focal epilepsy, one AED may be a sodium-channel blocking drug, e.g., lamotrigine, oxcarbazepine, carbamazepine, or lacosamide, and the second chosen from a different class, such as levetiracetam, zonisamide, or topiramate. For generalized epilepsy, the combination of lamotrigine and valproate may be more effective than other combinations and should be considered if monotherapy fails.

E. If seizures persist after trials of two appropriate AEDs (either separately or in combination) at therapeutic doses, the possibility of either misdiagnosis or of drug-resistant epilepsy should be considered. Referral for video electroencephalogram monitoring in an epilepsy monitoring unit is generally indicated in this scenario with the aims of (1) confirming the diagnosis of epilepsy rather than syncope or psychogenic events, (2) classifying epilepsy as focal or generalized, and (3) evaluating surgical options.

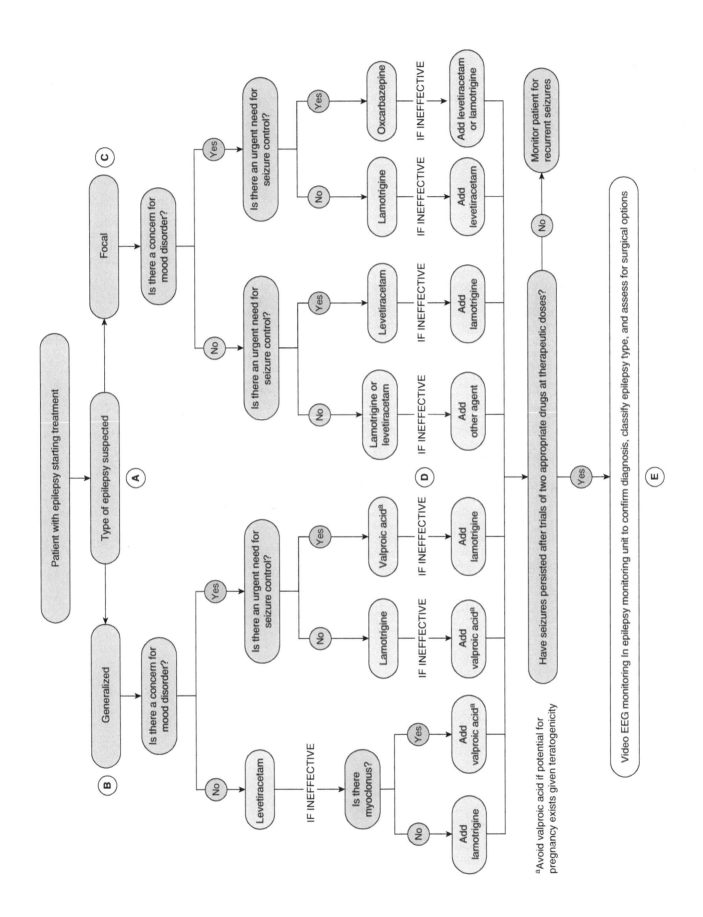

Drug-Resistant Epilepsy

Susanna O'Kula and Michael Gelfand

Most patients with epilepsy achieve seizure control with medications. However, about 30% of patients have drug-resistant epilepsy. Drug-resistant epilepsy, often known as medically intractable epilepsy, is defined as continued seizures despite adequate trials of two tolerated, appropriately chosen and dosed antiepileptic drugs (either as monotherapy or in combination). Early referral to an epilepsy center is recommended, as patients with drug-resistant epilepsy have higher rates of disability, injuries, and even death compared to those with well-controlled epilepsy.

A. Prior to categorizing epilepsy as drug-resistant, so-called "pseudo-resistance" should be excluded. This requires ensuring that (1) epilepsy is the correct diagnosis (ruling out syncope, sleep disorders, cardiac arrhythmias, and psychogenic nonepileptic seizures), (2) the selected antiepileptic medication is appropriate to the epilepsy type (generalized versus focal) and given at an adequate dose, and (3) poor or variable adherence to medication or provoking factors such as substance abuse are not thought to be the primary cause of continued seizures. Of note, intolerable side effects from an antiepileptic medication do not necessarily represent failure of efficacy, so more than two agents may need to be tried if the initial agents are limited by tolerability.

B. Patients with an identifiable seizure focus are potential candidates for resective surgery, which is more likely than continued medical therapy to lead to seizure freedom. Seizure remission rates are highest in cases when the lesion seen on magnetic resonance imaging (MRI) correlates with the anatomic focus identified on electroencephalogram (EEG). Counseling about the risk of sudden unexpected death in epilepsy (SUDEP), surgical risks, medication side effects, and cognitive and psychiatric morbidity associated with either surgical treatment or with continued uncontrolled seizures should be provided to the patient. The initial evaluation typically includes at least video EEG, high-resolution brain MRI, neuropsychological testing, and positron emission tomography (PET) scan. More extensive testing with ictal single photon emission computed tomography (SPECT), magnetoencephalography (MEG), functional MRI (fMRI), or other advanced imaging may be necessary as well.

C. If the epileptogenic zone (the optimal target for surgical resection to achieve seizure freedom) remains undefined after initial evaluation, more invasive monitoring can be considered. Intracranial EEG with electrode grids, strips, or stereotactically placed depth electrodes can aid in localization to identify the seizure focus in many cases. Intracranial EEG can also help to evaluate the proximity of seizure foci to "eloquent" cortex, to limit the risk of postoperative neurologic deficits.

D. If potentially curative resection or ablation are not considered good options due to inability to identify a single resectable focus or concern that resection would lead to unacceptable neurologic deficits, palliative options should be considered. Palliative surgery with incomplete resection of the epileptogenic zone may still provide significant benefit by decreasing the frequency or severity of seizures. Implanted devices including vagus nerve stimulation (VNS), responsive neurostimulation (RNS), and deep brain stimulation (DBS) to the anterior nucleus of the thalamus are generally not curative but do decrease seizure frequency, and may provide additional benefits in terms of mood or cognition.

E. For patients with drug-resistant generalized, or mixed, epilepsies, VNS, DBS, and a ketogenic diet, or other dietary therapy, may provide benefit. Corpus callostomy can prevent seizures starting in one hemisphere from spreading bilaterally and can thereby help prevent drop attacks such as those seen in Lennox-Gastaut syndrome.

REFERENCES

1. Kwan P, Arzimanoglou A, Berg AT, et al. Definition of drug resistant epilepsy: consensus proposal by the ad hoc Task Force of the ILAE Commission on Therapeutic Strategies. *Epilepsia.* 2010;51(6):1069–1077. https://doi.org/10.1111/j.1528-1167.2009.02397.x.
2. Nair DR. Management of drug-resistant epilepsy. *Continuum (Minneap Min).* 2016;22(1):157–172.

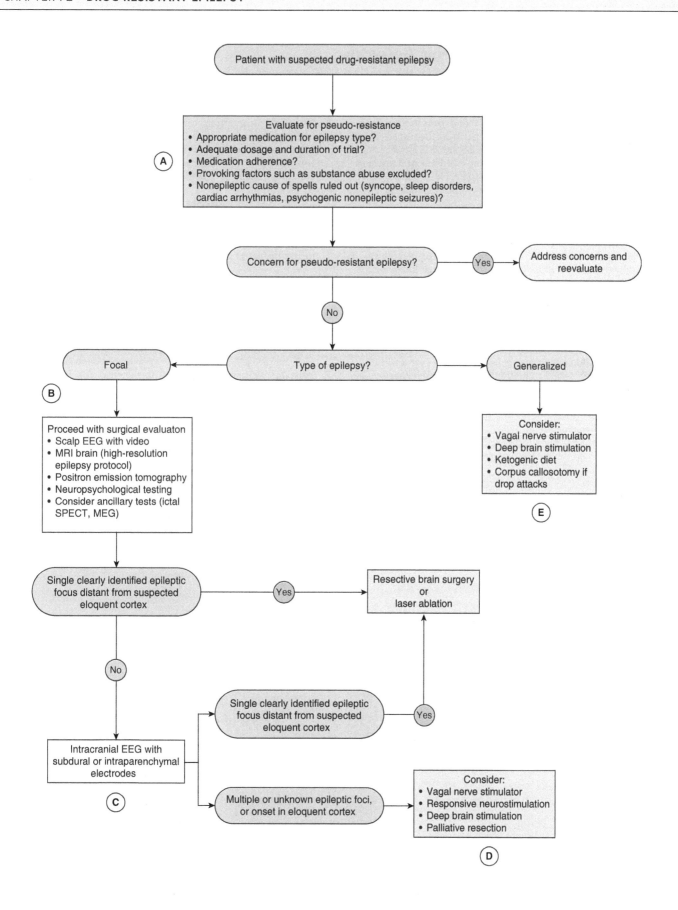

73 | Antiepileptic Drug Selection

Pouya Khankhanian and Michael Gelfand

In most cases, initial antiepileptic drug (AED) therapy is selected from a relatively short list of AEDs determined primarily by the suspected epilepsy syndrome, as previously described in Chapter 71. However, there are numerous alternative AEDs, and in many cases it is useful to consider individual patient features, such as demographics, medical comorbidities, and concomitant medications, when choosing therapy.

A. Many antiepileptic medications carry a risk of birth defects in pregnancy, but in most cases uncontrolled seizures carry a greater risk to the child. The teratogenic risk varies by drug, with lamotrigine felt to be the lowest risk and valproic acid the highest. When planning for a future pregnancy, transitioning to a lower-risk drug should be considered, and transition away from valproic acid in particular is usually advised. Caution should be exercised in switching drugs once pregnancy has occurred, however, due to the risk of breakthrough seizures.

B. Untreated patients with frequent tonic-clonic or disabling seizures require rapid treatment and are not good candidates for medications that require a long period of uptitration, most notably lamotrigine, but also topiramate and zonisamide.

C. Patients of Asian, South-Asian, and Indian descent who carry the HLA-B*15:02 genotype are at higher risk of Stevens-Johnson syndrome with carbamazepine, oxcarbazepine, and phenytoin. These medications should be avoided if genotype testing is positive or unknown.

D. There is evidence for a synergistic effect between valproic acid and lamotrigine in the syndrome of juvenile myoclonic epilepsy. Slow titration and frequent monitoring are recommended, as valproic acid will raise the serum level of lamotrigine.

E. Gabapentin, pregabalin, carbamazepine, and oxcarbazepine can be used to treat neuropathic pain. Topiramate, zonisamide, and valproic acid can be used to treat migraine. Lamotrigine may help with neuropathic pain, and for some patients may help with migraine, but a common side effect of lamotrigine is headache.

F. Lamotrigine, oxcarbazepine, valproic acid, and carbamazepine have varying degrees of mood-stabilizing effects. Levetiracetam can cause significant irritability, which may be improved with treatment with pyridoxine. Perampanel is also associated with significant adverse neuropsychiatric effects.

G. Elderly patients are at higher risk of side effects, particularly those related to cognition and balance. Medications are often started at lower doses in elderly patients. For elderly patients with no other significant medical comorbidity, lamotrigine, and levetiracetam are commonly used first-line agents. Lacosamide, zonisamide, and gabapentin are also considered well tolerated in this population.

H. Most medications may be used in patients with hepatic disease, although many require dosage adjustment and some agents are potentially hepatotoxic. In patients with mild renal disease, many agents can be used with appropriate dosage adjustment. Patients on hemodialysis often require more complex drug regimens with additional doses given immediately after dialysis.

I. In a patient on oral contraceptives, warfarin, or with a malignancy requiring chemotherapy or a chronic infection requiring long-term antimicrobials (e.g., human immunodeficiency virus, hepatitis B virus, or hepatitis C virus), consider the impact of drug interactions. These interactions may make contraception, chemotherapy, or antimicrobial therapy ineffective, or lead to subtherapeutic or dangerously supratherapeutic anticoagulant levels in the case of warfarin.

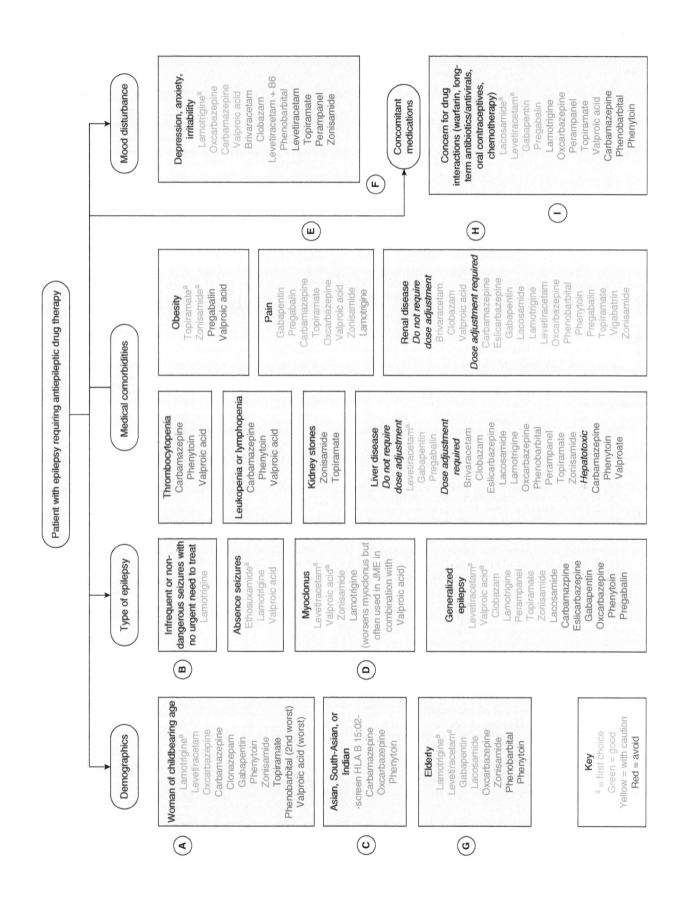

Patient with epilepsy requiring antiepileptic drug therapy

Demographics

A Woman of childbearing age
Lamotrigine[a]
Levetiracetam
Oxcarbazepine
Carbamazepine
Clonazepam
Gabapentin
Phenytoin
Zonisamide
Topiramate
Phenobarbital (2nd worst)
Valproic acid (worst)

C Asian, South-Asian, or Indian
-screen HLA B 15:02-
Carbamazepine
Oxcarbazepine
Phenytoin

G Elderly
Lamotrigine[a]
Levetiracetam[a]
Gabapentin
Lacosamide
Oxcarbazepine
Zonisamide
Phenobarbital
Phenytoin

Type of epilepsy

B Infrequent or non-dangerous seizures with no urgent need to treat
Lamotrigine

Absence seizures
Ethosuximide[a]
Lamotrigine
Valproic acid

Myoclonus
Levetiracetam[a]
Valproic acid[a]
Zonisamide
Lamotrigine
D (worsens myoclonus but often used in JME in combination with Valproic acid)

Generalized epilepsy
Levetiracetam[a]
Valproic acid[a]
Clobazam
Lamotrigine
Perampanel
Topiramate
Zonisamide
Lacosamide
Carbamazpine
Eslicarbazepine
Gabapentin
Oxcarbazepine
Phenytoin
Pregabalin

Medical comorbidities

Thrombocytopenia
Carbamazepine
Phenytoin
Valproic acid

Leukopenia or lymphopenia
Carbamazepine
Phenytoin
Valproic acid

Kidney stones
Zonisamide
Topiramate

Liver disease
Do not require dose adjustment
Levetiracetam[a]
Gabapentin
Pregabalin
Dose adjustment required
Brivaracetam
Clobazam
Eslicarbazepine
Lacosamide
Lamotrigine
Oxcarbazepine
Phenobarbital
Perampanel
Topiramate
Zonisamide
Hepatotoxic
Carbamazepine
Phenytoin
Valproate

Obesity
Topiramate[a]
Zonisamide[a]
Pregabalin
Valproic acid

Pain
Gabapentin
Pregabalin
Carbamazepine
Topiramate
Oxcarbazepine
Valproic acid
Zonisamide
Lamotrigine

H Renal disease
Do not require dose adjustment
Brivaracetam
Clobazam
Valproic acid
Dose adjustment required
Carbamazepine
Eslicarbazepine
Gabapentin
Lacosamide
Lamotrigine
Levetiracetam
Oxcarbazepine
Phenobarbital
Phenytoin
Pregabalin
Topiramate
Vigabatrin
Zonisamide

Mood disturbance

Depression, anxiety, irritability
Lamotrigine[a]
Oxcarbazepine
Carbamazepine
Valproic acid
Brivaracetam
Clobazam
Levetiracetam + B6
Phenobarbital
Levetiracetam
Topiramate
Perampanel
Zonisamide

E

F Concomitant medications

I Concern for drug interactions (warfarin, long-term antibiotics/antivirals, oral contraceptives, chemotherapy)
Lacosamide[a]
Levetiracetam[a]
Gabapentin
Pregabalin
Lamotrigine
Oxcarbazepine
Perampanel
Topiramate
Valproic acid
Carbamazepine
Phenobarbital
Phenytoin

Key
[a] = first choice
Green = good
Yellow = with caution
Red = avoid

74 Status Epilepticus

Angelica Maria Lee and Michael Gelfand

Status epilepticus (SE) can be categorized into convulsive and nonconvulsive status epilepticus (NCSE). Generalized convulsive status epilepticus is the most commonly encountered form of status epilepticus and is defined as: (1) clinical seizure activity lasting 5 minutes or longer; or (2) two or more seizures without full recovery of consciousness between them. NCSE is a persistent change in the level of consciousness or behavior associated with ongoing seizures on electroencephalogram (EEG), without convulsive activity. NCSE should be considered in patients who present after a prolonged generalized tonic-clonic seizure but do not return to baseline, and in patients who present with persistent confusion, abnormal behavior, or unexplained coma. It is often overlooked given the lack of motor manifestations. SE is a neurologic emergency associated with high morbidity and mortality, and urgent treatment is necessary. The prognosis depends both on the etiology and the duration of seizure activity. In some cases, treatment of the underlying cause of SE (e.g., autoimmune or infectious encephalitis, metabolic derangement) may be necessary to achieve successful seizure control.

A. The first phase of treatment comprises ensuring the airway is protected, ventilation is adequate, and the patient is hemodynamically stable. Immediate intubation is not always necessary, and use of paralytic drugs to assist intubation will confound the assessment of ongoing convulsive activity. The time of seizure onset should be determined in order to gauge the duration of SE, which impacts the decision of when to escalate therapy. Electrolytes and glucose should be assessed, and antiepileptic drug levels checked if the patient was taking these previously.

B. A benzodiazepine should be given as soon as possible; standard choices include either intravenous (IV) lorazepam if IV access is available or intramuscular (IM) midazolam otherwise. Adequate dosing (e.g., 4 mg of lorazepam or 10 mg of midazolam) is critical. This should be repeated after 5 minutes if seizures continue. In the prehospital setting where an IV line is not in place, midazolam IM has been demonstrated to be more efficacious than IV lorazepam because of speed and ease of administration. The patient's need for airway protection should be continually reassessed during treatment.

C. If the patient fails to respond to initial therapy, second-line therapy with an IV antiepileptic medication such as levetiracetam should be started. Valproic acid and phenytoin (or fosphenytoin) may be considered as alternatives; however, levetiracetam has a better side effect profile and fewer drug interactions. Levetiracetam is renally excreted, and dosing should be adjusted in patients with renal disease. IV phenytoin should be used with caution given the risk of infusion site reactions (purple glove syndrome) and cardiac arrhythmias, particularly with rapid infusion. These risks are reduced with fosphenytoin. If seizures abate, the antiepileptic drug given should be continued as maintenance therapy pending further evaluation. Noncontrast head computed tomography should be completed as soon as safe, particularly in patients without a well-established epilepsy diagnosis.

D. If convulsive seizures continue despite second-line therapy for a total duration of >30 minutes, midazolam should be started, typically given as a bolus followed by continuous infusion titrated to achieve cessation of seizure activity. Alternatives to midazolam include propofol and pentobarbital. The effectiveness of midazolam is reduced with prolonged use (>24 hours) and may require an increase in dosing. If not already performed, intubation is mandatory at this stage. Continuous EEG monitoring for subtle or subclinical continued seizures should be initiated if possible.

E. In the setting of NCSE, the benefit of midazolam or other anesthetic agents to control seizures must be weighed against the nontrivial risks of these therapies. The type and manifestations of NCSE should be considered. Patients with NCSE persisting after resolution of convulsive SE or those in coma should be treated more aggressively.

F. If refractory seizures continue, an infusion of propofol or pentobarbital can be considered. Continuous EEG monitoring should be considered mandatory at this stage and, if not available, transfer to facility capable of providing this should be considered. Propofol has a short half-life, but may lower blood pressure and, if used for more than 48 hours, can be associated with propofol infusion syndrome (rhabdomyolysis, congestive heart failure, lactic acidosis, and hypertriglyceridemia). Pentobarbital is typically used when a patient is weaned off another third-line agent, such as midazolam or propofol, after 24 to 48 hours. Pentobarbital has a long half-life and takes several hours to reach a therapeutic level. It is very effective at achieving a burst-suppression pattern on EEG, but it is associated with high morbidity because of the prolonged duration of pentobarbital-associated comas.

REFERENCE

1. Glauser T, Shinnar S, Gloss D, et al. Evidence-Based Guideline: Treatment of Convulsive Status Epilepticus in Children and Adults: Report of the Guideline Committee of the American Epilepsy Society. *Epilepsy Curr.* 16(1):48-61.

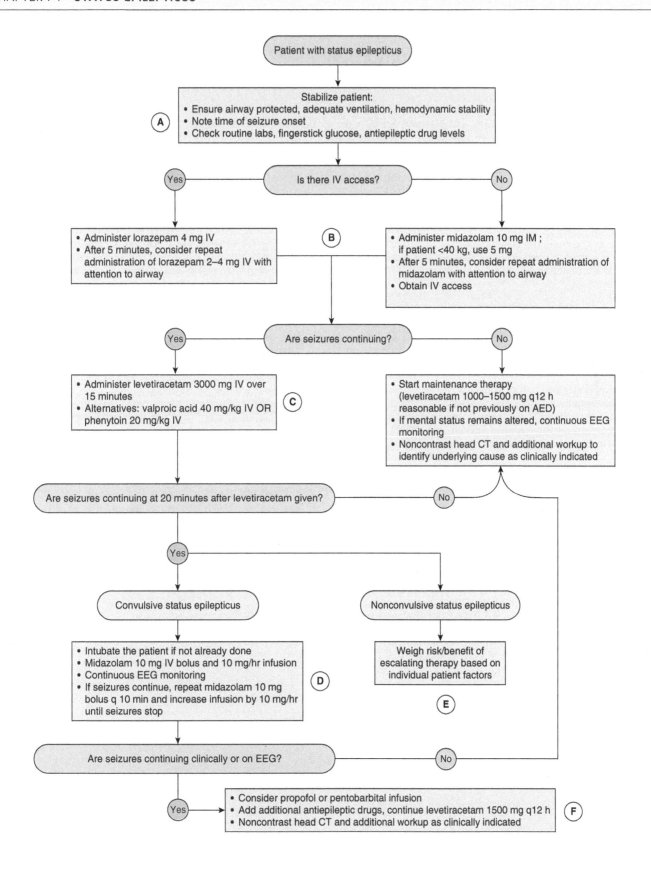

Patient with status epilepticus

(A) Stabilize patient:
- Ensure airway protected, adequate ventilation, hemodynamic stability
- Note time of seizure onset
- Check routine labs, fingerstick glucose, antiepileptic drug levels

Is there IV access?

Yes
- Administer lorazepam 4 mg IV
- After 5 minutes, consider repeat administration of lorazepam 2–4 mg IV with attention to airway

No
- Administer midazolam 10 mg IM ; if patient <40 kg, use 5 mg
- After 5 minutes, consider repeat administration of midazolam with attention to airway
- Obtain IV access

(B) Are seizures continuing?

Yes
(C)
- Administer levetiracetam 3000 mg IV over 15 minutes
- Alternatives: valproic acid 40 mg/kg IV OR phenytoin 20 mg/kg IV

No
- Start maintenance therapy (levetiracetam 1000–1500 mg q12 h reasonable if not previously on AED)
- If mental status remains altered, continuous EEG monitoring
- Noncontrast head CT and additional workup to identify underlying cause as clinically indicated

Are seizures continuing at 20 minutes after levetiracetam given?

No

Yes

Convulsive status epilepticus

Nonconvulsive status epilepticus

(D)
- Intubate the patient if not already done
- Midazolam 10 mg IV bolus and 10 mg/hr infusion
- Continuous EEG monitoring
- If seizures continue, repeat midazolam 10 mg bolus q 10 min and increase infusion by 10 mg/hr until seizures stop

(E) Weigh risk/benefit of escalating therapy based on individual patient factors

Are seizures continuing clinically or on EEG?

No

Yes
(F)
- Consider propofol or pentobarbital infusion
- Add additional antiepileptic drugs, continue levetiracetam 1500 mg q12 h
- Noncontrast head CT and additional workup as clinically indicated

Management of Comorbidities in Patients With Epilepsy

Etsegenet F. Tizazu and Michael Gelfand

A. Depression, bipolar disorder, anxiety, and psychosis are all more common in patients with epilepsy. If patients have symptoms or a history of depression, antiepileptic drugs (AEDs) with adverse mood effects (topiramate, levetiracetam, zonisamide, clobazam, perampanel, and phenobarbital) should be avoided whenever possible. Medications with favorable effects on mood ("mood stabilizers"), such as carbamazepine, lamotrigine, or valproate, are preferred. Withdrawal of these mood-stabilizing AEDs may also contribute to depressive symptoms. If treatment with an antidepressant is required, selective serotonin and serotonin norepinephrine reuptake inhibitors (SSRIs/SNRIs) are appropriate and safe. Clomipramine, maprotiline, amoxapine, and bupropion should be avoided due to risk of lowering the seizure threshold.

Anxiety is a common comorbid condition in patients with epilepsy. Symptoms of anxiety and panic may represent a seizure aura, and should be distinguished from a primary psychiatric cause. If the latter, SSRIs/SNRIs are a reasonable initial treatment options; long-term benzodiazepine use should be limited.

Psychosis occurs in 5%–10% of patients with epilepsy, most often in those with temporal lobe epilepsy. Psychosis in a patient with epilepsy may represent AED side effects, ictal or postictal psychosis, or a primary psychiatric disorder. AED changes should be made if appropriate. If psychosis is thought to be ictal or postictal, evaluation in an epilepsy-monitoring unit may be needed; in these cases improved seizure control is usually the best approach to limit recurrent episodes of psychosis. Postictal psychosis may require both improved seizure control as well as use of antipsychotic agents for acute symptom control during episodes. With the possible exception of ictal psychosis, treatment by a psychiatrist is needed, and initiation of antipsychotic medication is usually recommended. Use of some antipsychotics, particularly clozapine, should be limited due to risk for lowering seizure threshold.

B. Cognitive impairment is common in epilepsy, and can vary from subtle deficits to severe intellectual disability. Epilepsy-specific causes may include underlying disease, medication side effect, or increased duration or frequency of seizures. Ambulatory electroencephalogram may be needed for evaluation if increased seizure burden (including subclinical seizures) is suspected. If this is excluded, AEDs should be optimized. Among common AEDs, topiramate typically causes the most notable cognitive impairment, particularly at high dose or with rapid titration. Other potential contributing AEDs include zonisamide, phenobarbital, and benzodiazepines.

C. Obstructive sleep apnea (OSA) can be associated with increased seizure frequency. Use of AEDs that lead to weight loss, such as topiramate, and avoidance of those that lead to weight gain, such as valproate, may help decrease the severity of OSA. Of note, vagus nerve stimulation (VNS) has been shown to exacerbate sleep apnea, and sleep specialist consultation should be considered prior to VNS implantation if sleep apnea is present or suspected. Insomnia can be a side effect of AEDs, especially felbamate and lamotrigine. In these cases, dose medications earlier in the evening. AEDs with more sedating properties can be given with a higher dose in the evening than in the morning; this is especially valuable if seizures are primarily nocturnal. Use of extended-release formulations can help with both daytime fatigue and, with lamotrigine, insomnia. This can be done either using twice-daily dosing (to limit the effect of postdose peak) or once-daily dosing, typically given in the evening for potentially sedating medications. Similarly, medications given once daily, such as perampanel or zonisamide, should usually be given in the evening rather than the morning. Improved sleep hygiene, trial of melatonin, or referral to a sleep specialist should also be considered if AED adjustment fails to improve insomnia.

D. Headaches and epilepsy often coexist. Lamotrigine may trigger or exacerbate headache. Valproate, topiramate, and zonisamide generally improve headaches. Other common treatments for primary headaches, such as nortriptyline and propranolol, are reasonable once secondary causes of headache have been excluded.

REFERENCES

1. Sirven JI. Management of epilepsy comorbidities. *Continuum (Minneap Minn)*. 2016;22(1):191–203.
2. Adachi N, Kanemoto K, de Toffol B, et al. Basic treatment principles for psychotic disorders in patients with epilepsy. *Epilepsia*. 2003;54:19–33.
3. Kanner AM. The treatment of depressive disorders in epilepsy: what all neurologists should know. *Epilepsia*. 2013;54(suppl 1):3–12.

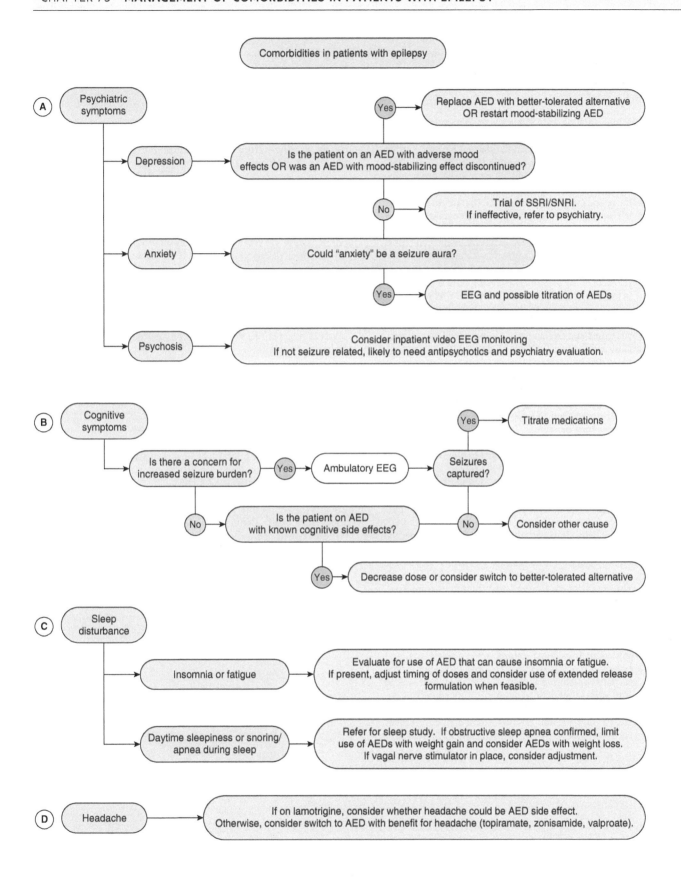

EEG Interpretation

Michael Gelfand

A. The initial step in evaluating an electroencephalogram (EEG) is to identify the recording montage. The typical initial montage is bipolar—each electrode is compared to a single adjacent electrode rather than to a common reference electrode—and longitudinal, indicating that comparisons are made sequentially along a chain progressing from anterior to posterior. There will usually be longitudinal chains covering both the lateral (temporal) and medial (parasagittal) regions over both the left and right hemispheres. Alternative montages may also be used. For example, using transverse rather than longitudinal bipolar may help to demonstrate sleep patterns, while referential montages may help to evaluate and localize possibly epileptic activity.

B. Next, identify the state of the patient. The waking state is most easily identified due to the presence of a posterior dominant rhythm (PDR), an 8–12 Hz "alpha" rhythm seen prominently in the posterior electrodes. Faster activity (beta) may be seen anteriorly. The PDR usually appears with eyes closed and attenuates or disappears with eyes open. Artifacts from muscle movement and eye blinks are often prominent. Sleep may be identified by several different features. Most notably, the PDR is absent, theta (4–8 Hz) or delta (<4 Hz) rhythms predominate, and muscle and eye blink artifacts disappear. Depending on the stage of sleep, vertex waves, sleep spindles, K complexes, positive occipital sharp transients (POSTS), slow waves, or artifacts from rapid eye movements may be seen.

C. The background should be classified as normal or abnormal; abnormal background patterns indicating mild-to-moderate diffuse cerebral dysfunction—for example, as seen in intoxication or mild renal dysfunction—may include slowing of the PDR to frequencies <8 Hz, disappearance of the anterior-to-posterior gradient of amplitude and frequency (known as "disorganization"), or absent PDR with diffuse theta or delta slowing. With obtundation or coma, the background may be interrupted intermittently by brief periods of much lower-amplitude signal ("discontinuity"). Finally, with severe global brain dysfunction, including after anoxic injury or with high-dose barbiturates, the background may be burst-suppressed, in which a low-voltage or flat pattern is only occasionally interrupted by a "burst" of activity, or is completely suppressed.

D. Focal slowing should be identified. This may include theta or delta frequencies seen asymmetrically, for example, over a single temporal lobe. Focal slowing indicates dysfunction in a specific region of the brain, although spatial resolution is limited. This may correlate to a structural injury such as infarction or tumor. It may also be seen in focal epilepsy, although it is not specific. One exception is unilateral, rhythmic delta slowing, for example, temporal intermittent rhythmic delta activity (TIRDA), which is frequently associated with focal epilepsy.

E. Epileptiform discharges may be either focal or generalized. The appearance of these may vary, but at a minimum they should be clearly distinct from the background and should have a physiologically plausible distribution ("field"). The morphology typically includes a negative (pointed *up*) "spike" or "sharp wave," or at times a polyspike, followed by a negative "slow wave." Generalized epileptiform discharges usually indicate generalized epilepsy. Discharges repeating at ~4–6 Hz are commonly seen in juvenile myoclonic epilepsy (JME), at ~3 Hz in childhood absence epilepsy (CAE), and at <3 Hz in Lennox-Gastaut syndrome (LGS). The location of a focal discharge helps to indicate the source of seizures, but is relatively imprecise. Epileptiform discharges must be distinguished from sharply contoured features without the typical epileptiform morphology. These "sharp transients," which often are less distinct from the background, often represent normal variants, and it is critical to avoid misidentifying them as epileptic in origin. In clinical practice, misidentification is common and may lead to an incorrect diagnosis of epilepsy.

F. Seizures are typically distinguished by a rhythmic pattern with a clearly identifiable start and end (i.e., standing out from background activity) and with evolution over time in frequency, spatial distribution, or morphology. Seizures may be clinical or subclinical. A seizure on an outpatient or routine EEG is effectively pathognomonic for epilepsy. A seizure on an inpatient EEG also usually suggests a diagnosis of epilepsy, but may also be seen with acute brain injury, and in the setting of persistently altered mental status should raise suspicion for nonconvulsive status epilepticus.

G. Rhythmic patterns and periodic discharges can vary widely in their appearance and significance. Generalized periodic discharges (GPDs) can be seen after anoxic brain injury or with nonspecific global dysfunction, and depending on morphology may be epileptic—"GPEDs"—or may indicate a metabolic abnormality, such as with so-called "triphasic waves." Lateralized periodic discharges (LPDs, often known as "PLEDs") usually indicate a high risk for seizures, but can also be seen in the setting of focal structural injury such as stroke. Terminology and understanding of these patterns both remain in flux, and they should typically be interpreted only in light of the complete clinical scenario.

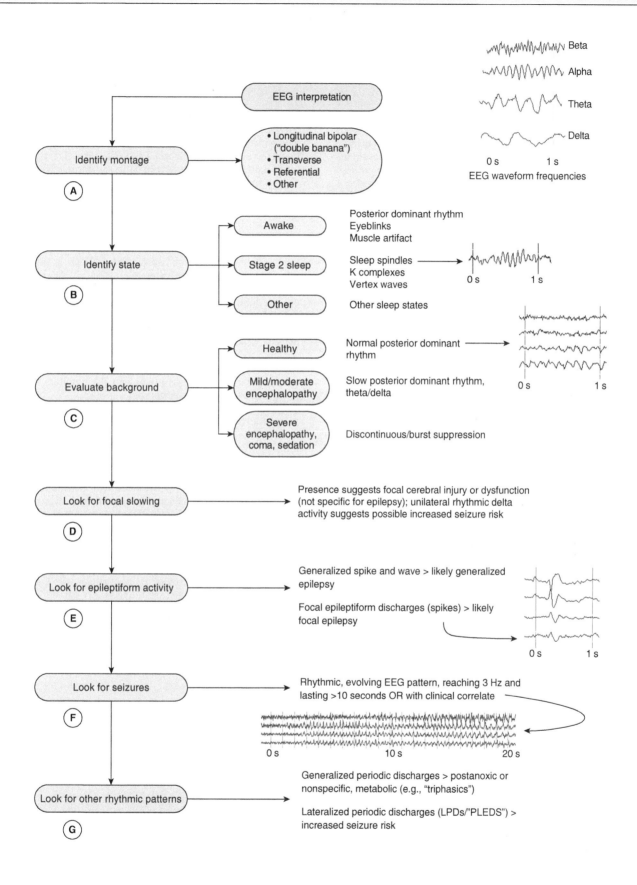

Hypersomnia

Charles J. Bae

Hypersomnia is the cardinal symptom of sleep disorders characterized by excessive daytime sleepiness, often resulting in increased sleep time or involuntary dozing. While insufficient sleep is the most common cause of excessive sleepiness, narcolepsy, circadian rhythm sleep disorders, sleep disordered breathing, insomnia, and medication effects are also implicated. The cause of hypersomnia can often be identified with a detailed clinical history, particularly noting comorbid systemic diseases or medications that may be contributing. Patients should be asked about sleep habits and schedules, what happens during the sleep period, and time periods they feel most awake and sleepy. It can be helpful to get collateral information from a family member or friend. An overnight polysomnogram (PSG) may be useful to diagnose sleep-disordered breathing or periodic limb movement disorder, and a daytime multiple sleep latency test (MSLT) can be done to objectively assess the degree of sleepiness in order to identify narcolepsy.

A. Insufficient sleep syndrome presents with daytime sleepiness due to chronic partial sleep deprivation. A typical patient sleeps less than 6 hours per night. Diagnosis can usually be made based on clinical history alone. An increase in total sleep time to at least 7–8 hours per night should be recommended.

B. Obstructive sleep apnea (OSA) is due to a recurrent collapse of the upper airway during sleep that is either partial (hypopnea) or complete (apnea). The severity of sleep apnea is defined by the apnea-hypopnea index (AHI), which is the number of times per hour of sleep that a respiratory event is present. An AHI <5 is considered to be normal, 5–14 mild, 15–30 moderate, and >30 indicates severe OSA. A sleep study, either overnight PSG or a home sleep apnea test, is needed to make a diagnosis of sleep apnea. Treatment options for OSA include weight loss, positional therapy, positive airway pressure (PAP) therapy, oral appliance therapy, and hypoglossal nerve stimulation. Patients with OSA who remain sleepy despite regular and effective use of PAP may benefit from alerting medications such as modafinil.

C. Periodic limb movement disorder (PLMD) is characterized by stereotyped leg movements during sleep that disturb sleep and thus cause daytime sleepiness. Periodic limb movements can be identified by PSG. A periodic limb movement frequency of >15 per hour of sleep suggests the diagnosis of PLMD. Treatment options include benzodiazepines, dopamine D2 agonists, alpha 2 delta ligands (e.g., gabapentin), and muscle relaxants. Asymptomatic periodic limb movements during sleep are common and do not require treatment.

D. Recurrent hypersomnia (also known as Kleine-Levin syndrome) is characterized by periods of excessive sleeping up to 20 hours a day, which lasts from 2–35 days. Between hypersomnia episodes, the patient is cognitively normal and not sleepy. Treatment options (all of limited utility) include stimulants and chronic lithium carbonate to prevent onset of a hypersomnia episode. Recurrent hypersomnia can be encountered in some women in association with menses.

E. Narcolepsy is associated with excessive daytime sleepiness, cataplexy, paralysis and hallucinations on sleep/wake transitions, and nocturnal sleep fragmentation. Cataplexy is the inappropriate loss of muscle tone with preservation of consciousness, which is triggered by a strong emotion, such as laughter; it is a feature of type 1 narcolepsy, but is absent in type 2 narcolepsy. Diagnosis of narcolepsy requires a positive MSLT: mean sleep latency (MSL) ≤8 minutes with two or more sleep onset rapid eye movement periods (SOREMPs). Treatment options directed at hypersomnolence include good sleep hygiene, scheduled short naps, daytime stimulants, and nighttime sodium oxybate. Sodium oxybate treats cataplexy in addition to sleepiness. Other treatment options for cataplexy include tricyclic antidepressants, selective serotonin reuptake inhibitors, and selective norepinephrine reuptake inhibitors

F. Idiopathic hypersomnia consists of excessive daytime sleepiness that is not explained by another sleep or medical disorder. MSLT shows an MSL ≤8 minutes and less than two SOREMPs. Treatment options include good sleep hygiene, short scheduled naps, or stimulants.

G. Delayed sleep phase syndrome is a circadian rhythm disorder characterized by habitual sleep and wake times that are delayed by at least 2 hours from the socially acceptable sleep period, resulting in sleep deprivation and subsequent daytime dysfunction. When these individuals are able to sleep on their preferred diurnal schedule, sleep deprivation does not occur and they do not experience daytime sleepiness. This sleep disorder is common in adolescents and young adults. Treatment can be either (1) phase delay with chronotherapy (delay sleep and wake times by 3 hours every day until the desired sleep and wake times are achieved), or (2) phase advance with melatonin in the evening and bright light exposure in the morning. Other circadian rhythm sleep disorders (e.g., shift work sleep disorder, jet lag, advanced sleep phase syndrome, non–24-hour sleep-wake disorder) can also be associated with daytime sleepiness.

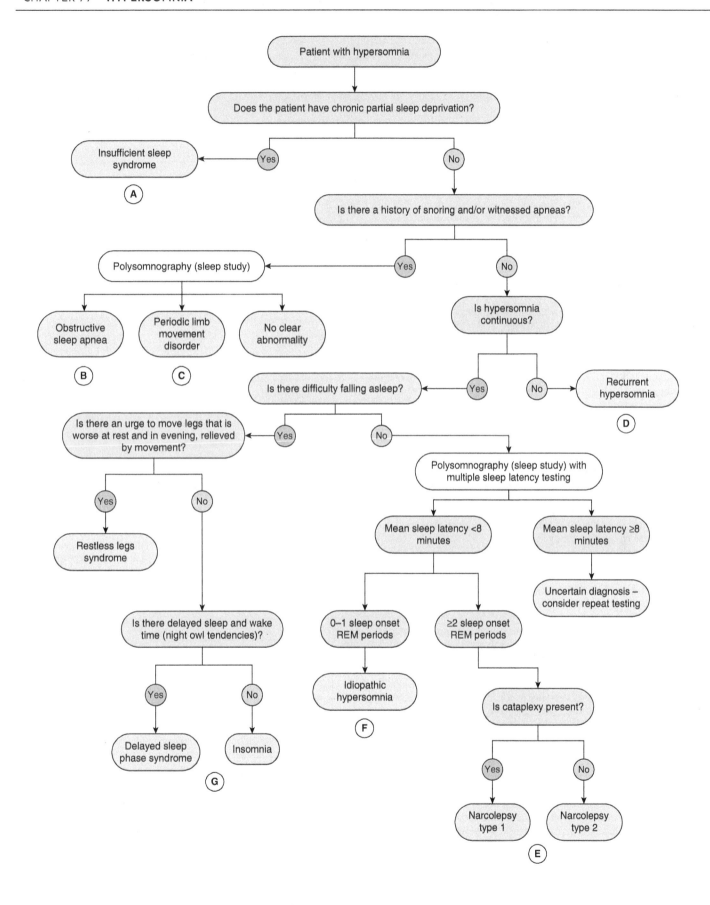

Insomnia

Jessica Oehlke, Ilene M. Rosen, and Philip Gehrman

Insomnia is a near universal experience, but can be extremely disruptive when frequent and persistent. Insomnia is often driven by the development of maladaptive behaviors and thoughts surrounding the sleep disturbance. Such behaviors include naps, irregular sleep schedules, or excessive time in bed. Typical maladaptive thoughts include excessive worry about the inability to sleep or concern about the impact of the sleep disturbance on daytime function. These behaviors and thoughts can perpetuate the insomnia cycle. Patients with insomnia should be distinguished from "short sleepers" who average less than 6 hours of sleep per night but lack any sleep disturbances or functional impairment, and from those who lack an adequate opportunity for sleep but, when given sufficient time and circumstances to sleep, achieve normal sleep without disruptions or impairment.

A. Short-term insomnia is often due to a precipitating event or identifiable stressor, such as a change in environment or schedule, or medical or psychiatric illness. Often as the precipitating event resolves or diminishes, so does the insomnia. If there are maladaptive behaviors or thoughts surrounding the sleep disturbance, cognitive behavioral therapy for insomnia (CBT-I) can be helpful. Depending on the degree of distress or impairment, short-term hypnotic use may be appropriate.

B. Environmental factors, such as noise, light, uncomfortable temperatures, or safety concerns, may contribute to insomnia, with improvement when these factors are addressed.

C. Stimulants can interfere with sleep and cause insomnia, including caffeine, nicotine, amphetamines, and cocaine. Activating antidepressants, such as bupropion, and other medications such as corticosteroids, can also interfere with sleep. Withdrawal from hypnotics, anxiolytics, and sedating substances such as alcohol or marijuana may cause rebound insomnia.

D. Insomnia is frequently comorbid with psychiatric, medical, and other sleep disorders. If comorbid disorders are present, treatment should focus on the underlying condition as well as the insomnia as there is likely a reciprocal relationship between the two.

E. Obstructive sleep apnea, parasomnias, periodic limb movements, and narcolepsy may present with insomnia complaints due to nighttime awakenings or fragmented sleep. Restless legs syndrome may present with difficulty falling asleep, but this disorder can be differentiated from sleep-onset insomnia by the clinical history. Circadian rhythm sleep-wake disorders such as advanced sleep-wake phase disorder, delayed sleep-wake phase disorder, and shift work disorder should be considered in the setting of insomnia complaints. Advanced sleep-wake phase disorder should be differentiated from insomnia with early morning awakening, as individuals with an advanced endogenous circadian rhythm tend to go to bed early and wake up early but otherwise sleep normally, unlike someone with insomnia. Early morning awakening may also be common in individuals with depression. Delayed sleep-wake phase disorder can present as sleep-onset insomnia if an individual attempts to go to bed earlier than their endogenous circadian clock. However, when allowed to have a later bedtime and wake time, these individuals sleep normally without difficulty falling asleep.

TABLE 78.1	MEDICATIONS COMMONLY USED TO TREAT INSOMNIA		
Medication	Starting dose	Usual dose	Considerations
Nonbenzodiazepine Receptor Agonists			
Zolpidem	5 mg	5–10 mg	Sleep-onset insomnia
Zolpidem extended-release	6.25 mg	6.25–12.5 mg	Sleep-onset and maintenance insomnia
Eszopiclone	1mg	1–3 mg	Sleep-onset and maintenance insomnia
Zaleplon	5 mg	10–20 mg	Sleep-onset insomnia
Melatonin Receptor Agonists			
Ramelteon	8 mg	8 mg	Sleep-onset insomnia
Selective Histamine Receptor Antagonist			
Doxepin	3 mg	3–6 mg	Sleep maintenance insomnia
Dual Orexin Receptor Antagonist			
Suvorexant	5 mg	10–20 mg	Sleep-onset and maintenance insomnia
Benzodiazepine Receptor Agonists			
Temazepam	7.5 mg	7.5–30 mg	Sleep-onset and maintenance insomnia
Other Medications			
Amitriptyline	10 mg	10–100 mg	Comorbid depression or chronic pain
Trazodone	25 mg	25–100 mg	Comorbid depression or substance use
Mirtazapine	7.5 mg	7.5–30 mg	Comorbid depression
Quetiapine	25 mg	25–200 mg	Comorbid psychosis or mania
Gabapentin	100 mg	100–900 mg	Comorbid pain or alcohol use
Melatonin	0.3 mg	0.3–10 mg	Circadian rhythm disorders or dementia

F. CBT-I is the first-line treatment for chronic or persistent insomnia. CBT-I is a nonpharmacological therapy that targets both the maladaptive behaviors and thoughts that contribute to chronic insomnia; it has more durable long-term benefits after treatment completion compared to hypnotic medications. If CBT-I is not effective, available, or feasible, pharmacotherapy for insomnia can be considered (Table 78.1). Hypnotic medications for insomnia can be associated with side effects, drug-drug interactions, dependency, and habituation. If needed, hypnotic medications should be used on a short-term basis and supplemented with CBT-I when possible.

REFERENCES

1. Sateia MJ, Buysse DJ, Krystal AD, Neubauer DN, Heald JL. Clinical practice guideline for the pharmacologic treatment of chronic insomnia in adults: an American Academy of Sleep Medicine clinical practice guideline. *J Clin Sleep Med.* 2017;13(2):307–349.
2. Winkelman JW. Insomnia disorder. *N Engl J Med.* 2015;373(15):1437–1444.

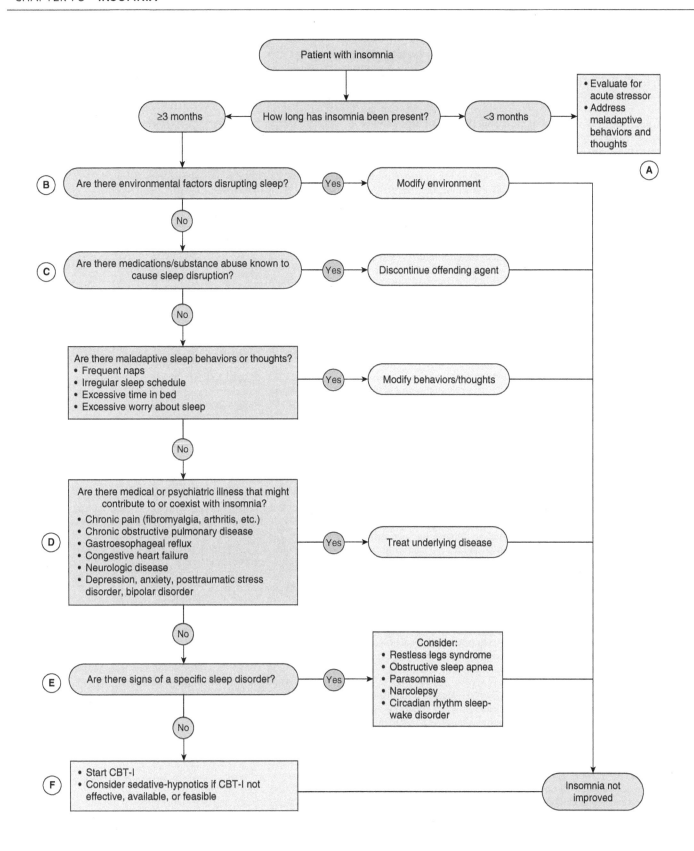

Patient with insomnia

How long has insomnia been present?

≥3 months → <3 months → • Evaluate for acute stressor
• Address maladaptive behaviors and thoughts

A

B Are there environmental factors disrupting sleep? Yes → Modify environment

No

C Are there medications/substance abuse known to cause sleep disruption? Yes → Discontinue offending agent

No

Are there maladaptive sleep behaviors or thoughts?
• Frequent naps
• Irregular sleep schedule
• Excessive time in bed
• Excessive worry about sleep

Yes → Modify behaviors/thoughts

No

D Are there medical or psychiatric illness that might contribute to or coexist with insomnia?
• Chronic pain (fibromyalgia, arthritis, etc.)
• Chronic obstructive pulmonary disease
• Gastroesophageal reflux
• Congestive heart failure
• Neurologic disease
• Depression, anxiety, posttraumatic stress disorder, bipolar disorder

Yes → Treat underlying disease

No

E Are there signs of a specific sleep disorder? Yes → Consider:
• Restless legs syndrome
• Obstructive sleep apnea
• Parasomnias
• Narcolepsy
• Circadian rhythm sleep-wake disorder

No

F • Start CBT-I
• Consider sedative-hypnotics if CBT-I not effective, available, or feasible

Insomnia not improved

Restless Legs Syndrome

Charles Cantor and David Raizen

The cardinal feature of restless legs syndrome (RLS) is an urge to move the limbs, often accompanied by uncomfortable sensations, which come on in the evening and nighttime, and which are relieved by moving the limbs. A family history of RLS, history of periodic leg movements during sleep (seen in ~90% of patients with RLS), and symptomatic improvement with dopamine agonist medications are supporting features. In cases where the history is unclear, a sleep study assessing for the presence of periodic limb movements of sleep may be useful.

A. Antihistamines, caffeine, nicotine, and selective serotonin receptor inhibitors (SSRIs), selective norepinephrine inhibitors (SNRIs), and tricyclic antidepressants (TCAs) may exacerbate symptoms of RLS. Bupropion, mirtazapine, and trazodone are antidepressants considered "safe" for RLS. Although the pathophysiology of RLS is not fully understood, overt iron deficiency or a relative deficiency of brain iron have been implicated, possibly through downstream effects on dopaminergic transmission. For this reason, patients should be evaluated for iron deficiency. Treat for ferritin <75 mcg/mL with ferrous sulfate 325 mg bid + vitamin C (to aid iron absorption) or other iron formulations that give the equivalent dose of elemental iron (total of 130–195 mg of elemental iron daily). Consider polysomnography if comorbid obstructive sleep apnea (OSA) is suspected, since OSA can cause further sleep fragmentation and make management of RLS more difficult.

B. Various forms of counterstimulation (limb-rubbing, stretching, and other movements) provide transient, and in some cases sufficient, relief for some patients.

C. First-line treatments for RLS include dopamine agonists (pramipexole, ropinirole, rotigotine) or alpha 2 delta ligands (gabapentin, extended-release gabapentin, pregabalin, gabapentin enacarbil) (Table 79.1). The choice of drugs can be guided by comorbidities. Consider an alpha 2 delta ligand for patients with pain, ropinirole for patients with renal insufficiency, and rotigotine patch for patients who do not tolerate oral agents. Note that only pramipexole, ropinirole, rotigotine, and gabapentin enacarbil are approved by the Federal Drug Administration for treatment of RLS, though many other medications are used off label. For long-term follow-up, observe for side effects. With dopamine agonists, these include nausea, loss of efficacy, compulsive behaviors, and augmentation (see section D); alpha 2 delta ligands can cause sedation, weight gain, depression, and edema.

D. If symptoms recur after a period of stability, reevaluate for modifiable risk factors and iron deficiency as described above. If dopamine agonists or alpha 2 delta ligands are ineffective after dose adjustment or if side effects occur, switch to the other drug class; if this is ineffective, switch to a long-acting agent within the drug class. Combined therapy with drugs in different classes may be considered in difficult-to-treat cases if side effects are not limiting. Other important considerations specific to dopamine agonists are loss of efficacy and augmentation. Augmentation refers to a paradoxical worsening of RLS symptoms seen with long-term use of dopaminergic agents. This is manifested by more diffuse somatic involvement (typically arms in addition to legs) and the development of symptoms earlier in the day. It is usually treated by switching an alpha 2 delta ligand or an opioid.

TABLE 79.1 DOSING AND TITRATION OF MEDICATIONS FOR RESTLESS LEGS SYNDROME			
Drug	Starting dose	Titration	Maximum dose
Ferrous sulfate	325 mg bid	Take with vitamin C	
Vitamin C	250 mg bid	Taken with iron supplement	
Ropinirole	0.25 mg qhs	Increase 0.25 mg q3–4 d	4 mg
Pramipexole	0.125 mg qhs	Increase 0.125 mg q3–4 d	1 mg
Gabapentin	100 mg qhs	Increase in 100–300 mg increments	1200 mg tid or qhs
Codeine	30 mg qhs	Increase in 30 mg increments	30 mg tid
Oxycodone	2.5 mg qhs	Increase in 2.5–5 mg increments	10 mg tid
Methadone	2.5–5 mg qhs	Increase in 2.5–5 mg increments	15 mg bid
Pregabalin	25–50 mg qhs	Increase in 50 mg increments	300 mg
Gabapentin enacarbil	300 mg	Increase in 300 mg increments	1200 mg at 6.00 p.m.
Rotigotine patch	1 mg	Increase in 1 mg increments daily	3 mg

E. Patients who have developed symptoms in the daytime or evening as well as at bedtime may benefit from the use of longer-acting medications. These include extended-release forms of pramipexole and ropinirole, the rotigotine patch, gabapentin enacarbil, and long-acting gabapentin formulations.

F. For patients with refractory symptoms or side effects on dopamine agonists and alpha 2 delta ligands, use of an opioid can be considered. These medications are generally effective in treating RLS; however, they should be used only in selected patients who have been educated about their risks and appropriate use. Treatment generally starts with a low-potency opioid (e.g., codeine). If this is ineffective, oxycodone may be used. For severe around-the-clock RLS symptoms unresponsive to combinations of drugs listed above, treat with methadone, starting at 2.5–5 mg nightly or twice a day.

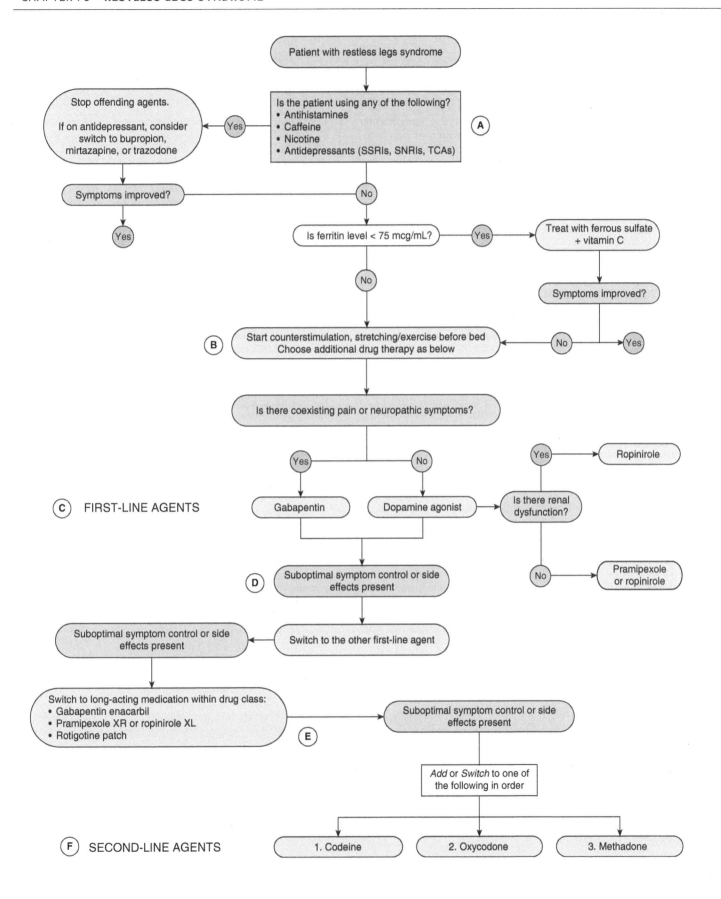

Parasomnias

Alice Cai and Charles J. Bae

Parasomnias are unwanted events or experiences that occur during sleep, during the transition from wake to sleep, or during arousals from sleep. Parasomnias may result from a mixed or unstable state of consciousness where certain areas of the brain are awake and others are asleep. There are two types of parasomnias: those that occur during the rapid eye movement (REM) stage of sleep and those in non–rapid eye movement (NREM) stages of sleep (Table 80.1).

A. REM-sleep behavior disorder (RBD) is a type of REM parasomnia. A cardinal feature is the loss of REM atonia, resulting in dream enactment during REM sleep. The presenting symptom is most often injury to the patient and/or bed partner. Patients should be asked if they can recall their dreams and actions, and are often able to recall violent dream content. Movements may be complex and involve shouting, reaching out, kicking, punching, running, or even dancing. However, walking is not common, and leaving the room is rare. Eyes typically remain closed during the event. A prodrome can exist of sleep talking, limb twitching, or jerking during sleep. Autonomic changes are uncommon, in contrast with disorders of arousal from NREM sleep such as sleep terrors. Three-quarters of patients have concurrent periodic limb movements during NREM sleep. RBD usually affects those over 50 years of age; men are affected more than women. Over 80% of patients with RBD will be diagnosed with a synucleinopathy (Parkinson's disease, dementia with Lewy bodies, multiple system atrophy) within 10 years. Patients should be asked if they have anosmia, constipation, or orthostasis; follow-up cognitive testing and neurologic exams are indicated to monitor for signs of neurodegeneration. RBD can also be associated with stroke, head injury, posttraumatic stress disorder, and depression. Medications associated with RBD include venlafaxine, serotonin selective reuptake inhibitors, mirtazapine, tricyclic antidepressants, selegiline, and rarely beta blockers and acetylcholinesterase inhibitors. Polysomnography (PSG) is required for diagnosis, and shows evidence of increased REM sleep muscle tone (REM sleep without atonia). Management of RBD involves modifying the sleep environment, including placing the mattress on the floor, having the patient and their bed partner sleep in a separate bed or room, and removing dangerous objects from the vicinity. Melatonin (6–18 mg qhs.) is a common first-line treatment with few side effects. Clonazepam is also frequently used (0.5–2.0 mg qhs.), but caution should be exercised in patients with dementia, gait dysfunction, or obstructive sleep apnea. If synucleinopathy is present, acetylcholine receptor inhibitors (e.g., donepezil, rivastigmine) may be helpful. Pramipexole may be used in RBD with periodic limb movements.

B. Pseudo-RBD is an NREM parasomnia that mimics features of RBD. This should be considered in patients younger than age 50, and in whom the dream content is not very violent. There also may be a strong suspicion for obstructive sleep apnea (OSA) based on a history of snoring and witnessed apneas. PSG is indicated for diagnosis (demonstrating normal REM-sleep atonia) and to assess for OSA. Treating OSA is typically effective at treating the abnormal sleep behaviors.

C. Other NREM parasomnias include sleepwalking, sleep terrors, confusional arousals, sleep eating disorder, and sexomnia. These are more prevalent in younger adults, and may be normal in children. During sleepwalking, the patient has blunted responses to questions. They may engage in inappropriate complex activity such as climbing out of a window. There is amnesia of the event, and the patient is confused during the episode. Sleep terrors are heralded by a scream with intense fear and signs of autonomic arousal. Bolting from bed can occur. These are similar to but not the same as nightmares, which may also involve complex dream imagery followed by an arousal, but do not involve dream enactment. Sleep-related abnormal sexual behaviors can occur, as can sleep driving, smoking, or eating. Electroencephalogram (EEG) may not correlate well to the event; in sleep eating, the EEG pattern is predominantly awake, but the patient has an altered level of consciousness. In sleepwalking, there is a classic EEG pattern of high-voltage delta with mixes of delta, theta, and alpha. NREM parasomnias also are diagnosed with PSG—some patients have significant arousals out of slow wave sleep. These can be precipitated by lack of sleep, use of sedative/hypnotics, and other sleep disorders.

D. Nocturnal seizures can be complex, and patients may have multiple different behaviors, making them difficult to differentiate from parasomnias, especially the nocturnal frontal lobe epilepsies. Seizures are usually stereotyped and repetitive, can be associated with tachycardia and hypertension, and are followed by a postictal confusional state. Patients are amnestic to the events. A PSG with a full 10–20 EEG montage is needed to look for evidence of epileptiform activity.

TABLE 80.1 CHARACTERISTICS OF PARASOMNIAS				
	RBD	Pseudo-RBD	NREM-behavior disorders	Nocturnal seizures
Population affected	>50 years old, males	< 50 years old	<35 years old, can be normal in children	
Timing of onset	Often during the second part of the night (during REM sleep)	Anytime	Within 2 hours of sleep onset (during NREM sleep)	Occur least frequently during REM sleep
Movement type	Complex, dream enactments	Simple or complex	Automatic, basic, disinhibited	Sudden repetitive movements
Post-event confusion	No, often good recall of violent dream content	No	Yes (confusional arousals, amnesia)	Yes
Walking, exiting room	Rare	Rare	Cardinal feature of sleepwalking	Sometimes (wandering in postictal state with subsequent amnesia)
Autonomic features	None	None	Tachycardia, mydriasis, tachypnea, diaphoresis in sleep terror	Yes (tachycardia, hypertension)

NREM, Non–rapid eye movement; *RBD,* REM-sleep behavior disorder; *REM,* rapid eye movement.

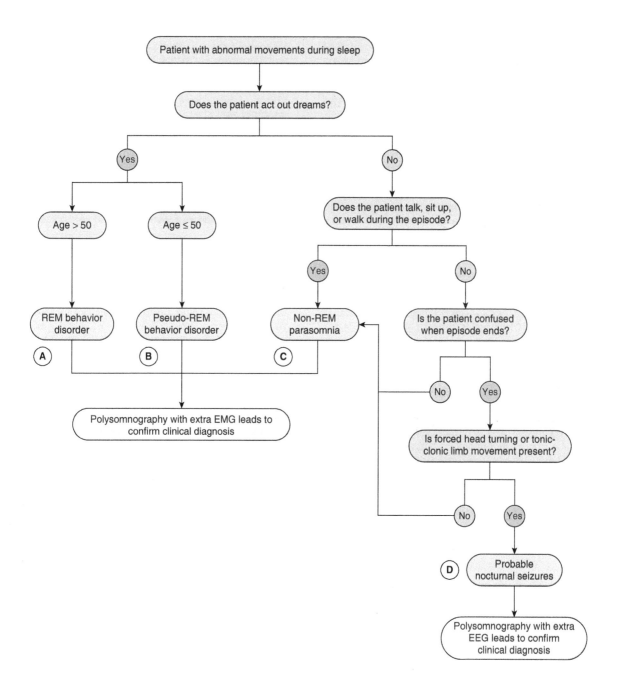

Abnormal Involuntary Movements

David Coughlin and Andres Deik

A. Paroxysmal kinesogenic dyskinesia (PKD) is characterized by sudden onset of abnormal hyperkinetic movements (dystonia, chorea, ballism, athetosis, or a combination of these) triggered by movement. Mutations in the *PRRT2* gene are a common cause, but other gene mutations have been described. In paroxysmal non-kinesogenic dyskinesia (PNKD) movements can be triggered by caffeine or alcohol, or can occur spontaneously. Patients can be tested for the *MR1* gene, although it is likely that mutations in yet undiscovered loci may account for some cases of PNKD. Epilepsy and functional movement disorders should always be in the differential diagnosis of patients thought to have PNKD.

B. There are few movement disorders that persist or happen exclusively during sleep. Bruxism is characterized by clenching or grinding of the teeth and/or by bracing or thrusting of the mandible. Propriospinal myoclonus is characterized by repetitive, stereotyped truncal jerks that may affect the hips and knees. Of note, many cases of propriospinal myoclonus are thought to be functional in nature. Periodic limb movements of sleep are stereotyped and intermittent movements of the ankle or knee joints. Rapid eye movement (REM)–sleep behavior disorder (RBD) is a parasomnia characterized by loss of REM sleep–associated atonia, which results in motor activity during dreaming and carries significant risk for future development of a synucleinopathy (Parkinson disease, Lewy body dementia, or multiple system atrophy). Hypnagogic myoclonus is a form of physiologic myoclonus that can occur in healthy individuals, just like hiccups or a startle response.

C. Movements that happen constantly throughout the daytime tend to be either twitch-like or choreiform. Twitch-like movements are likely to be myokymia, fasciculations, or myoclonus. Each of these movements has an electromyographic signature, and neurophysiologic studies can be used to distinguish them. Myokymia can occur in multiple sclerosis and Guillain-Barré syndrome, and after radiation therapy. Fasciculations can be a benign finding, but can also be caused by radiculopathies, entrapment neuropathies, or motor neuron disease. Myoclonus can be seen in a variety of scenarios, including genetic conditions such as myoclonus dystonia, medication side effects, and metabolic derangements (classically uremia or liver failure), and in many neurodegenerative diseases.

D. Chorea, athetosis, and ballism fall within a spectrum of hyperkinesias. Chorea consists of irregular, nonstereotyped, dance-like spontaneous movements. Huntington disease is the most common cause of generalized chorea in adults, whereas in childhood, Sydenham chorea is a common cause. In athetosis, the movements are slower and have a writhing or twisting motion, often involving the fingers. Ballism, on the other hand, is a severe form of chorea where there is violent flinging of the limbs, and is often limited to one side of the body. Hemiballism or hemichorea may be an acute presentation or delayed sequela of stroke.

E. Dystonia is due to sustained or intermittent muscle contractions causing abnormal, often repetitive movements, postures, or both. These abnormal movements are typically patterned and twisting, and may be tremulous. Other signs of dystonia include the presence of a sensory trick (improvement in movements caused by a tactile stimulus) and the presence of directionality (tendency of a dystonic body part to twist in a certain direction).

F. Tics are sudden, stereotyped movements that are often accompanied by an urge to perform the movement and a sense of relief once the movement is performed. Tics can be motor or vocal: the former are often simple movements of a body part (blinking, neck extension, grimacing, shoulder shrugging) whereas the latter is any action that causes a sound. Most tics are brief, but they can also be prolonged and ritualistic. These are known as a complex motor tics, and can be seen in patients with Tourette syndrome.

G. Functional (or psychogenic) movement disorders are common, disabling, and at times difficult to diagnose and treat. A careful history and examination may demonstrate features diagnostic of a functional movement disorder and eliminate the need for ancillary testing. Functional movements can resemble organic abnormal movements (tremor is the most common example), or be bizarre, unpredictable, and unclassifiable. Their phenomenology may change throughout the course of the examination, or be stereotyped. They may be episodic or nearly continuous. Distraction and suggestibility on examination, and entrainment (change in the frequency of a tremor during activation of the contralateral limb) are highly suggestive of a functional cause.

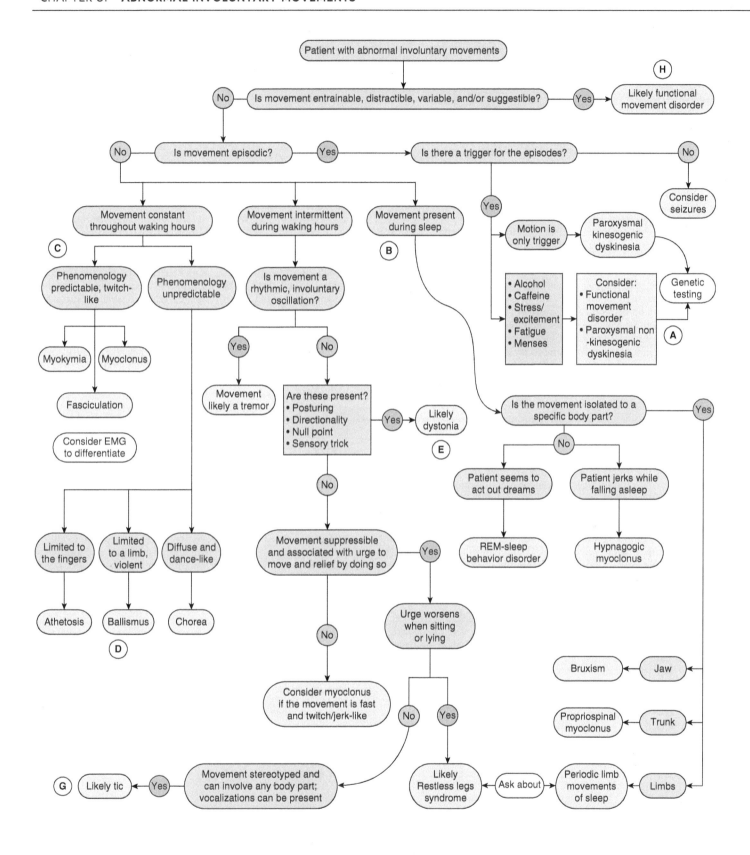

Chorea

David Coughlin and Andres Deik

Chorea is an irregular, often jerky, flowing movement that moves between different body parts. Chorea can often be observed throughout the examination at rest and posture and can be exacerbated by action and while walking.

A. There are a few specific clinical events that can precipitate chorea. Hemichorea can arise as a presentation of acute stroke but can also occur in the subsequent weeks during recovery. 'Post-pump' chorea occurs rarely after extracorporeal membrane oxygenation (ECMO). Chorea has also been described after global hypoxic-ischemic injury.

B. Uptitration of dopaminergic medications in patients with Parkinsonism can cause choreiform movements abruptly, both in Parkinson disease and the atypical Parkinsonian syndromes. Tardive dyskinesia from dopamine blockade causes orobuccal choreiform movements. Illicit drugs including cocaine, methamphetamine, synthetic cannabinoids, and others can cause acute chorea as part of their toxidromes.

C. Many of the metabolic causes of chorea are treatable, so a thorough workup is essential. Hyperglycemia can cause chorea and is associated with bilateral basal ganglia hyperintensities on magnetic resonance imaging (MRI) T1 sequences. Liver failure of any cause can lead to hepatocerebral degeneration because of inability to metabolize certain heavy metals. Wilson disease is a specific metabolic disorder due to inability to excrete copper that results in chorea and also liver failure. Polycythemia vera is known to cause chorea, presumably due to "sludging" in lenticulostriate vessels leading to hypoxia in the basal ganglia.

D. Sydenham chorea after streptococcal infection is likely the most common cause of chorea in children.[1] Immune-mediated vasculitides that cause chorea include lupus and antiphospholipid antibody syndrome. Several paraneoplastic syndromes can include chorea as part of their neurologic phenotype.

E. Toxic exposure causing chorea is rare but has been ascribed to manganese, mercury, and carbon monoxide toxicity. Creutzfeldt-Jakob disease can cause a subacute progressive chorea. Other cerebral infections have also been described.

F. If investigations for acquired causes of chorea have been unrevealing, genetic causes should be considered. Sporadic mutations, anticipation, and nonpaternity can all lead to a presentation of genetic chorea without a significant family history. Huntington disease (HD) is by far the most likely entity given population carrier rates of intermediate length *huntingtin* expansions.

G. Chorea with an autosomal dominant inheritance pattern is highly likely to be due to HD and therefore testing for this entity should occur first. If negative, there are several HD phenocopies.[2] *C9orf72* hexameric repeat expansions have emerged as a cause of hereditary chorea. The same repeat expansion is also a common cause of familial and sporadic amyotrophic lateral sclerosis and frontotemporal dementia. A brain MRI with iron deposition is highly suggestive of neuroferritonopathy, the only autosomal dominant neurodegeneration with brain iron accumulation (NBIA) syndrome. HD-like 2 (HDL 2 due to expansion mutations in *JPH3*) is common in African populations. Further testing may be guided by associated symptoms and signs. Dementia and epilepsy are described in Huntington disease-like 1 (HDL 1 due to mutations in the *PRNP* gene), dentatorubral-pallidoluysian atrophy (DRPLA due to expansion mutations in *ATN1*) and spinocerebellar ataxia type 17 (SCA-17). Otherwise, SCA 1–3 have been described as causing chorea. *ADCY5* mutations have recently been associated with childhood onset chorea, facial myokymia, and other movement disorders. Patients with mild, minimally progressive chorea with childhood onset without other neurologic features may have a mutation in the *TITF-1* gene leading to benign hereditary chorea (BHC).

H. The majority of NBIAs are inherited in an autosomal recessive fashion (e.g., those due to mutations in *PANK2*, *PLA2G6*, *C19orf12*, *FA2H*, *ATP13A2*, *COASY*, *CP*, and *DCAF17*).[3] Aceruloplasminemia can also cause iron deposition on MRI, and also has the additional features of low ceruloplasmin, copper, and iron. Acanthocytosis can be seen in chorea acanthocytosis. Wilson disease should be ruled out if not done already. Lastly, chorea has been described in ataxia telangiectasia and Friedrich ataxia. X-linked inherited genetic choreas are rare. One of the NBIAs is X-linked inherited beta-propeller protein-associated neurodegeneration (BPAN) due to mutations in *WDR45*. McCleod syndrome is another of the core neuroacanthocytosis syndromes. Chorea is a less common manifestation of Lubag disease (DYT3: X-linked dystonia Parkinsonism due to mutations in *TAF1*) and has been described in female carriers of the mutation.

REFERENCES

1. Gilbert DL. ed. Acute and chronic chorea in childhood. *Semin Pediatr Neurol.* 2009;16(2):71–76.
2. Hensman Moss DJ, Poulter M, Beck J, et al. C9orf72 expansions are the most common genetic cause of Huntington disease phenocopies. *Neurology.* 2014;82(4):292–299.
3. Gregory A, Hayflick S. Neurodegeneration with Brain Iron Accumulation Disorders Overview. In: Adam MP, Ardinger HH, Pagon RA, Wallace SE, Bean LJH, Stephens K, et al., editors. *GeneReviews®.* Seattle WA: 1993–2020, University of Washington, Seattle.

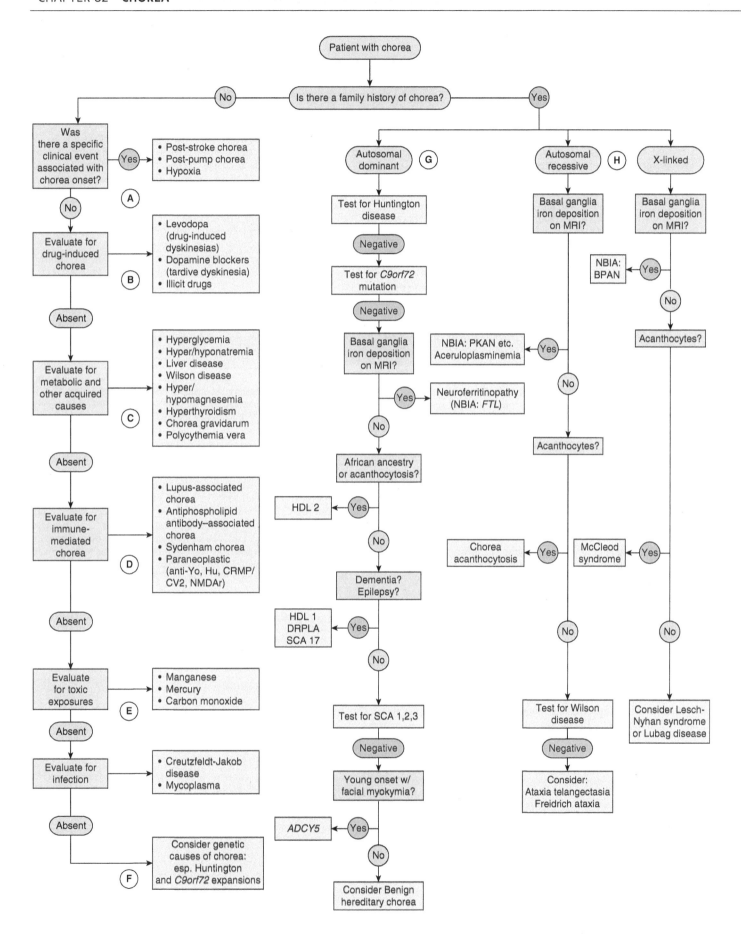

Tremor

David Coughlin and Andres Deik

A. Tremor is defined as "an involuntary, rhythmic, oscillatory movement of a body part."[1] Tremor is typically assessed when the patient is relaxed and distracted, with arms outstretched in posture, and when performing finger-to-nose testing to assess components of resting, postural, and intention tremors. Other movement disorders can resemble tremor, including myoclonus, polyminimyoclonus, and athetosis. Myoclonus is a fast, jerky movement that can arise spontaneously, with activity, or in response to a stimulus. Trains of myoclonus can mimic fast, low-amplitude tremor. Electrophysiologic studies (e.g., electromyogram/nerve conduction studies [EMG/NCS]) are necessary at times to establish an accurate diagnosis. Polyminimyoclonus is seen often in patients with multiple system atrophy and is characterized by irregular, small-amplitude myoclonic movements of the hands and/or fingers in posture. Athetosis can also involve the fingers, but it is slower and characterized by an inability to keep them in a certain position. Pseudoathetosis, which has an identical phenomenology, is seen in patients with impaired joint position sense. Functional movement disorders should also be considered and are distinguished based on clinical examination.

B. Both cerebellar tremor and rubral tremor are often of sudden onset and high amplitude, and present in a combination of rest and posture. Cerebellar tremors are slower (<4 Hz), worse with intention, and are accompanied by other signs of ataxia. Rubral tremor is also slow, often irregular, and can occur at rest, posture, and intention. These patients should undergo brain magnetic resonance imaging as focal lesions, such as stroke or multiple sclerosis, are frequent causes. If the tremor is distractible or entrains to the frequency of distracting maneuvers, functional tremor should be considered.

C. Parkinsonism is defined by the presence of bradykinesia and one or more of the following symptoms: rigidity, tremor, or postural instability. The most common form of tremor in these patients is rest tremor (a tremor that emerges seconds after a limb is allowed to rest completely and disappears with activation). Patient with Parkinsonian rest tremors may also exhibit tremor with posture and/or intention, but the resting component is often the most prominent. Resting tremors can also be seen in patients with dystonia or advanced essential tremor (ET), so identifying bradykinesia and other features of Parkinsonism is necessary to establish a diagnosis. In patients with subtle or questionable bradykinesia, an [I-123] ioflupane dopamine transporter (DAT) single proton emission computerized tomography (SPECT) scan can identify the nigrostriatal dopaminergic deficit associated with Parkinsonian syndromes. The ligand is directed against the dopamine reuptake transporter on the presynaptic side of the terminal end of the nigrostriatal pathway.

D. Patients with rest tremor without other signs of Parkinsonism typically have a dystonic tremor, defined as tremor in a limb affected by dystonia. Dystonic tremors are often jerky and irregular and can resemble myoclonus or coarse essential tremor. Distinguishing dystonic tremor from other tremor types can be challenging, but presence of the following can be helpful: (1) directionality—a tendency of the affected limb to move in a certain direction upon positioning of the limb in the opposite direction; (2) null point—significant tremor improvement when the limb is positioned in the direction in which it tends to move; and (3) the presence of a sensory trick—improvement in tremor severity by light tactile stimulation of the affected body part.

E. All patients with a prominent postural tremor should be screened for causes of tremor, including exposure to medications or substances, comorbid medical diseases, or anxiety. Patients with ET may also find the same factors exacerbate their tremor. It can be difficult to distinguish enhanced physiologic tremor from ET, particularly early in the course of the disease.

F. Most patients with isolated prominent postural tremor are thought to have an enhanced physiologic tremor. These patients have a tremor that is fast frequency, low amplitude, and most visible when holding the arms outstretched.

G. Patients with ET may exhibit additional subtle neurologic signs of uncertain significance (such as impaired tandem gait, questionable dystonic posturing, or memory impairment); these patients have been recently defined as having "ET plus".[1] Patients with action tremor for <3 years who do not have signs of dystonia or Parkinsonism are defined as having an indeterminate tremor.[1] Patients with prominent postural and intention tremor in ET often have the appearance of slight resting tremor, which may be due to incomplete relaxation. Occasionally DAT scan may be necessary to exclude a developing Parkinsonian disorder.

REFERENCE

1. Bhatia KP, Bain P, Bajaj N, et al. Consensus Statement on the classification of tremors. From the task force on tremor of the International Parkinson and Movement Disorder Society. *Mov Disord.* 2018;33(1):75–87.

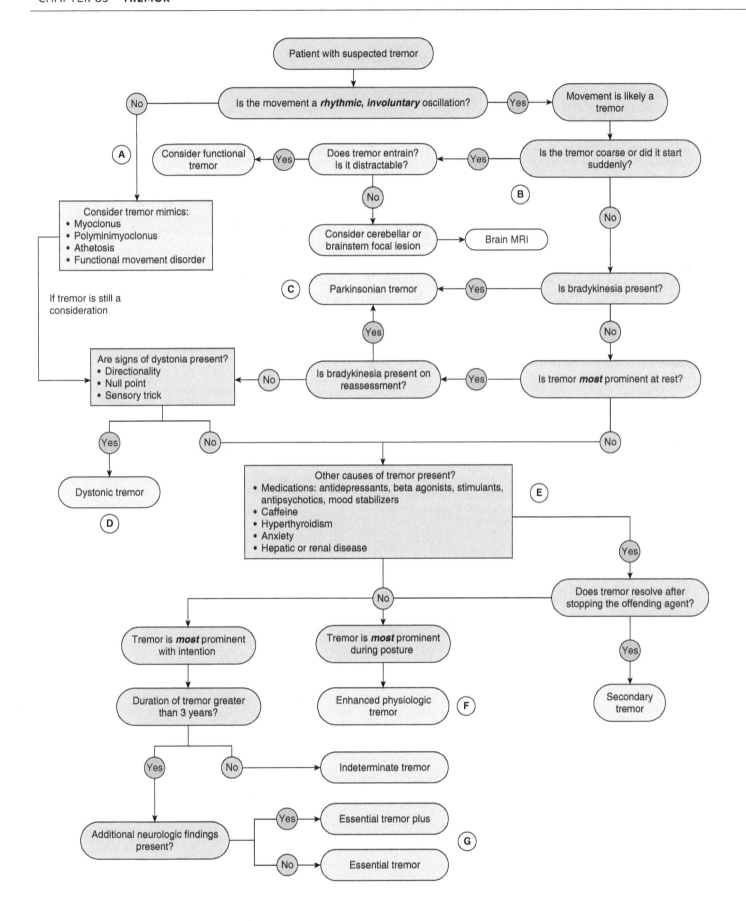

Treatment of Essential Tremor

David Coughlin and Andres Deik

A. Certain patients with mild tremor may only need tremor control for short, specific periods of time (for example, while giving a speech or going to dinner with friends). In such cases, propranolol (10–20 mg, immediate-release form) can be used as needed; if ineffective or causing side effects, alprazolam 0.25–1 mg can be tried. Daily medication may be required when as-needed medication fails.

B. Propranolol (extended release 80–160 mg daily) and primidone (typically 50–250 mg daily) are first-line agents for the management of essential tremor. Both have demonstrated efficacy in clinical trials.[1] Agent selection depends largely on the patient's preference and comorbidities. For patients with diabetes, asthma, or cardiac disease, primidone may be preferred. However, primidone can be sedating and may not be ideal for younger, employed patients; it also increases the risk of osteoporosis with long-term use. When no relevant comorbidities are present, propranolol is preferred due to its more favorable side-effect profile.

C. When first-line agents do not provide sufficient tremor control or are poorly tolerated, second-line agents can be considered either as monotherapy or as adjunctive agents. Benzodiazepines, including clonazepam and alprazolam, have been shown to be effective, but can cause sedation and carry the potential for abuse. Clonazepam (0.5–2 mg twice daily) is generally preferred given its longer duration of action. If benzodiazepines are unsuccessful, then topiramate (25–100 mg twice daily) can be tried. Side effects include cognitive slowing, weight loss, paresthesias, and, in certain populations, an increased rate of nephrolithiasis. Gabapentin may also be considered, though efficacy in clinical trials has been mixed. Finally, the β-blockers atenolol or sotalol can be considered as alternatives to propranolol, but have not been well studied.

D. While medical management is effective in some patients, approximately one-third of them discontinue medications due to either side effects or lack of efficacy. If a patient has failed first- and second-line agents, or has contraindications to their use but is not willing to consider surgical management, botulinum toxin injections can be considered. These can be effective in dampening head, voice, and limb tremors, but injections need to be repeated quarterly and rarely provide complete tremor remission.[2-4]

E. Deep brain stimulation (DBS) is a neurosurgical procedure in which electrodes are implanted in the brain and connected to programmable pulse generators that are implanted subcutaneously. For essential tremor, the electrodes are placed in the ventral intermediate nucleus of the thalamus. DBS is a well-established, efficacious treatment option for ET that significantly improves quality of life.[5] For patients with bilateral tremor who are cognitively intact, bilateral DBS is suggested. For patients with dementia or mild cognitive impairment, unilateral lead implantation is preferred, to decrease the possibility of worsening cognition.

F. Magnetic resonance–guided focused ultrasound (FUS) is a noninvasive procedure in which ultrasound beams are arranged to converge on a specific target within the brain, causing the tissue to heat until a permanent lesion is generated.[6] Currently, FUS is only approved in the United States for unilateral lesioning (and therefore results in unilateral tremor control) and can be appropriate for patients with cognitive impairment, or for patients with unilateral predominant tremor.

REFERENCES

1. Zesiewicz TA, Elble RJ, Louis ED, et al. Evidence-based guideline update: Treatment of essential tremor: report of the Quality Standards Subcommittee of the American Academy of Neurology. *Neurology.* 2011;77(19):1752–1755.
2. Jankovic J, Schwartz K, Clemence W, Aswad A, Mordaunt J. A randomized, double-blind, placebo-controlled study to evaluate botulinum toxin type A in essential hand tremor. *Mov Disord.* 1996;11(3):250–256.
3. Warrick P, Dromey C, Irish JC, Durkin L, Pakiam A, Lang A. Botulinum toxin for essential tremor of the voice with multiple anatomical sites of tremor: a crossover design study of unilateral versus bilateral injection. *Laryngoscope.* 2000;110(8):1366–1374.
4. Wissel J, Masuhr F, Schelosky L, Ebersbach G, Poewe W. Quantitative assessment of botulinum toxin treatment in 43 patients with head tremor. *Mov Disord.* 1997;12(5):722–726.
5. Flora ED, Perera CL, Cameron AL, Maddern GJ. Deep brain stimulation for essential tremor: a systematic review. *Mov Disord.* 2010;25(11):1550–1559.
6. Elias WJ, Lipsman N, Ondo WG, et al. A randomized trial of focused ultrasound thalamotomy for essential tremor. *N Engl J Med.* 2016;375 (8):730–739.

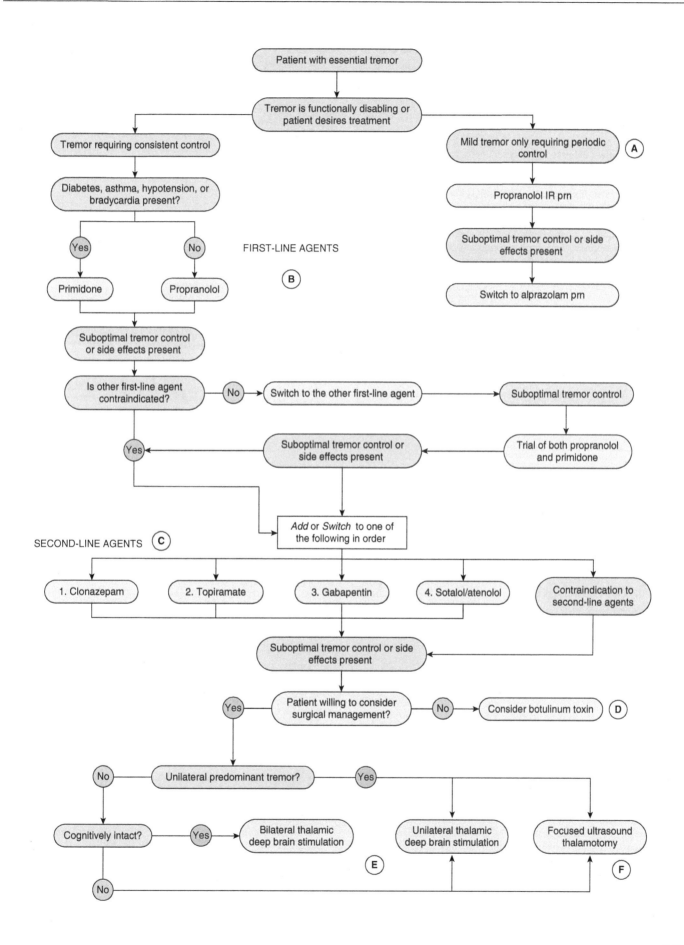

Treatment of Parkinson's Disease

Andres Deik and David Coughlin

A. Aerobic exercise may be neuroprotective, and should be recommended for all Parkinson disease (PD) patients.

B. Cognitively intact patients under age 65 years can try a monoamine oxidase type B inhibitor (MAOBI) or a dopamine agonist (DA) for the management of mild rigidity, bradykinesia, and gait changes (Table 85.1). MAOBIs tend to be well tolerated but can cause hypertension and nonspecific dizziness, and selegiline can cause insomnia; they also can cause serotonin syndrome when used in combination with other serotoninergic medications. MAOBIs are relatively weak symptomatic medications, have a narrow dosing range, and are rarely used as monotherapy. Oral ropinirole and pramipexole, and transdermal rotigotine, are the most commonly used DAs. Side effects include hypersomnolence, leg edema, compulsivity, hypotension, and psychosis.

C. Patients under 65 years old with tremor-predominant PD may try trihexyphenidyl, a powerful anticholinergic. Side effects include dry eyes, xerostomia, trouble urinating, and confusion. If this fails, consider amantadine, which can be used as monotherapy or as an adjunct to levodopa, and may be appropriate for cognitively intact elderly patients. Amantadine and trihexyphenidyl should be avoided in all patients with cognitive impairment, regardless of age; levodopa should be the first-line agent for these patients.

D. Carbidopa/levodopa should be the first line of treatment for patients who are older than 65 years, cognitively impaired, or with moderate or severe symptoms.

E. Patients with advanced PD may notice that levodopa doses provide benefit for shorter periods of time. Symptom breakthrough is known as "off" time. Options for managing off time include (1) increasing each levodopa dose, (2) shortening the interval between levodopa doses, or (3) adding an adjunctive agent. Adjunctive agents include DAs and inhibitors of dopamine breakdown (MAOBIs and the catechol-o-methyl transferase [COMT] inhibitor entacapone). The main side effects of entacapone are diarrhea and a reddish discoloration of the urine. A minority of patients will experience sudden, severe, sometimes unpredictable off periods. Subcutaneous apomorphine rescue doses may be useful in these cases, but nausea, lightheadedness, and headaches are common side effects. Treating off time with any of these strategies may trigger or worsen levodopa side effects, including dyskinesias, psychosis, hypotension, or hypersomnolence. If these therapies fail, are contraindicated, or symptoms remain inadequately managed, a time-release long-acting form of carbidopa/levodopa can be tried. As opposed to immediate release and older extended-release formulations, the time-release formulation contains dissolvable beads with different durations of effect.

F. Psychiatric side effects (paranoia, delusions, or visual hallucinations) and dyskinesias can limit the titration of dopaminergic medications. DAs are more likely than carbidopa/levodopa to cause hallucinations. When motor symptoms do not allow a reduction in carbidopa/levodopa, hallucinations can be managed with pimavanserin (a novel, highly selective inverse agonist and antagonist of the serotonin 5-HT$_{2A}$ receptors), clozapine, or quetiapine. Relatively low doses of quetiapine can manage hallucinations effectively, but somnolence is reported frequently, and Parkinsonian symptoms can worsen at high doses. Pimavanserin, in contrast, does not worsen Parkinsonism. Clozapine is an effective antipsychotic, but its use is limited by somnolence and the need for frequent screening for agranulocytosis. Dyskinesias can be managed with amantadine. Patients unable to tolerate amantadine (or with refractory dyskinesias) may benefit from deep brain stimulation (DBS) surgery. DBS can also benefit PD patients who are intolerant of higher doses of dopaminergic medications.

TABLE 85.1 DOSING AND TITRATION OF MEDICATIONS FOR PARKINSON DISEASE

Medication	Starting dose	Titration	Max dose
MAOBIs			
Rasagiline	0.5 mg daily	Increase to 1 mg daily in 2 weeks	1 mg daily
Selegiline	5 mg daily	Increase to 5 mg bid after 2 weeks	5 mg twice daily
Safinamide	50 mg daily	Increase to 100 mg daily after 2 weeks	100 mg daily
Dopamine Agonists			
Ropinirole	ER: 2 mg daily IR: 0.25 mg tid	ER: Increase by 2 mg every week IR: increase by 0.25 mg tid increments weekly	24 mg total daily dose
Pramipexole	ER: 0.375 mg daily IR: 0.125 mg tid	ER: increase by 0.375 mg every week IR: Increase by 0.125 mg tid increments weekly	4.5 mg total daily dose
Rotigotine	2 mg patch, apply daily	Increase by 2 mg patch every week	8 mg patch
Apomorphine	0.2 mL (2 mg) SC tid prn	May increase by 0.1 mL (1 mg) per dose every 3 days until single dose effectively rescues OFF period	Max single dose 0.6 mL (6 mg) Do not exceed 2 mL (20 mg) in a single day
Carbidopa/levodopa			
	IR: 25/100 mg daily ER: 25/100 mg daily	Increase 1/2 tablet weekly for IR formulations; Increase 1 tablet weekly for ER formulations	Limited by side effects
Other			
Amantadine	IR: 100 mg daily ER: 137 mg qhs	IR: Increase by 100 mg each week ER: increase to 274 mg qhs after 1 week	IR: 100 mg tid ER: 274 mg qhs
Trihexyphenidyl	0.5 mg daily	Add 0.5 mg weekly in bid or tid manner	4 mg tid Limited by side effects
Antipsychotics			
Quetiapine	25 mg qhs	Increase by 25 mg weekly	300 mg daily
Pimavanserin	34 mg daily	None	34 mg daily
Clozapine	25 mg daily	Increase by 25 mg weekly	450 mg bid

IR, Immediate release; *ER*, extended release; *MAOBI*, monoamine oxidase type B inhibitor; *SC*, subcutaneous.

G. DBS, in which an electrode is placed stereotactically into the deep brain nuclei and connected via a subcutaneous wire to an implanted pulse generator, can improve tremor, rigidity, bradykinesia, dyskinesias, off time, and, in some cases, walking in patients with PD. Ideal candidates are cognitively intact, have a normal magnetic resonance imaging examination, and have levodopa-responsive symptoms. An alternative to DBS is the carbidopa/levodopa enteral suspension pump, in which a gel formulation of carbidopa/levodopa is delivered directly to the small bowel via a jejunal feeding tube, reducing motor fluctuations.

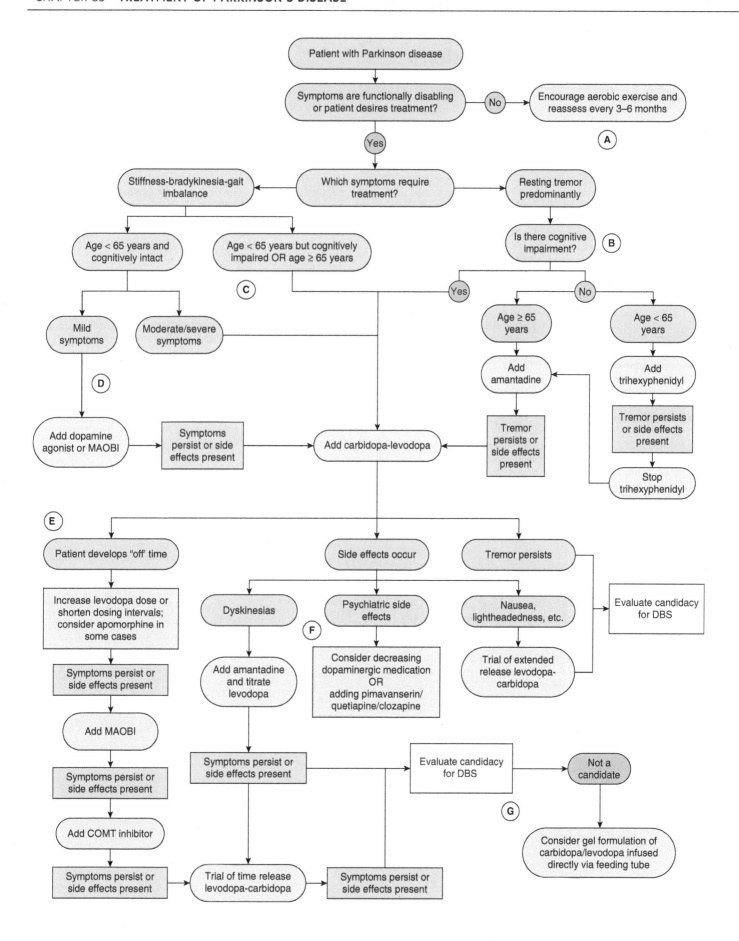

Treatment of Dystonia

David Coughlin and Andres Deik

Dystonia is characterized by sustained or intermittent muscle contractions causing abnormal, often repetitive, movements, postures, or both. Dystonic movements are typically patterned and twisting, and may be tremulous. Dystonia is often initiated or worsened by voluntary action and associated with overflow muscle activation.[1] It may involve just one body part (as with cervical dystonia), be present with one specific action (as with writer's cramp or musician's dystonia), or involve multiple areas of the body and be constant. Examination should focus on demonstrating the movement or posture in question to better characterize it. It may be useful to ask the patient to perform specific tasks such as writing or playing an instrument if they report this triggers the dystonic movement.

A. Dopa-responsive dystonia (DRD) is a genetic form of dystonia that improves significantly with levodopa therapy. Unlike patients with Parkinson disease, patients with DRD do not develop dyskinesias or motor fluctuations, and the beneficial effect of levodopa can last throughout their lifetime. Typical patients with DRD are young patients with a gait disorder from lower limb dystonia that improves with sleep and that worsens as the day goes by. This phenomenon is known as diurnal fluctuation. The most common cause of DRD is GTP cyclohydrolase 1 deficiency, but deficiencies in tyrosine hydroxylase, sepiapterin reductase, and other enzymes that are involved in the biosynthesis of dopamine can cause a similar phenotype.[2]

B. The distribution of dystonia symptoms guides selection of initial therapy. Patients with multifocal or generalized dystonia should be offered deep brain stimulation (DBS) surgery early in the course of their disease to prevent the development of disabling contractures that can limit the benefit this therapy can provide. Patients with focal or segmental dystonia, however, may respond to oral medications or botulinum toxin injections, and should try these strategies before pursuing a surgical option.

C. Injected botulinum toxins provide highly specific inhibition of presynaptic neurotransmitter (acetylcholine) release. This results in chemical denervation of the muscle injected, the effect lasting on average about 3 months. With repeated use, botulinum toxin can rarely lead to the formation of neutralizing antibodies that limit efficacy; when this happens, switching to a different type of botulinum toxin can help to recover clinical benefit.[3] Botulinum toxin injections can provide significant symptom relief and spare patients from the systemic side effects of oral medications; however, they can cause problematic muscle weakness.

D. Oral medications useful for treating dystonia include the anticholinergic trihexyphenidyl, the benzodiazepine clonazepam, and in some cases muscle relaxants such as baclofen, cyclobenzaprine, and tizanidine. Trihexyphenidyl tends to be poorly tolerated by the elderly and those with cognitive impairment, and should be avoided in these populations. It also causes dry eyes, dry mouth, constipation, urinary retention, glaucoma, forgetfulness, and confusion. Benzodiazepines, however, cause dose-related sedation and have a potential for abuse. Muscle relaxants are frequently limited by the side effect of somnolence.

E. DBS can help patients with any form of dystonia, but is most successful in the treatment of certain genetic forms of dystonia (e.g., DYT1 due to *torsinA* mutations and DYT11 typically due to *SGCE* mutations) and focal dystonias such as cervical or task-specific dystonia. Whereas genetic testing can be helpful to predict the success of the procedure in certain populations, it is not a preoperative requirement if patients are otherwise good surgical candidates and have failed (or are not likely to respond) to other treatment modalities. Potential complications of DBS include dysarthria, gait changes, Parkinsonism, hardware-related infections, and perioperative bleeding. The most common surgical target in these patients is the globus pallidus pars interna, but there is literature to suggest the subthalamic nucleus is an acceptable alternative.[4]

REFERENCES

1. Albanese A, Bhatia K, Bressman SB, et al. Phenomenology and classification of dystonia: a consensus update. *Mov Disord.* 2013;28(7):863–873.
2. Wijemanne S, Jankovic J. Dopa-responsive dystonia—clinical and genetic heterogeneity. *Nat Rev Neurol.* 2015;11:414–424.
3. Walker TJ, Dayan SH. Comparison and overview of currently available neurotoxins. *J Clin Aesthet Dermatol.* 2014;7(2):31–39.
4. Hu W, Stead M. Deep brain stimulation for dystonia. *Transl Neurodegener.* 2014;3(1):2.

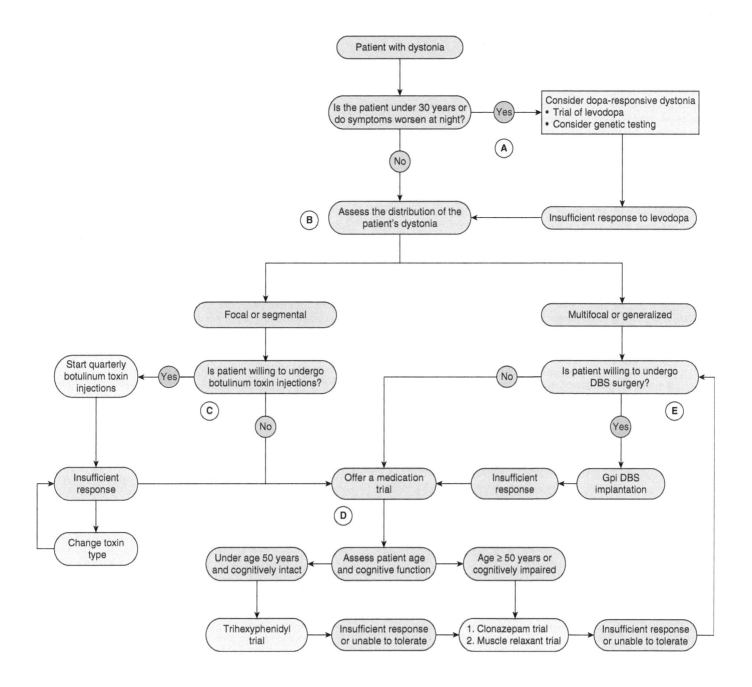

Treatment of Tics

David Coughlin and Andres Deik

A. Patients with simple motor tics can sometimes achieve acceptable symptom control with botulinum toxin injections, particularly if the areas injected involve the face (e.g., blinking tics, or tics involving the mouth or lower face). The main side effects include pain at the injection sites and excessive, undesired weakness of the area injected. Conservative dose escalation through subsequent injection trials is recommended.

B. Clonidine and other α-agonists like guanfacine can be successful in controlling tics in children (Table 87.1). They tend to cause sedation, but at times this side effect is desired in children with comorbid hyperactivity or agitation.

C. Clonazepam is a long-acting benzodiazepine that can be useful in the treatment of many different hyperkinetic movement disorders including tics. The main side effect of clonazepam is dose-related sedation, and the minimum dose that is effective should be used. Clonazepam, like all other benzodiazepines, has a potential for tolerance and abuse.

D. Topiramate is an antiepileptic that has been used successfully in some patients with tics. Side effects includes paresthesias, nephrolithiasis (it should be avoided in patients with a history of kidney stones), weight loss, and reversible cognitive impairment; the latter limits its use in elderly patients.

E. Potent dopamine receptor blockers like risperidone can be highly effective in the treatment of tics, even in severe cases. Unfortunately, the use of this class of medications is associated with the development of metabolic syndrome, sedation, drug-induced parkinsonism, and tardive dyskinesias.

F. Tetrabenazine is a VMAT2 inhibitor that depletes presynaptic dopamine reserves. Because of this, it is a powerful anti-tic medication. Unfortunately, the side effects of tetrabenazine limit its use, including depression (which can be severe at times and trigger suicidal ideation), sedation, and drug-induced parkinsonism. Newer VMAT2 inhibitors, such as valbenazine and deutetrabenazine, have become commercially available in the United States for the treatment of tardive dyskinesia and may have a role in treating tics.[1]

G. Patients with the most refractory cases of tics, particularly patients with complex motor tics or tics leading to self-injury, may be candidates for deep brain stimulation targeting the thalamus or globus pallidus pars interna.[2]

REFERENCES

1. Jankovic J. Dopamine depleters in the treatment of hyperkinetic movement disorders. *Expert Opin Pharmacother.* 2016;17(18):2461–2470.
2. Jankovic J. Therapeutic developments for tics and myoclonus. *Mov Disord.* 2015;30(11):1566–1573.

TABLE 87.1 MEDICATIONS USEFUL IN TREATMENT OF TICS			
Medication	**Starting dose**	**Titration**	**Max dose**
Guanfacine	1 mg qhs	Increase by 1 mg every week, can be used qhs or bid	4 mg daily
Clonidine	0.1 mg daily	Increase 0.1 mg weekly	0.2 mg tid
Topiramate	25 mg daily	Increase by 25 mg weekly in bid fashion	100 mg bid
Clonazepam	0.5 mg daily	Increase by 0.5 mg weekly in bid fashion	2 mg bid
Risperdal	0.5 mg daily	Increase by 0.5 mg weekly in bid fashion	3 mg bid
Tetrabenazine	12.5 mg daily	Increase by 12.5 mg weekly in tid fashion	75 mg tid

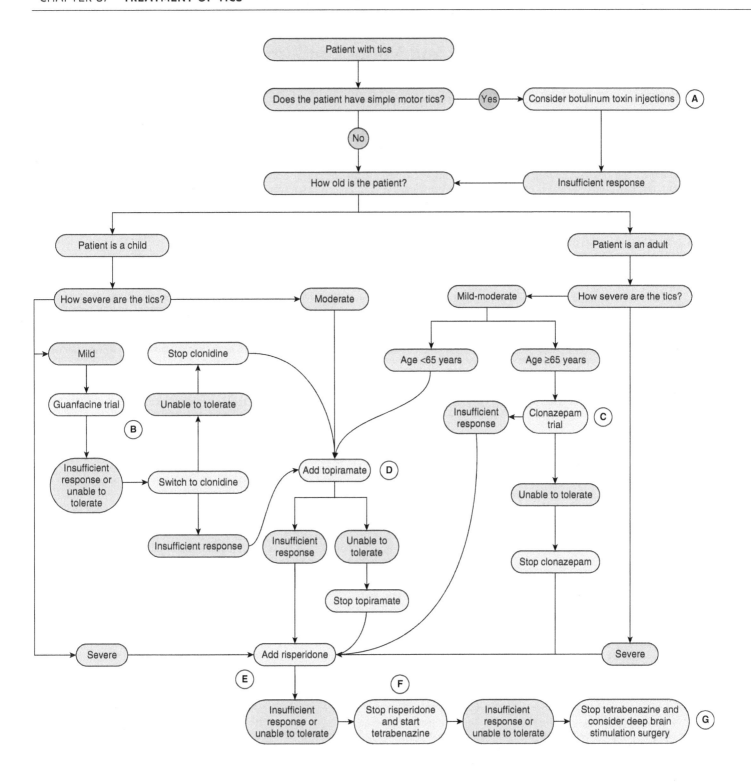

Electromyography and Nerve Conduction Studies

Colin Quinn and Raymond S. Price

Electrophysiologic study of the peripheral nervous system typically involves nerve conduction studies (NCS) and needle examination of the muscle (electromyography; EMG). NCS/EMG is useful to localize a lesion (root/plexus/nerve/neuromuscular junction/muscle) and may also characterize the specific pathology (e.g., demyelinating vs. axonal pathology). Note that the presence of multiple coexisting pathologies— for example, a myopathy in conjunction with diabetic neuropathy—will limit the applicability of this algorithm.

A. When reviewing NCS, sensory responses are examined first. In the setting of sensory symptoms or findings of sensory loss on examination, normal sensory responses localize the lesion proximal to the dorsal root ganglion (DRG) of the sensory neuron. Lesions distal to the DRG cause disconnection between the distal sensory axon and the cell body, resulting in Wallerian degeneration. This results in low amplitude or absent sensory responses. In radiculopathy or central nervous system lesions, the DRG and the distal axon are preserved, resulting in normal sensory responses.

B. In patients with weakness but no sensory symptoms and normal sensory responses, localization can be narrowed to the lower motor neuron cell bodies, motor nerves, neuromuscular junction (NMJ), or muscle.

C. While rare, isolated demyelination of the motor neurons (multifocal motor neuropathy; MMN) may clinically mimic anterior horn cell disease. MMN causes slowly progressive asymmetric weakness, typically beginning in the upper extremities. Anti-GM1 bodies are seen in some but not all patients. Conduction block is the demyelinating feature most frequently described.

D. The prototypical postsynaptic NMJ disorder is myasthenia gravis, which typically presents with fluctuating weakness and bulbar or ocular symptoms (e.g., double vision). In generalized myasthenia gravis, 2-Hz repetitive stimulation demonstrates decremental motor response amplitudes in ~80% of patients. With each successive stimulation in the first second, less acetylcholine is released, resulting in the reduced motor amplitudes.

E. Diffuse reduction of motor response amplitudes with spared sensory responses suggests either diffuse motor neuron dysfunction without sufficient collateral sprouting, as can be seen in advanced amyotrophic lateral sclerosis, or a presynaptic disorder of the NMJ such as Lambert-Eaton myasthenic syndrome (LEMS). LEMS is an autoimmune disease often associated with small cell lung cancer. LEMS presents with leg greater than arm weakness without significant muscle atrophy along with autonomic dysfunction, such as dry mouth. Testing for presynaptic disorders should be performed in all patients with diffusely reduced motor amplitudes. Similar to postsynaptic NMJ disorders, slow (2 Hz) repetitive stimulation produces a decrement in motor response amplitudes; however, LEMS can be distinguished by a >100% increase in the amplitude of the motor response following a brief period of exercise (10 seconds) of the affected muscle.

F. In patients with normal NCS and needle EMG, most peripheral nervous system issues can be excluded. One exception is myasthenia gravis with limited generalized symptoms (e.g., ocular myasthenia).

G. Myopathic features include small amplitude motor units with early recruitment. On a physiologic basis these small units are explained by the loss of myocytes that contribute to the electrical potential of a motor unit. Loss of myocytes results in ineffective force generation by individual motor units, resulting in early recruitment of several units to generate the required force.

H. Denervation on needle EMG manifests as reduced motor unit recruitment and abnormal spontaneous muscle activity in the form of fibrillation potentials and positive sharp waves. Reduced motor unit recruitment results from the loss of motor neurons and manifests as an increase in the firing frequency of the remaining motor neurons; this finding is present immediately. Fibrillation potentials and positive sharp waves start several weeks after denervation. While often associated with neurogenic disease, fibrillation potentials and positive sharp waves can also be seen in myopathic processes with fiber splitting, resulting in partial denervation of the affected myocytes (e.g., inflammatory myopathies). Chronic reinnervation results in large amplitude motor units, as remaining motor neurons will collaterally sprout to denervated myocytes. These findings appear several months after a denervating injury.

I. On motor NCS, there are two measures of conduction speed: (1) the speed of conduction between the distal stimulation site and the muscle, assessed by distal motor latency; and (2) the speed of conduction between stimulation sites, assessed by conduction velocity. In focal nerve compression, only one of these two parameters will be abnormal, localizing the site of compression. For example, the median distal motor latency would be prolonged in moderate carpal tunnel syndrome, but the median nerve conduction velocity would be normal.

J. Conduction speed is determined by the presence of myelin and large diameter axons. The electrophysiologic criteria for demyelination is shown in the flowchart. Conduction block is defined as ≥50% reduction of the proximal amplitude compared to the distal amplitude. Loss of large-diameter axons will result in mildly slowed conduction but will not meet criteria for demyelination.

K. When multiple compressive neuropathies are seen, consider diabetic polyneuropathy, amyloidosis, and, if a family history is present, hereditary neuropathy with liability to pressure palsies (HNPP).

L. The involvement of multiple nerves in an asymmetric, non–length-dependent pattern is referred to as mononeuropathy multiplex and requires assessment for autoimmune and inflammatory conditions. A mononeuropathy outside of typical compression site or multiple mononeuropathies in one limb should prompt consideration of a mass lesion or brachial neuritis.

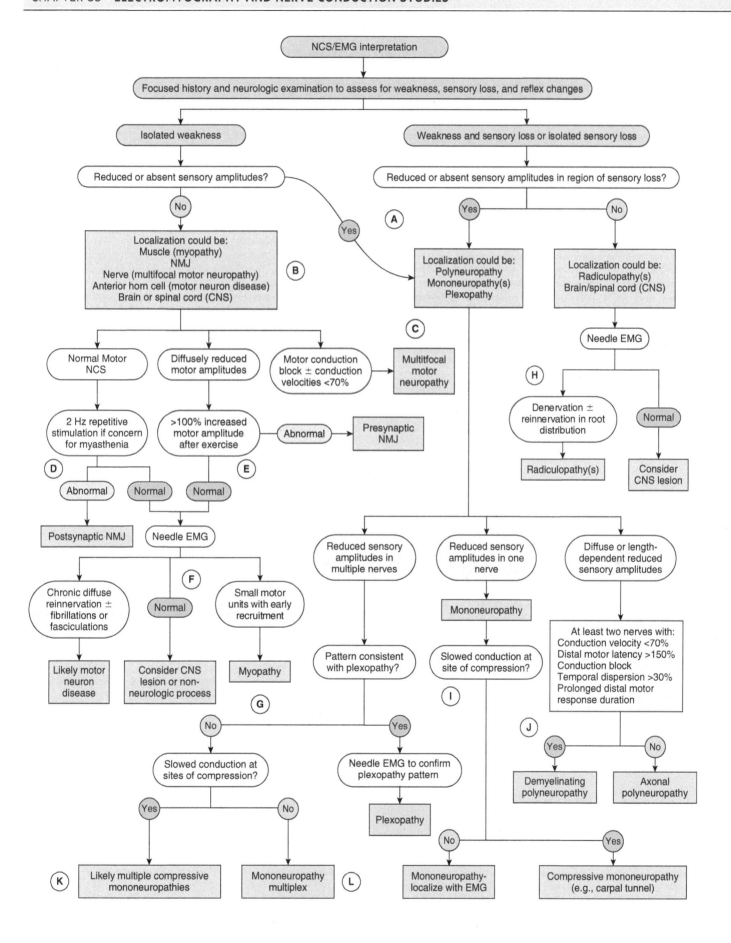

Distal Symmetric Polyneuropathy

Colin Quinn and Raymond S. Price

Polyneuropathy that involves the distal aspects of the limbs (at least initially) in a symmetric pattern is a common neurologic presentation. Sometimes referred to as a "stocking-glove" distribution, the most typical symptoms are numbness and tingling, which can take on a dysesthetic and painful quality in some patients. Symptoms tend to slowly progress in a length-dependent manner. When motor involvement occurs, it is typically milder than sensory symptoms.

A. Some causes of distal symmetric polyneuropathy may be apparent from the history. Most prominent of these is diabetes, which is the most common identifiable cause of polyneuropathy. Heavy, chronic alcohol use and numerous drugs have also been implicated. Chemotherapeutic agents, particularly platinum-containing agents, amiodarone, and oversupplementation of vitamin B6 (pyridoxine), are common offending agents. In chemotherapy-associated polyneuropathy, patients commonly note sensory disturbances near the latter portion of treatment, which continues to worsen for a period of time after the treatment cessation ("drift" or "coasting"). A family history of polyneuropathy, particularly at a young age, suggests a genetic cause. Most known hereditary neuropathies are dominantly inherited (e.g., Charcot-Marie-Tooth disease). It is important when inquiring about family history to focus not just on diagnosed polyneuropathy but also on functional symptoms (difficulty walking/falls) or other details (high arches and hammertoes) that may not have been diagnosed as neuropathy in previous generations. It is usually desirable to test a panel of genetic mutations associated with polyneuropathy rather than testing single genes when screening for familial neuropathies.

B. The duration of diabetes should be considered in comparison to the severity of disease. For example, if a patient has a severe neuropathy with recent onset of diabetes, other causes should be considered. It is reasonable to check a B12 level in all diabetic or alcoholic patients with neuropathy to exclude coexistent B12 deficiency.

C. Young age, rapid progression over a short period of time, very severe symptoms, and predominant motor involvement are unusual in common mild or idiopathic polyneuropathies and are "red flags" indicating the need for more detailed investigation. This will typically include electromyography (EMG) and nerve conduction studies to characterize the type of neuropathy, and extensive blood testing to identify an etiology. When these red flags are absent, a more basic, limited investigation consisting of testing for undiagnosed diabetes (Hgb1AC and/or 2-hour glucose tolerance test), B12 deficiency, and paraprotenemia (serum protein electrophoresis [SPEP] with immunofixation) is typically sufficient.

D. If the B12 level is in the low-normal range, a methylmalonic acid (MMA) level should be sent. An elevated MMA in this setting may indicate relative B12 deficiency.

E. Vasculitic neuropathies are caused by an immune-mediated attack on blood vessels supplying nerves. Vasculitic neuropathies can be seen in isolation or with systemic vasculitis. While often associated with an asymmetric pattern, a significant minority present with a distal symmetric polyneuropathy. Most patients experience pain and paresthesias in the affected nerves. Sedimentation rate and C-reactive protein are elevated in most patients with vasculitic neuropathy but are not specific. An antineutrophil cytoplasmic antibody (ANCA) is a more specific serum test seen in patients with some systemic vasculitides. The presence of other rheumatologic markers may suggest vasculitis in the setting of another rheumatologic condition.

F. Amyloidosis is caused by the deposition of protein fibrils that aggregate in tissues. Amyloid neuropathy can be familial or acquired. In primary amyloid, an immunoglobulin light chain is deposited in the tissues. Secondary amyloid related to other chronic rheumatologic disease is not associated with neuropathy. Familial amyloidosis is most commonly caused by transthyretin (TTR) gene mutations, though there are other known genetic causes. TTR amyloid is a target of new specific therapies, such as inotersen and patisiran, and it is therefore important to identify patients with TTR mutations.

G. Polyneuropathies related to heavy metal exposures are a frequent concern of patients but an atypical cause of neuropathy. Specific occupations and systemic symptoms such as gastrointestinal symptoms may raise suspicion for a toxic exposure. Lead neuropathy can be seen in children who ingest lead-based paints and can cause progressive weakness affecting the wrist and finger extensors with relative preservation of sensation.

H. Paraneoplastic neuropathies occur in patients with a variety of cancers. Anti-Hu (Antineuron nuclear antigen [ANNA1]) is most commonly seen with small cell lung cancer (SCLC) and is associated with distal sensory polyneuropathies or pure non–length-dependent sensory ganglionopathies. Collapsing response mediator protein 5 (CRMP-5) antibodies are associated with SCLC and thymoma. Amphiphysin is associated with SCLC and breast cancer. In addition to polyneuropathy these antibodies are associated with various central nervous system syndromes including encephalomyelitis, limbic encephalitis, and cerebellar degeneration.

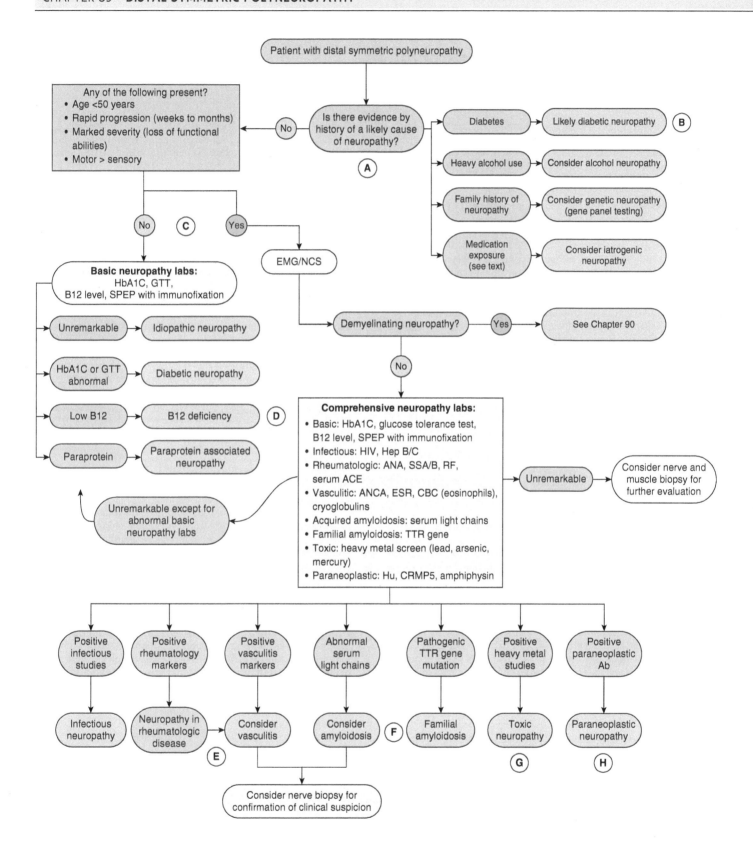

Demyelinating Neuropathies

Noah Levinson and Christyn Edmundson

Nerve conduction studies (NCSs) can determine whether a neuropathy is due to injury to the nerve axon (axonal neuropathy) or to the myelin sheath (demyelinating neuropathy). As the number of conditions that cause demyelinating neuropathy is quite limited, this distinction is clinically important and helps focus the diagnostic evaluation. While specific electrophysiologic findings vary between hereditary and acquired demyelinating neuropathies, slowed conduction velocities (<70% normal) and prolonged distal motor latencies (>150% normal) are characteristic features in both.

A. Diffusely and uniformly slowed nerve conduction velocities strongly suggest an inherited demyelinating neuropathy. In contrast, variably slowed conduction velocities, conduction block, or abnormal temporal dispersion suggest an acquired process. Acute axonal injury or nerve transection can electrodiagnostically mimic conduction block before Wallerian degeneration of the distal axon occurs. This is known as "pseudoconduction block" and can be clarified by repeating NCS after several days or weeks.

B. Charcot-Marie-Tooth disease (CMT) refers to a group of hereditary sensory and motor polyneuropathies categorized by electrophysiologic findings (demyelinating or axonal) and clinical and genetic features. Features that raise suspicion for a hereditary neuropathy include foot deformities (i.e., pes cavus, hammertoes) and a family history of similar neuropathies. CMT1A, which is caused by a duplication in the *PMP22* gene, accounts for ~70% of hereditary demyelinating neuropathies. There is no disease-modifying therapy currently available for any form of CMT, and treatment consists primarily of supportive care such as bracing and physical therapy.

C. Hereditary neuropathy with liability to pressure palsies (HNPP) causes a polyneuropathy with intermediate conduction velocities, as well as multiple demyelinating mononeuropathies at sites of common nerve entrapment (i.e., median neuropathies at the wrists, ulnar neuropathies at the elbows, and common peroneal neuropathies at the fibular heads). HNPP is caused by *PMP22* deletion (allelic with CMT1A). As with CMT, there is no disease-specific treatment.

D. In patients with demyelinating neuropathies with hereditary features, genetic testing can provide a definitive diagnosis. The exact testing strategy (i.e., testing for a single gene mutation, a panel of genetic tests, whole exome sequencing) depends on local cost and availability of different approaches. Thorough genetic testing will uncover a responsible gene mutation in up to 90% of patients with hereditary demyelinating neuropathies.

E. In addition to HNPP, multiple demyelinating mononeuropathies at sites of common nerve entrapment should prompt consideration of transthyretin (*TTR*) hereditary amyloidosis. *TTR* hereditary amyloidosis often causes an axonal polyneuropathy in addition to multiple compression neuropathies, and is also associated with cardiac and renal disorders. Identification of *TTR* amyloid is essential given effective disease-modifying therapy (patisiran and inotersen).

F. Guillain-Barré syndrome (GBS) is a clinically heterogeneous group of acute inflammatory neuropathies. The most common subtype is acute inflammatory demyelinating polyneuropathy (AIDP), a rapidly progressive demyelinating polyneuropathy causing ascending weakness and numbness. Axonal GBS variants have similar clinical characteristics but lack demyelinating findings on NCS. Often preceded by a mild viral or diarrheal illness, GBS is thought to be related to antigenic molecular mimicry of proteins found on nerve axons or the myelin sheath. Cytoalbuminologic dissociation (elevated protein with normal white blood cells) in the cerebrospinal fluid (CSF) supports a diagnosis of GBS, but may be absent early in the disease course. While a variety of disorders can mimic GBS clinically, fewer conditions produce both rapidly progressive sensorimotor symptoms and the peripheral demyelination seen on NCS in AIDP. These include human immunodeficiency virus (HIV)-related inflammatory demyelinating polyradiculoneuropathy, diphtheritic neuropathy, polyneuropathy associated with immune checkpoint inhibitors (including nivolumab, pembrolizumab, and nivolumab), hexacarbon or arsenic toxicity, and, rarely, atypical cases of lymphomatous neuropathy. By definition, AIDP is a monophasic illness with slow recovery over weeks to months. Treatment with intravenous immunoglobulin (IVIG) or plasmapheresis improves recovery. Disease relapse or clinical worsening more than 8 weeks after symptom onset should prompt consideration of chronic inflammatory demyelinating polyneuropathy (CIDP).

G. A number of conditions cause a more chronically progressive demyelinating neuropathy. CIDP typically causes slowly progressive, relatively symmetric, weakness and numbness. Weakness is typically more prominent than sensory loss and involves both proximal and distal muscles. As in AIDP, CSF cytoalbuminologic dissociation helps confirm the diagnosis, though both HIV and immune checkpoint inhibitors can cause CIDP associated with elevated CSF protein and leukocytes. Initial treatment should consist of corticosteroids or IVIG; plasmapheresis may also be used. If refractory, rituximab, cyclophosphamide, and azathioprine may be considered. Consider testing refractory patients for anti-neurofascin antibodies; when present, consider rituximab therapy. Multifocal acquired demyelinating sensory and motor polyneuropathy (MADSAM), a variant of CIDP, presents with asymmetric weakness and numbness, and multifocal motor neuropathy (MMN), which is associated with anti-GM1 antibodies, present with pure motor symptoms, most prominent in the upper extremities. Some chronic demyelinating neuropathies are associated with serum paraproteins, and are often refractory to traditional CIDP treatment (see Chapter 91).

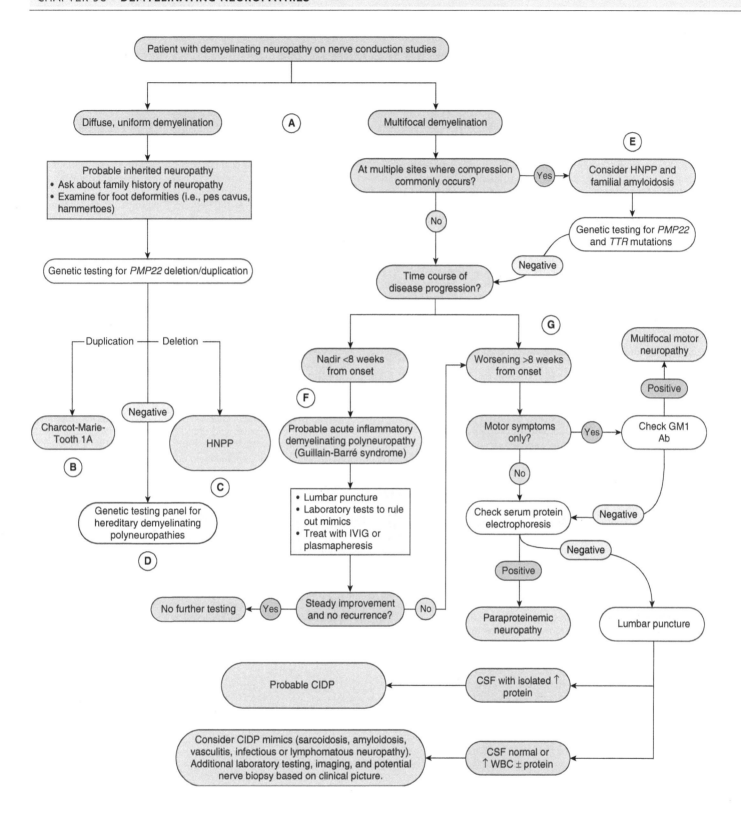

Paraprotein-Associated Neuropathies

Colin Quinn and Raymond S. Price

Neuropathies associated with monoclonal gammopathies (paraproteinemias) are relatively uncommon. Paraprotein subtypes most frequently associated with polyneuropathy include heavy chains (IgM, IgA, and IgG) and light chains (kappa or lambda). Determining whether a paraproteinemia is clinically significant requiring specific treatment or is an unrelated finding can be complex. Hematologic consultation is often necessary to determine whether the paraprotein is the consequence of hematologic malignancy.

A. Nerve conduction studies are helpful in differentiating demyelinating from axonal neuropathies. Disorders resulting in loss of myelin result in prolonged distal latencies greater than 150% of normal, slowing of conduction velocity to less than 70% of normal, and partial conduction block. Pure axonal neuropathies cause reduced or absent sensory and/or motor responses with normal or mildly slowed conduction velocities or prolonged distal latencies.

B. IgA M-proteins generally require further evaluation with bone marrow biopsy regardless of their concentration.

C. Light chain paraproteins occur when a monoclonal protein is produced without an associated heavy chain component; these can form into fibrils, which may be deposited in tissues causing multisystem disease as seen in AL amyloidosis. This fibril deposition may be seen on a fat pad or nerve and muscle biopsy. If there is a high clinical suspicion, AL amyloid should still be considered even with negative biopsies. Not all light chain overproduction results in amyloidosis. As seen with heavy chain overproduction, light chain paraproteins may be produced in monoclonal gammopathy of undetermined significance (MGUS) or in clonal plasma cell disorders. Light chain ratios are often helpful to determine the presence of a true monoclonal protein from polyclonal immune responses or impaired light chain excretion due to renal dysfunction.

D. IgG paraproteins are most commonly associated with MGUS, but all heavy and light chain subtypes can be produced at low levels without clear systemic effects as seen in MGUS. The majority of patients with MGUS have a monoclonal protein of less than 1.0 g/dL; by definition, all MGUS patients have a monoclonal protein concentration less than 3.0 g/dL. The particular concentration of monoclonal protein chosen here for further workup (1.5 g/dL) is somewhat arbitrary, and evaluation should be planned in partnership with a hematologist. All patients with suspected MGUS should undergo an evaluation for "CRAB" signs: hyperCalcemia, Renal insufficiency, Anemia, and Bone lesions.

E. Waldenstrom macroglobulinemia (WM) is a disorder of lymphoplasmacytic cell proliferation and IgM protein production. Most patients with WM present with nonspecific fatigue, though they may demonstrate weight loss, bleeding (e.g., nose bleeds), hepatomegaly, or splenomegaly. The neuropathy associated with WM is sensory predominant and typically unresponsive to immune modulation or chemotherapy.

F. Type 1 cryoglobulinemia produces symptoms related to vascular occlusion in the setting of cryoprecipitation. These symptoms include skin necrosis, livedo reticularis, and ischemia of the digits. A significant minority of these patients develop a peripheral neuropathy, which typically presents as mononeuropathy multiplex.

G. POEMS is an acronym for Peripheral neuropathy, Organomegaly, Endocrinopathy, Monoclonal gammopathy, and Skin changes. Most patients do not have all of these clinical features. A diagnosis of POEMS requires the presence of peripheral neuropathy and a monoclonal protein along with one other major criteria (sclerotic bone lesions, Castleman disease or elevated vascular endothelial growth factor [VEGF]) and one minor criteria (organomegaly, extravascular volume overload, endocrinopathy, skin changes, papilledema, or thrombocytosis/polycythemia). The monoclonal heavy chain subtype is typically IgG or IgA. IgM heavy chains are rare in POEMS. The light chain is almost always lambda. Isolated sclerotic bone lesions can be treated with radiation whereas more diffuse disease is treated with chemotherapy with or without hematopoietic cell transplantation.

H. CANOMAD syndrome (Chronic Ataxic Neuropathy, Ophthalmoplegia, IgM paraprotein, cold Agglutinins, and Disialosyl antibodies) results in sensory ataxia and ophthalmoplegia. Polyclonal IgM antibodies that react with disialosyl epitopes of gangliosides are common. Additionally, most patients have IgM monoclonal antibodies.

I. Distal acquired demyelinating symmetric (DADS) neuropathy is characterized by insidiously progressive predominant sensory symptoms with minimal or no weakness. Sensory symptoms can be severe and cause a sensory ataxia. On examination there is sensory loss along with areflexia. Nerve conduction studies often demonstrate absent sensory responses with prolongation of the distal motor latencies, though there may be other signs of demyelination. Approximately two-thirds of patients with a DADS phenotype have a monoclonal protein, which is overwhelmingly IgM kappa, and these patients appear refractory to immunomodulatory treatment. Approximately 50% of patients with IgM kappa DADS have myelin-associated glycoprotein (MAG) antibodies. Patients with a DADS phenotype without a monoclonal protein appear to have a similar response rate to chronic inflammatory demyelinating polyneuropathy.

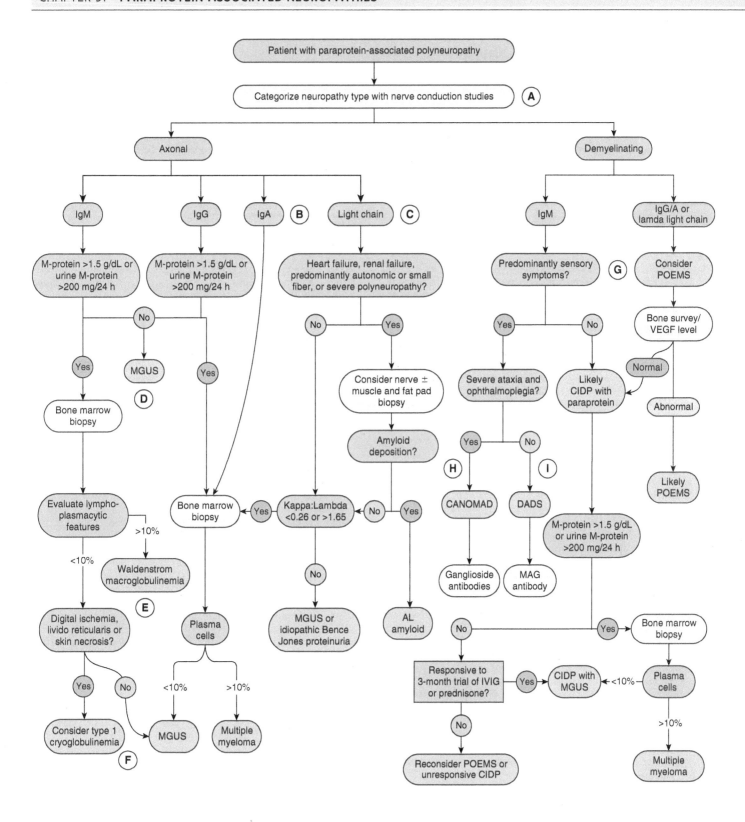

Mononeuropathy Multiplex

Noah Levinson and Raymond S. Price

Mononeuropathy multiplex (sometimes referred to as mononeuritis multiplex) is defined as lesions affecting two or more nerves that cannot be explained by a single root or plexus injury. The involvement of multiple nerves is usually in an asymmetric, non–length-dependent pattern and develops subacutely. If this process continues with additional individual nerve involvement, it can progress to appear clinically and electrophysiologically identical to a more common polyneuropathy. An extensive evaluation for the etiology of mononeuropathy multiplex should be performed, as treatable autoimmune and inflammatory causes are frequently identified.

A. Nerve conduction studies and electromyography (NCS/EMG) should be performed in all patients with suspected mononeuropathy multiplex to confirm the pattern of nerve injury and to characterize the specific nerve pathology (e.g., demyelinating vs. axonal).

B. In a patient with multiple mononeuropathies at common sites of compression (e.g., ulnar neuropathy at the elbow) and a family history of polyneuropathy, hereditary neuropathy with liability to pressure palsies (HNPP) and familial amyloidosis should be considered. HNPP is caused by a deletion of the *PMP22* gene and would be suggested by moderate diffuse slowing of the motor conduction velocities that do not meet criteria for demyelination. Familial amyloidosis, which is most commonly caused by a transthyretin mutation, would be suspected in patients with autonomic dysfunction or systemic disease (e.g., cardiac abnormalities).

C. Neurolymphomatosis is the direct invasion of nerve roots or peripheral nerves by lymphoma cells. Depending on the extent of involvement, this can present as an individual mononeuropathy, radiculopathy, or mononeuropathy multiplex. In bone marrow transplant patients, graft-versus-host disease occurs when the transplanted immune cells attack organs of the bone marrow recipient. The skin, gastrointestinal tract, and liver are the most commonly affected organs, but rarely peripheral nerves can also be injured in this disease. Diagnosis of these conditions requires nerve biopsy.

D. Leprosy is rare in the United States, but should be considered as a cause of axonal mononeuritis multiplex in endemic areas in Mexico, Central America, South America, and Africa. In tuberculoid leprosy, nerve injury usually occurs around skin lesions. In lepromatous leprosy, nerve injury can be much more diffuse.

E. Lead toxicity is a very rare cause of neuropathy in adults. It has an unusual pattern that is classically an isolated motor neuropathy with a predilection for extensor muscles of the arms and legs. Gasoline and certain adhesives contain n-hexane, a chemical that is toxic to peripheral nerves. Chronic sniffing, or huffing, of these substances classically causes a motor-predominant axonal multifocal neuropathy.

F. Primary vasculitides frequently cause neuropathy in addition to other end-organ injury, and neuropathy often occurs early in the course of systemic vasculitis. Subacute onset and rapid progression of symptoms, severe pain, and the presence of concurrent systemic complaints suggest vasculitis. Peripheral nervous system involvement most commonly occurs in small and medium-vessel primary vasculitides, which include polyarteritis nodosa (PAN), granulomatosis with polyangiitis (formerly Wegner's granulomatosis), microscopic polyangiitis, and eosinophilic granulomatosis with polyangiitis (formerly Churg-Strauss syndrome). Treatment is typically high-dose steroids and cyclophosphamide. A secondary vasculitic neuropathy can be caused by cryoglobulinemia and numerous autoimmune diseases, most commonly lupus, rheumatoid arthritis, Sjögren syndrome, and Behçet disease. Treatment is targeted to the underlying autoimmune condition. Patients with peripheral nerve injury from either primary or secondary vasculitides will likely also need physical therapy, bracing, and neuropathic pain management for the nerve injury.

G. Nonsystemic vasculitic neuropathy is an isolated vasculitis of the peripheral nerves without other end-organ involvement. These patients must be carefully monitored because up to 10% of these patients will eventually develop systemic vasculitis. Nerve and muscle biopsy is necessary for diagnosis. Biopsy of both muscle and nerve is recommended to increase the diagnostic yield of the biopsy. Treatment is similar to systemic vasculitis with high-dose oral steroids and cyclophosphamide.

H. Amyloidosis should be suspected in patients with autonomic dysfunction or systemic disease such as cardiac abnormalities or renal failure. Serum protein electrophoresis with immunofixation may show elevated serum free light chains. Amyloid deposition may be seen on a fat pad or nerve and muscle biopsy.

I. Isolated demyelination of the motor neurons (multifocal motor neuropathy, MMN) may clinically mimic anterior horn cell disease. MMN causes slowly progressive asymmetric weakness, typically beginning in the upper extremities. Anti-GM1 bodies are seen in some but not all patients.

J. Acquired demyelinating neuropathies can rarely cause mononeuropathy multiplex. Guillain-Barré syndrome is classically symmetric, but a small subset of patients may have asymmetric features. When chronic inflammatory demyelinating polyneuropathy presents as mononeuropathy multiplex, this variant is known as multifocal acquired demyelinating sensory and motor polyneuropathy (MADSAM). The key to distinguishing these disorders from vasculitis is evidence of multifocal demyelinating features on the NCS.

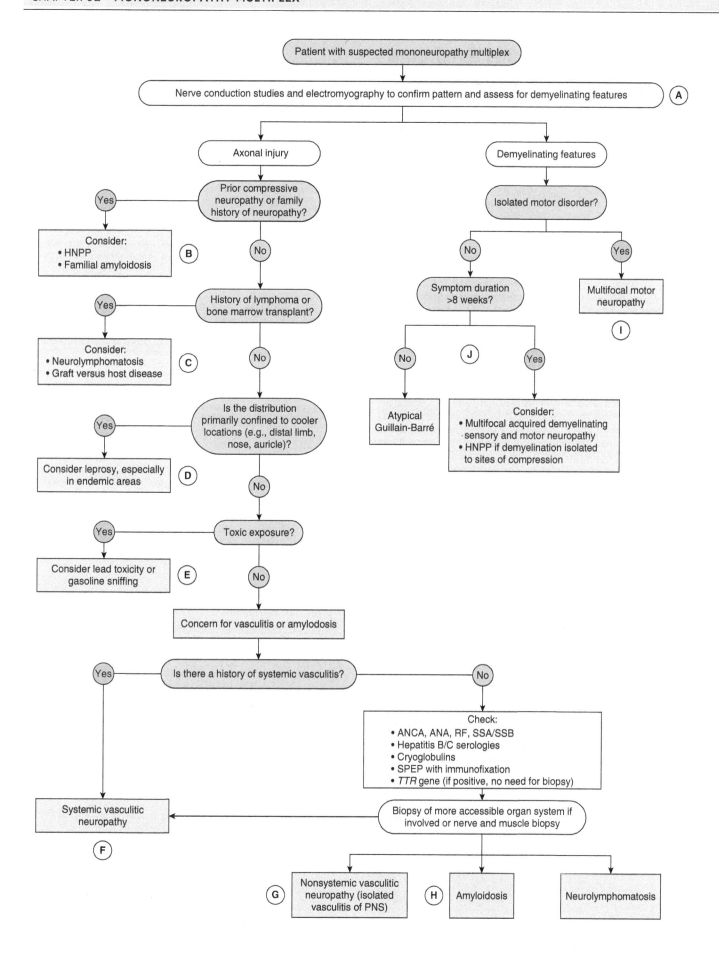

Carpal Tunnel Syndrome

Colin Quinn and Raymond S. Price

Carpal tunnel syndrome (CTS) refers to symptomatic compression of the median nerve in the wrist as it passes through the carpal tunnel, which is bounded by the carpal bones and the transverse carpal ligament. In CTS, a combination of compression and inflammation results in demyelination and eventually axonal injury of the median nerve. The resulting median neuropathy at the wrist is the most common mononeuropathy seen clinically. Hand paresthesias are one of the hallmark symptoms of CTS; weakness in median-nerve-innervated intrinsic hand muscles is seen in more severe cases. The palmar cutaneous branches of the median nerve arise prior to the carpal tunnel, and therefore it is only the digital branches going to the thumb, index, middle, and half of the ring finger that are affected in CTS. Despite this specific distribution of median nerve sensory changes, many patients are unable to localize their symptoms in the hand and may even describe paresthesia in the forearm where there is no median sensory innervation.

A. While there are multiple intrinsic hand muscles innervated by the median nerve after it passes through the carpal tunnel, the abductor pollicis brevis (APB) muscle is the most useful to assess clinically. The APB is easily inspected for atrophy and weakness: atrophy can be seen in the lateral portion of the thenar eminence, and weakness is seen with thumb abduction. When weakness is present, confirmation of the diagnosis with nerve conduction studies/electromyography (NCS/EMG) is appropriate. In patients with isolated paresthesias or numbness in a clear distribution of the median nerve but without weakness, a trial of conservative management is reasonable prior to performing further testing. This typically consists of a "cock-up" wrist splint at night, which places the wrist in mild extension and maximizes the space within the carpal tunnel, thereby decompressing the median nerve.

B. Definitive diagnosis of CTS requires electrophysiologic testing with EMG/NCS. In CTS, reduced median nerve sensory conduction across the wrist is frequently identified on a standard median sensory study from the index finger. However, the most sensitive finding for CTS is reduced mixed median nerve sensory conduction after palmar stimulation, which assesses median sensory conduction through the carpal tunnel across a smaller distance. To ensure that the reduced median conduction velocity is secondary to CTS and not a more diffuse process such as an axonal or demyelinating polyneuropathy, it should be compared to ulnar sensory conduction across the wrist. In more severe CTS, motor involvement will be apparent on EMG/NCS. For the median motor study, the median distal motor latency assesses the time required for motor conduction through the carpal tunnel to the APB muscle, which can be prolonged in moderate-severe CTS. Note that the median motor conduction velocity will remain normal in CTS because that velocity assesses median motor conduction in the forearm and not through the carpal tunnel.

C. The complete absence of responses on median sensory and motor NCS indicates median nerve pathology but does not reveal the location of the median nerve injury. In these instances, a more complex NCS can be done (such as an ulnar/median lumbrical comparison study) to more clearly localize the lesion. Additionally, needle examination of median innervated muscles proximal (e.g., flexor pollicis longus) and distal (e.g., APB) to the carpal tunnel can be informative.

D. In patients with mild to moderate CTS, intracarpal steroid injections are given with the goal of reducing inflammation affecting the median nerve. Such injections have demonstrated symptomatic benefit with a variable duration of relief. Unfortunately, most patients experience an eventual return of their symptoms.

E. Carpal tunnel release surgery involves incision of the transverse ligament and can be performed as an open or endoscopic procedure. Good symptom relief is seen in approximately three-quarters of patients after surgery.

REFERENCE

1. Jarvik JG. Surgery versus non-surgical therapy for carpal tunnel syndrome: a randomised parallel-group trial. *Lancet.* 2009;374(9695):1074–1081.

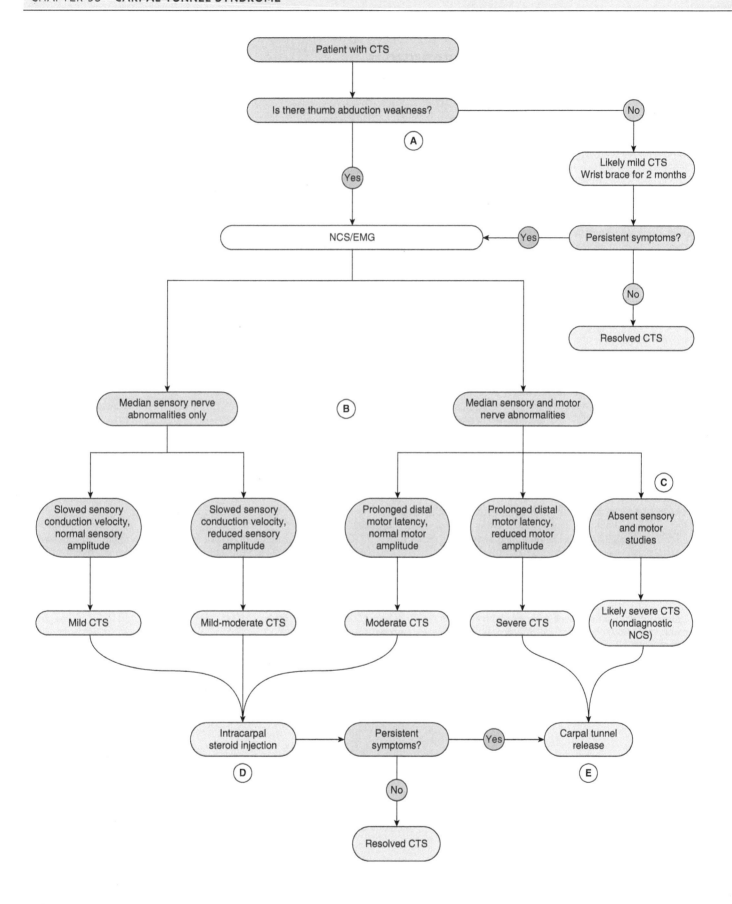

Brachial Plexus Syndromes

Raymond S. Price

The brachial plexus is formed from the C5–C8 and T1 nerve roots. It is divided into three trunks: the upper trunk is formed by the junction of the C5 and C6 nerve roots, the middle trunk is a continuation of the C7 nerve root, and the lower trunk is formed by the junction of the C8 and T1 nerve roots. Each trunk gives off an anterior and posterior division. The posterior divisions from each trunk form the posterior cord, which terminates in the axillary and radial nerves. The anterior division from the upper and middle trunk join to form the lateral cord, which terminates in the musculocutaneous nerve and half of the median nerve. The anterior division of the lower trunk continues as the medial cord, which terminates in the ulnar nerve and the other half of the median nerve. Brachial plexus syndromes are an uncommon cause of arm weakness and numbness. As a general rule, it is much more likely that a patient with these symptoms has a cervical radiculopathy (or multiple cervical radiculopathies) or multiple mononeuropathies. Nevertheless, brachial plexus syndromes are important to identify as the likely etiologies and evaluation are different from either radiculopathy or mononeuropathy.

A. A brachial plexus cord lesion can usually be distinguished from a cervical radiculopathy based on the clinical examination; however, it is usually not possible to distinguish a cervical radiculopathy from a brachial plexus trunk lesion. In the latter scenario, nerve conduction studies and needle electromyography (NCS/EMG) would be indicated to confirm the clinical localization of a brachial plexus cord lesion or to distinguish a brachial plexus trunk lesion from a cervical radiculopathy. NCS should demonstrate normal sensory responses in the setting of radiculopathy. In an upper trunk or lateral cord injury, the lateral antebrachial and median sensory responses should be abnormal. In a middle trunk or posterior cord injury, the radial sensory response should be abnormal. In a lower trunk or medial cord injury, the medial antebrachial and ulnar sensory responses should be abnormal.

B. Trauma is a frequent cause of brachial plexus injury, particularly motorcycle accidents.

C. Brachial plexus injury, particularly involving T1 fibers in the lower trunk, is a known complication of coronary artery bypass grafting surgery. It is felt to occur due to stretching or compressive injury during the operation. This injury can result in the unusual NCS findings of a preserved ulnar sensory amplitude with a reduced medial antebrachial cutaneous sensory amplitude.

D. Radiation plexopathy is a delayed complication of radiation. Patients typically present with insidiously progressive painless weakness. Clinical myokymia or myokymic discharges on EMG can be seen in a subset of patients.

E. In classic neuralgic amyotrophy (also known as brachial neuritis or Parsonage Turner syndrome), the patient has severe pain that spontaneously resolves. After the pain resolves, arm weakness is noted. Numbness is either absent or minimally present in a patchy distribution. Persistent pain with weakness should prompt reconsideration of the diagnosis with a particular focus on cervical radiculopathy or a mass lesion. The pattern of weakness is unusual in neuralgic amyotrophy in that it does not localize well to a particular portion of the brachial plexus or a single nerve root. There is a predilection for the pronator teres, flexor digitorum profundus, and infraspinatus muscles, in addition to the deltoid, serratus anterior, triceps, and trapezius. While there is no specific treatment, the acute pain in brachial neuritis should be treated symptomatically and may require narcotic pain medications. Weakness typically spontaneously improves by around 3 months after onset.

F. Neurogenic thoracic outlet syndrome, in which the lower trunk of the brachial plexus is compressed by bone or fibrous tissue, is rare. NCS will show a reduced ulnar sensory amplitude and medial antebrachial sensory amplitude as well as denervation of the ulnar and median-innervated hand muscles on needle EMG. Cervical x-rays can be done to assess for a cervical rib or elongated C7 transverse process, and magnetic resonance imaging of the chest to assess for a fibrous band. Treatment consists of surgical decompression, such as removal of a cervical rib or lysis of a fibrous band.

G. For most patients, brachial neuritis is a monophasic event. Rarely, patients can have recurrent brachial neuritis or a family history of brachial neuritis. In these patients, a genetic etiology should be considered. The most common genetic mutation in hereditary neuralgic amyotrophy is the *SEPT9* mutation. Many but not all patients have associated facial dysmorphisms including hypotelorism or epicanthal folds.

H. Local mass lesions can compress or invade the brachial plexus causing neurologic dysfunction. Typical causes are breast cancer or lymphoma. Slowly progressive symptoms over weeks-months and persistent pain should raise concern for a mass lesion.

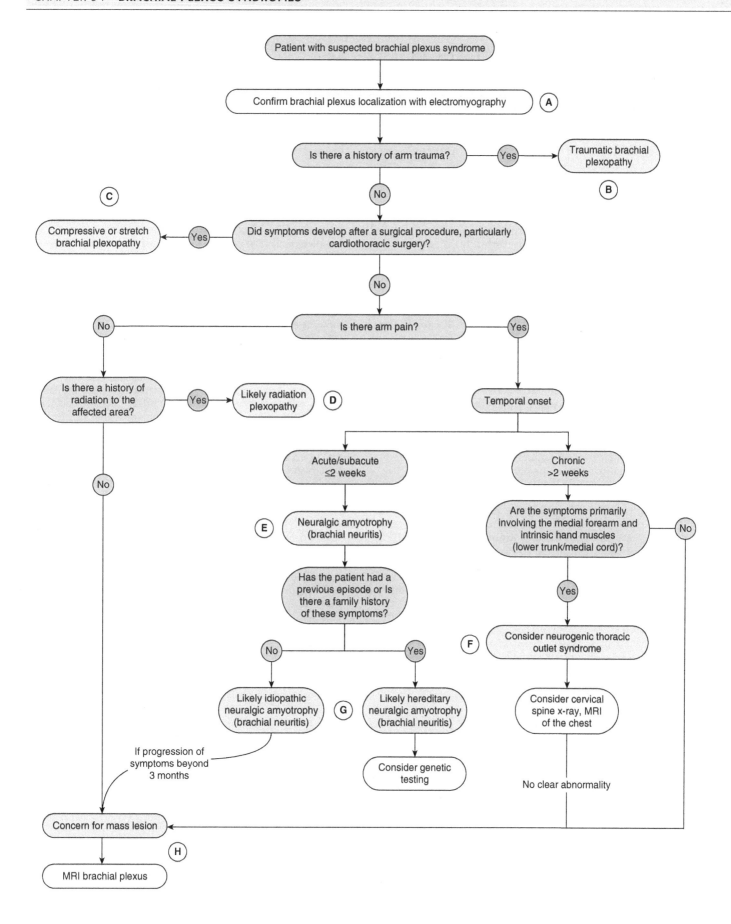

Lumbosacral Plexus Syndromes

Noah Levinson and Christyn Edmundson

The lumbosacral plexus is formed from the L1–S3 nerve roots. It is divided into an upper component (the lumbar plexus), which innervates hip flexion, hip adduction, and knee extension, and a lower component that innervates hip extension, hip abduction, knee flexion, and all ankle and toe movements. Lumbosacral plexus syndromes are an uncommon cause of leg weakness and numbness. As a general rule, it is much more likely that a patient with these symptoms has a lumbosacral radiculopathy (or multiple radiculopathies) or multiple mononeuropathies. Nevertheless, lumbosacral plexus syndromes are important to identify, as the causes and evaluation differ from that with radiculopathy or mononeuropathy.

A. While an L5 or S1 radiculopathy can usually be distinguished from a lower lumbosacral plexus lesion based on the clinical examination, an upper lumbosacral plexus lesion (lumbar plexus) usually cannot be differentiated from an L3 or L4 radiculopathy. Nerve conduction studies and needle electromyography (NCS/EMG) are necessary to confirm the localization to the lumbosacral plexus. NCS shows normal sensory responses in the setting of radiculopathy, whereas in a lumbosacral plexus lesion the amplitude of the saphenous sensory response is reduced when the upper portion is involved and the amplitudes of the sural and superficial peroneal sensory responses are reduced when the lower portion is involved.

B. An ischemic lumbosacral plexopathy should be considered following any surgical procedure that requires cross-clamping of the aorta, such as aortic aneurysm repair or kidney transplant.

C. Radiation plexopathy typically arises months to years after local radiation therapy. Symptoms progress slowly for years, and these patients often have minimal or no pain, which distinguishes it from other causes of plexopathy. The finding of myokymia on needle EMG is seen in some cases, though the absence of myokymia does not exclude radiation plexopathy.

D. Malignancies most often involve the lumbosacral plexus by direct tumor extension. The most commonly involved tumors arise from local tissues: colorectal, ureteral, bladder, cervical, uterine, ovarian, vaginal, testicular, penile, and prostate carcinomas and retroperitoneal or pelvic sarcomas. Distant malignant spread can also occur with common cancers, such as breast and lung carcinoma. Lymphoma can directly infiltrate the plexus or cause compression injury.

E. Inflammatory serologies should include Sjogren's Syndrome anti-RO/anti-LA antibodies (SSA/SSB), antinuclear antibody (ANA), and anti-neutrophil cytoplasmic autoantibody (ANCA); erythrocyte sedimentation rate (ESR), C-reactive protein (CRP), angiotensin-converting enzyme (ACE), and serum protein electrophoresis (SPEP) with immunofixation should also be tested. Testing for human immunodeficiency virus (HIV), Epstein-Barr virus (EBV), cytomegalovirus (CMV), varicella-zoster virus (VZV), syphilis, Lyme disease (if in an endemic area), and tuberculosis should be considered. Cerebrospinal fluid (CSF) should be evaluated, including cytology and flow cytometry.

F. Diabetic amyotrophy, also known as diabetic radiculoplexus neuropathy or Bruns-Garland syndrome, typically presents as severe asymmetric pelvic and leg pain followed by weakness in the proximal leg, though symptoms may also involve distal muscles. It is often seen in diabetic patients with recent improvement in glycemic control or who have had weight loss. Symptoms usually progress over several weeks and may spread to involve the contralateral limb. Improvement is gradual and incomplete in most patients. While the underlying mechanism is uncertain, some evidence suggests nerve damage due to ischemic microvasculitis. CSF protein may be elevated in patients with diabetic amyotrophy, though mild CSF protein elevation can also be seen in unaffected diabetic patients. There are no proven treatments for diabetic amyotrophy, though brief corticosteroid tapers are used by some providers to address severe neuropathic pain. Neuropathic pain agents are often used, and brief treatment with narcotic analgesics may be considered in the acute phase of the illness.

G. Rarely, atypical presentations of inflammatory disorders, direct infection, or latent effects of infectious agents may cause lumbosacral plexopathy. Such inflammatory disorders include vasculitides and sarcoidosis or, even less commonly, Sjögren syndrome, systemic lupus, and mixed connective tissue disease. Amyloidosis has also been implicated in rare cases. Infectious etiologies include HIV, EBV, CMV, VZV, Lyme disease, tuberculosis, and syphilis. Local abscess formation can also lead to direct compressive effects on the lumbosacral plexus.

H. Idiopathic lumbosacral radiculoplexus neuropathy is similar to diabetic amyotrophy with respect to its pathophysiology, clinical features, prognosis, and management. CSF protein may be elevated in some, though not all, cases.

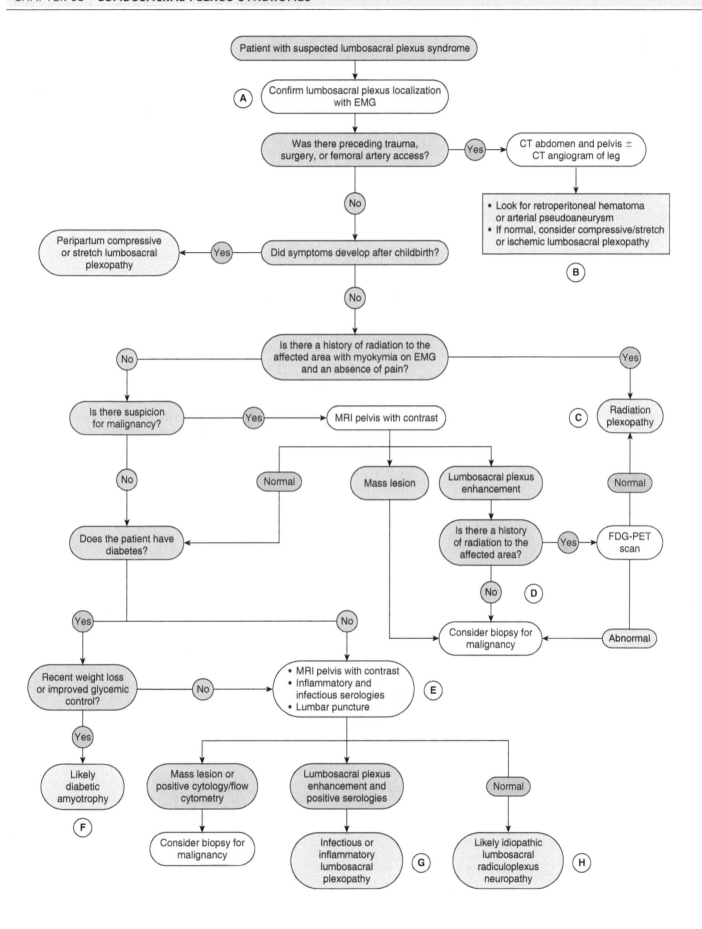

Motor Neuron Disease

Colin Quinn and Raymond S. Price

Motor neuron disease refers to a disease process affecting one or both of the two neurons in the motor circuit: (1) the upper motor neurons (UMNs), which originate in the primary motor cortex and project through the corticospinal tract; and (2) the lower motor neurons (LMNs), which originate in the anterior horn of the spinal cord and project peripherally to the skeletal muscle. A motor neuron process should be considered in patients with isolated weakness (no associated sensory symptoms), and particularly in those with LMN signs such as atrophy or fasciculations.

A. The presence of hyperreflexia indicates involvement of the UMN pathways either in the brain or spinal cord. Hyperreflexia in the setting of weakness and atrophy is seen in most patients with amyotrophic lateral sclerosis (ALS). However, a structural spinal cord lesion can cause LMN signs at the level of the lesion due to anterior horn cell involvement and UMN signs below the lesion due to corticospinal tract involvement. For example, a C6 spinal cord lesion may cause ipsilateral biceps atrophy and hyperreflexia in the leg. The combination of cervical and lumbar spine disease can cause LMN signs at both levels and UMN signs below the cervical spine lesion. To identify the cause of UMN signs, neuroimaging should be performed at every level rostral to the highest level of clinical UMN findings. For example, if hyperreflexia is present only in the legs, magnetic resonance imaging (MRI) of the brain and cervical and thoracic spine should be performed, whereas only MRI of the brain and cervical spine would be indicated in a patient with arm and leg hyperreflexia.

B. A diagnosis of clinically definite ALS requires (1) clinical UMN signs in at least three of the following four regions: bulbar, cervical, thoracic, and lumbar; (2) clinical or electrophysiologic LMN signs in three of these four regions; and (3) no alternative explanation. A diagnosis of clinically probable ALS has the same requirements, but only two regions need be clearly involved. Unexplained hyperreflexia and a single region of motor neuron injury are concerning but not diagnostic for ALS. Such patients should be followed closely with serial examinations to assess for progression.

C. In a patient with diffuse weakness, hyperreflexia, unremarkable imaging, and diffuse active on chronic denervation on electromyography (EMG) with normal sensory responses, ALS is the likely diagnosis.

D. Hereditary spastic paraparesis (HSP) typically presents with slowly progressive weakness and UMN findings in the lower extremities. Complicated HSP may involve systems beyond the corticospinal tracts including LMN and sensory pathways. Adrenomyeloneuropathy (AMN) is an X-linked disorder often manifesting in early adulthood with gait impairment. Adrenal insufficiency, sexual dysfunction, and neurogenic bladder may also be present. Serum very long chain fatty acid levels are elevated in AMN. Sequencing of the *ABCD1* gene provides definite diagnosis.

E. While rare, isolated demyelination of the motor neurons (multifocal motor neuropathy [MMN]) is a frequent consideration in the differential of motor neuron diseases, since it can be treated with intravenous immunoglobulin or plasma exchange. Clinically, MMN causes slowly progressive asymmetric weakness, most typically beginning in the upper extremities. The disorder is more common in men. Anti-GM1 bodies are seen in some but not all patients with MMN. Conduction block is the demyelinating feature most frequently described in MMN.

F. In a patient with diffuse weakness, normal or reduced reflexes, normal sensory responses on NCS, and diffuse active and chronic denervation on needle EMG, motor neuron disease and polyradiculopathies from a subarachnoid process are both diagnostic possibilities. A lumbar puncture should be performed to evaluate for malignancy (cytology and flow cytometry), albuminocytologic dissociation (elevated protein) as may be seen in chronic inflammatory demyelinating polyneuropathy (CIDP), or a pleocytosis as may be seen in infectious (e.g., human immunodeficiency virus or inflammatory (e.g., sarcoidosis) polyradiculitis.

G. Kennedy disease (spinal-bulbar muscular atrophy) is a slowly progressive X-linked disorder of the androgen receptor that causes progressive weakness, atrophy, and fasciculations, particularly of the proximal limbs and bulbar muscles. Patients often have a tremor and facial twitching. Sensory symptoms are often not a prominent complaint, but NCS typically reveals absent or severely reduced sensory responses. Genetic testing provides definitive diagnosis.

H. If the lumbar puncture is normal, the most likely diagnosis is progressive muscular atrophy (PMA), which is an exclusively LMN form of ALS. Approximately a quarter of patients with PMA will eventually develop some UMN signs, typically within 2 years of disease onset.

I. Late-onset Tay Sachs (LOTS) disease is a rare disorder that can be misdiagnosed as PMA, since it also presents with predominantly LMN signs. However, patients with LOTS often have an accompanying cerebellar ataxia and psychiatric symptoms (e.g., bipolar disorder and psychotic symptoms). LOTS is an autosomal recessive disorder caused by mutations in the *HEXA* gene, resulting in reduced hexosaminidase A activity. Brain MRI commonly demonstrates cerebellar atrophy.

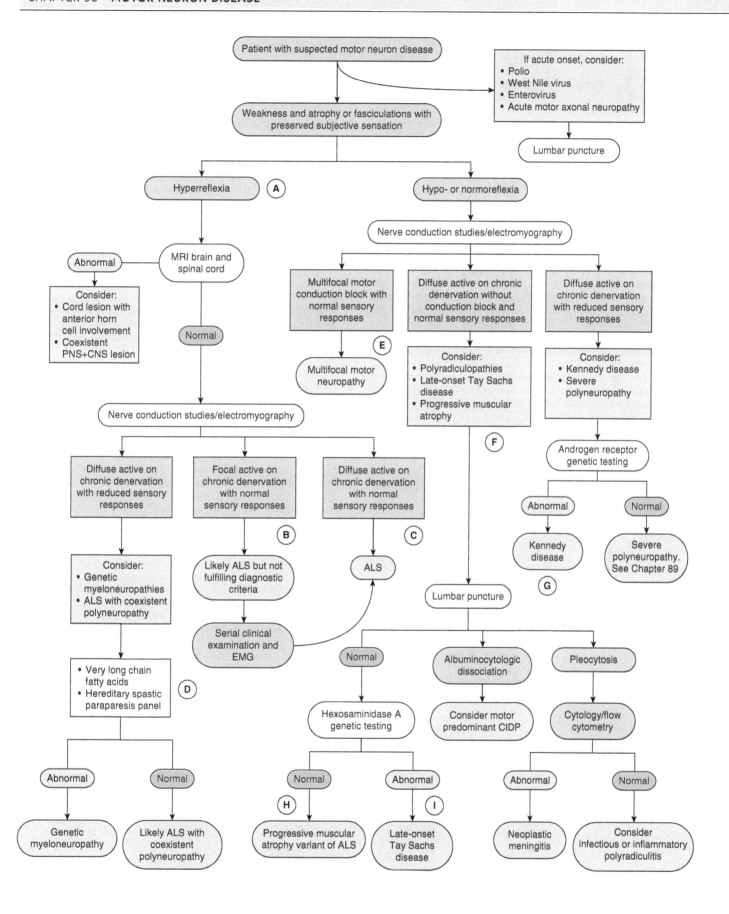

Myasthenia Gravis: Diagnosis

Christyn Edmundson

Myasthenia gravis (MG) is an autoimmune disorder caused by antibodies directed against the postsynaptic neuromuscular junction of skeletal muscle. MG is characterized by fluctuating weakness that worsens with activity and improves with rest. In ocular MG, weakness is limited to periocular muscles, resulting in fluctuating ptosis and double vision. In generalized MG, weakness may also involve limb muscles, respiratory muscles, or pharyngeal muscles.

A. Anti–acetylcholine receptor (AChR) antibodies are present in about 85% of patients with generalized MG and in 40%–50% of patients with ocular MG. Anti–muscle-specific kinase (MuSK) antibodies are found in 40%–50% of patients with generalized MG who lack anti-AChR antibodies. Anti-LRP4 antibodies are present in a small subset of patients, but the clinical utility of testing for these antibodies is unclear. Patients who lack detectable antibodies but have evidence of MG on ancillary tests are termed "seronegative."

B. Slow repetitive nerve stimulation (RNS) at a rate of 2–3 Hz may produce a decrement in motor response amplitudes in both pre- and postsynaptic neuromuscular junction disorders. A decrement is considered significant when the drop in amplitude is >10%. In patients with generalized MG, a decrement with slow RNS is seen in ∼80%. The sensitivity of slow RNS is much lower in patients with ocular MG. Decrement may also be seen in patients with congenital myasthenic syndrome, Lambert-Eaton myasthenic syndrome (LEMS), or botulism, and occasionally in patients with motor neuron disease.

C. Single fiber electromyography (SFEMG) is the most sensitive test for myasthenia gravis (90% sensitive in generalized MG, 80%–95% sensitive in ocular MG). However, SFEMG is not specific for MG and may be abnormal in other disorders of the neuromuscular junction, myopathies, neuropathies, or motor neuron diseases.

D. LEMS is a presynaptic disorder of neuromuscular transmission characterized by antibodies directed against voltage-gated calcium channels (VGCC). LEMS can be a paraneoplastic disorder, most frequently associated with small cell lung cancer or a primary autoimmune disorder. Patients present most frequently with proximal muscle weakness and reduced reflexes. Strength and reflexes often improve after brief exercise (postexercise facilitation), but weakness often worsens with protracted exercise. Ptosis, diplopia, and oropharyngeal symptoms may be present, but are less common and less prominent than in MG. Autonomic dysfunction is common in patients with LEMS. In LEMS, motor response amplitudes are reduced at baseline. High-frequency (10–50 Hz) RNS or repeat testing of motor response amplitude after brief, maximal exercise that produces an increment in amplitude >100% of baseline is considered diagnostic of a presynaptic neuromuscular junction disorder. In patients with clinical features and electrodiagnostic findings suggestive of LEMS, serum anti-P/Q-type VGCC antibodies should be sent to confirm the diagnosis. All patients with LEMS should undergo a thorough evaluation for malignancy.

E. Functional neurologic disorders are a diagnosis of exclusion, but may be considered if a thorough and appropriate examination and workup fails to disclose an organic cause of symptoms.

F. Congenital myasthenic syndromes (CMSs) are caused by genetic defects in proteins that facilitate neuromuscular junction transmission. Unlike LEMS or MG, these are not disorders of autoimmunity. Most individuals with CMS are affected at birth or soon after, but milder forms may present in childhood or adolescence with fatigable limb or oculobulbar weakness. CMS can be difficult to diagnose and often requires genetic testing.

G. Thymic tumors, primarily thymoma, are present in up to 15% of patients with anti-AChR antibody-positive MG, and these patients should have mediastinal imaging with chest computed tomography (CT). If thymoma is identified, resection is indicated, which may improve MG symptoms. Though less likely to be revealing, CT chest to assess for thymoma should also be performed in patients with seronegative MG. Patients with anti-MuSK antibody–positive MG are not at increased risk of thymoma.

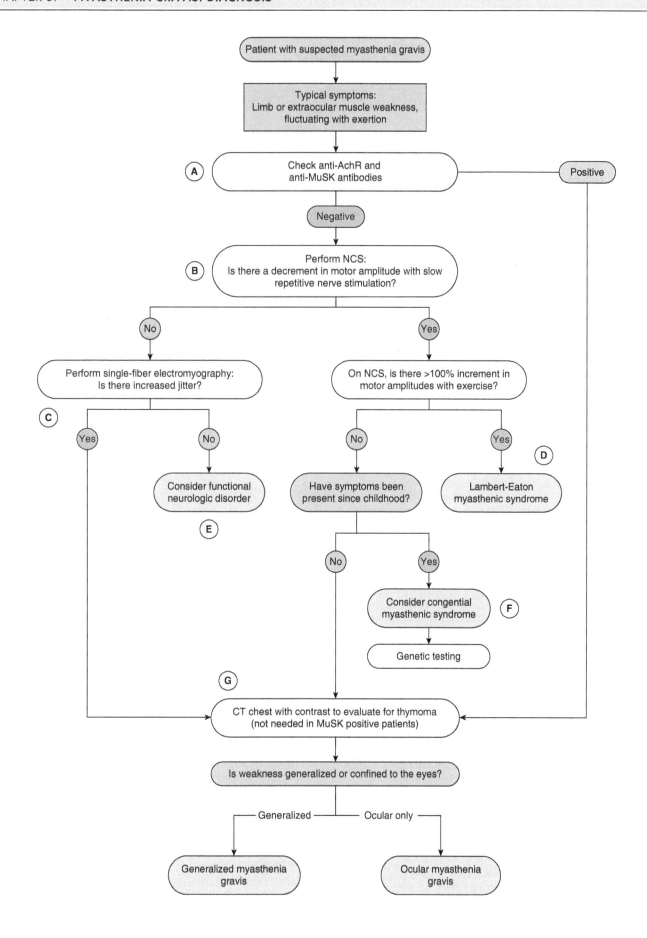

Patient with suspected myasthenia gravis

Typical symptoms:
Limb or extraocular muscle weakness,
fluctuating with exertion

(A) Check anti-AchR and
anti-MuSK antibodies

Positive

Negative

(B) Perform NCS:
Is there a decrement in motor amplitude with slow
repetitive nerve stimulation?

No

Yes

Perform single-fiber electromyography:
Is there increased jitter?

On NCS, is there >100% increment in
motor amplitudes with exercise?

(C)

Yes

No

No

Yes

(D)

Consider functional
neurologic disorder

Have symptoms been
present since childhood?

Lambert-Eaton
myasthenic syndrome

(E)

No

Yes

Consider congential
myasthenic syndrome

(F)

Genetic testing

(G)

CT chest with contrast to evaluate for thymoma
(not needed in MuSK positive patients)

Is weakness generalized or confined to the eyes?

Generalized

Ocular only

Generalized myasthenia
gravis

Ocular myasthenia
gravis

Myasthenia Gravis: Treatment

Christyn Edmundson

A. Myasthenic crisis is a life-threatening, rapid worsening of myasthenia gravis (MG) leading to respiratory failure requiring intubation or non-invasive ventilation. Impending crisis is rapid clinical worsening that could lead to crisis in days to weeks. Respiratory function must be closely monitored in patients with worsening myasthenic symptoms, as rapid deterioration can occur (see Chapter 60). Myasthenic crisis (or impending crisis) should be treated with either intravenous immunoglobulin (IVIg, 2 g/kg per day for 5 days) or plasmapheresis (three to five exchanges over 1–2 weeks), with the choice of therapy based on comorbidities and institutional availability. Plasmapheresis is probably more effective in patients with anti–muscle-specific kinase (MuSK) antibodies. Corticosteroids (prednisone 1 mg/kg daily) or nonsteroidal immunosuppressive therapies (such as azathioprine) may be started to control MG after the effects of IVIg or plasmapheresis have worn off. However, high-dose oral corticosteroids may transiently worsen myasthenic symptoms shortly after initiation so, in patients not already intubated, should generally be avoided until several days after initiation of IVIg or plasmapheresis. Alternatively, they may be started at a low dose (e.g., prednisone 10–20 mg daily) and gradually increased by no more than 5 mg every 3–5 days (Table 98.1).

B. Pyridostigmine, an acetylcholinesterase inhibitor, improves transmission across the neuromuscular junction and offers symptomatic improvement to many patients. Side effects include respiratory secretions, diarrhea, and muscle twitching. In patients with significant symptoms, corticosteroids or nonsteroidal immunosuppressant agents (IS) may be started concurrently.

C. Thymoma is present in ~15% of patients with acetylcholine receptor (AChR) antibody-positive MG, and very rarely in patients with seronegative MG. When thymoma is present, MG may be considered a paraneoplastic disease. Thymomas are typically benign, but rarely invasive thymic carcinoma is present. Thymoma should be removed as soon as considered safe given MG disease activity. Treatment with IVIg or plasmapheresis may be required to adequately control respiratory and/or bulbar symptoms prior to surgery. Resection may improve disease control, although this is not always the case. In patients with generalized MG and positive anti-AChR antibodies, thymectomy improves outcome and should be performed regardless of the presence of thymoma. However, because the effect on disease activity is delayed, it should be performed only when MG symptoms are well controlled. Thymectomy is typically not recommended in patients over age 60 years, although there is no firm upper age limit. Patients with MuSK antibodies do not have an increased risk of thymoma.

D. Remission in MG is defined as the absence of symptoms or signs of MG, other than weakness of eye closure. Minimal manifestation status is defined as the absence of symptoms or functional limitations, but some weakness on muscle examination. Both are considered reasonable goals of treatment.

E. Oral corticosteroids, typically prednisone, should be used in all MG patients who have not met treatment goals with pyridostigmine, unless there is a contraindication (i.e., nonhealing wound, brittle diabetes mellitus). Transient worsening in MG symptoms occurs in ~50% of patients within several days of starting high-dose corticosteroids. To avoid this, outpatient steroids should be started at a low dose, such as prednisone 10–20 mg daily and gradually increased by no more than 5 mg every 3–5 days until reaching a dose of 1 mg/kg daily. Alternate daily dosing (i.e., prednisone 40 mg every other day in lieu of 20 mg daily) may reduce corticosteroid side effects.

TABLE 98.1 MEDICATIONS COMMONLY USED IN MYASTHENIA GRAVIS			
Medication	Starting dose	Titration	Maximum dose
First-line Therapies			
Pryridostigmine	30 mg tid	Add 30 mg per dose q5–10 days. Extended release form can be added 180 mg qhs.	1500 mg daily; doses >120 mg q3–4 h often cause side effects
Prednisone	10–20 mg daily	Increase no faster than 5 mg q3–5 d	1 mg/kg daily or 100 mg daily
Steroid-sparing Immunosuppressants			
Azathioprine	50 mg daily	Increase by 50 mg q1–2 wk	3 mg/kg daily
Cylcosporine	100 mg bid	Increase by 0.5 mg/kg per day q2–4 wk to achieve trough serum level 75–150 ng/ml	3–6 mg/kg divided bid
Mycophenolate mofetil	500 mg bid	Increase by 500 mg bid q2–4 wk	1000–1500 mg bid
Tacrolimus	3 mg daily or 0.1 mg/kg per day in 1–2 divided doses	Titrate to achieve a trough concentration of 7–8 ng/mL	–

F. Patients with anti-MuSK antibody-positive MG who have an unsatisfactory response to corticosteroids may respond particularly well to rituximab, so this should be considered as an early therapeutic option in these patients.

G. A nonsteroidal IS should be added to corticosteroids when steroid side effects develop, response is inadequate, or the dose cannot be reduced due to symptom relapse. Nonsteroidal agents used in MG include azathioprine (typically the first-line nonsteroidal agent), mycophenolate mofetil, methotrexate, cyclosporine, and tacrolimus.

H. Once patients achieve treatment goals, corticosteroids should be gradually tapered, though a low dose may be necessary long term. For nonsteroidal IS, once treatment goals are reached, these agents should be continued for 6–24 months, then gradually weaned to no more frequently than every 3–6 months.

I. Refractory MG is defined as disease in which symptoms have not improved after use of corticosteroids and at least two other nonsteroidal IS agents at an adequate dose for an adequate duration, or have side effects that limit functioning. Chronic IVIg or plasmapheresis, cyclophosphamide, eculizumab, or rituximab may be considered in such patients.

REFERENCE

1. Sanders DB, Wolfe GI, Benatar M, et al. International consensus guidance for management of myasthenia gravis: executive summary. *Neurology*. 2016;87:419–425.

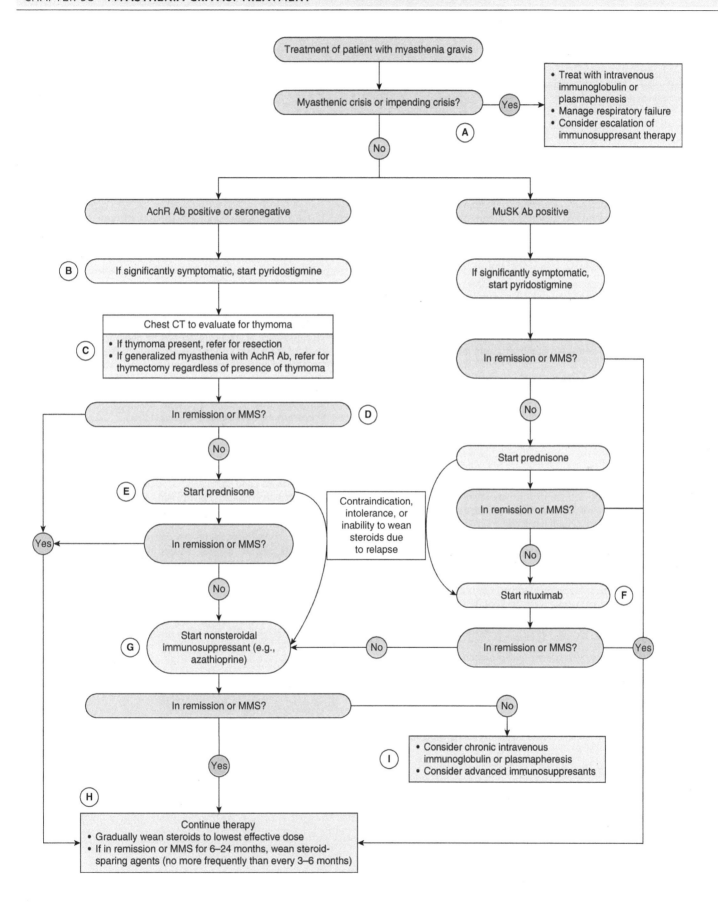

Myopathy

Colin Quinn and Raymond S. Price

Myopathy, a disorder of muscle, should be suspected in patients with weakness without numbness. The diagnosis is supported by elevated creatine kinase (CK) levels, although a normal CK does not exclude myopathy. Electromyography (EMG) can be a useful diagnostic tool, with the limitation that mild myopathies may appear normal, and chronic myopathies may appear neuropathic on EMG. The temporal course of symptom onset (acute/subacute vs. chronic) is important to focus the diagnostic evaluation. When present, a family history of myopathy may directly suggest the likely diagnosis.

Acute or Subacute Myopathy

A. Typical skin findings in dermatomyositis (DM) include erythema of sun exposed areas (e.g., face and chest), purple discoloration around the eyes ("heliotrope" rash), papules on the fingers (Gottron papules), and dry, cracked skin on the lateral surface of the fingers ("mechanic's hands"). Calcium deposits in the skin ("calcinosis cutis") are rare in adults but commonly seen in children. The combination of weakness and any of the above suggests DM. Skin or muscle biopsy can be diagnostic. Skin biopsy typically demonstrates perivascular lymphocytes and vacuoles in the basal keratinocyte layer, and muscle biopsy demonstrates perivascular inflammation, perifascicular atrophy, and membrane attack complex deposition on capillaries. DM is frequently associated with malignancy; cancer screening should be performed at diagnosis and over the subsequent 2 years.

B. Sporadic inclusion body myositis is an acquired myopathy typically seen in older adults with a fairly distinct pattern of long finger flexor and/or quadriceps weakness. Patients may report difficulty climbing stairs or opening jars. Dysphagia is common. Characteristic changes on biopsy include rimmed vacuoles, inclusions, and the presence of inflammatory cells. NT5c1A antibodies are seen in 60%–70% of patients.

C. Chronic exposure to high-dose corticosteroids can cause insidiously progressive proximal weakness in addition to systemic Cushingoid features. The serum CK and EMG are usually normal. Characteristic changes on biopsy include atrophy of type 2 muscle fibers.

D. Critically ill patients with systemic inflammatory response syndrome or hyperglycemia are at increased risk of developing an acute myopathy, which often manifests as proximal weakness and difficulty weaning from the ventilator. The serum CK may be elevated but is often normal. Nerve conduction studies may demonstrate prolonged distal compound muscle action potential duration or the muscle may be electrically inexcitable. There is frequently coexistent critical illness neuropathy.

E. Consider toxic myopathies in patients presenting with acute/subacute weakness, elevated CK, and exposure to a potential offending agent. Statins are a common offender and may cause either a toxic or immune-mediated necrotizing myopathy (IMNM; see section H). Immune-mediated myopathies may also be seen with check-point inhibitor antineoplastic agents.

F. Inherited myopathies occasionally present more acutely and can mimic an acquired myopathy.

G. Sporadic late-onset nemaline myopathy is a rare acquired myopathy presenting with rapid onset of proximal muscle weakness with normal or mildly elevated CK. The diagnosis is confirmed by the presence of nemaline bodies on muscle biopsy. Patients frequently also have a monoclonal gammopathy. Cardiac involvement is common.

H. Necrotizing myopathies are defined by necrotic muscle fibers with scant inflammation and may be immune mediated or due to toxic exposures. Signal recognition particle (SRP) and anti–HMG-CoA are the antibodies most commonly associated with IMNMs. IMNMs are often refractory to treatment and may require more aggressive immunomodulatory therapy. Like dermatomyositis, necrotizing myopathies are frequently associated with malignancy; cancer screening should be performed at diagnosis and over the subsequent 2 years.

I. Polymyositis is uncommon, and necrotizing myopathy, inclusion body myositis, and inherited myopathy are frequently misdiagnosed as polymyositis. Polymyositis is defined by characteristic changes on biopsy, including endomysial inflammation composed of CD8 T cells and macrophages invading nonnecrotic fibers. Polymyositis can be associated with malignancy but less frequently than dermatomyositis or necrotizing myopathy; cancer screening should be performed at diagnosis and over the subsequent 2 years.

J. In patients with a presumed inflammatory myopathy that is unresponsive to treatment, reconsider the diagnosis. Inherited myopathies mimicking an acquired myopathy will not respond to treatment.

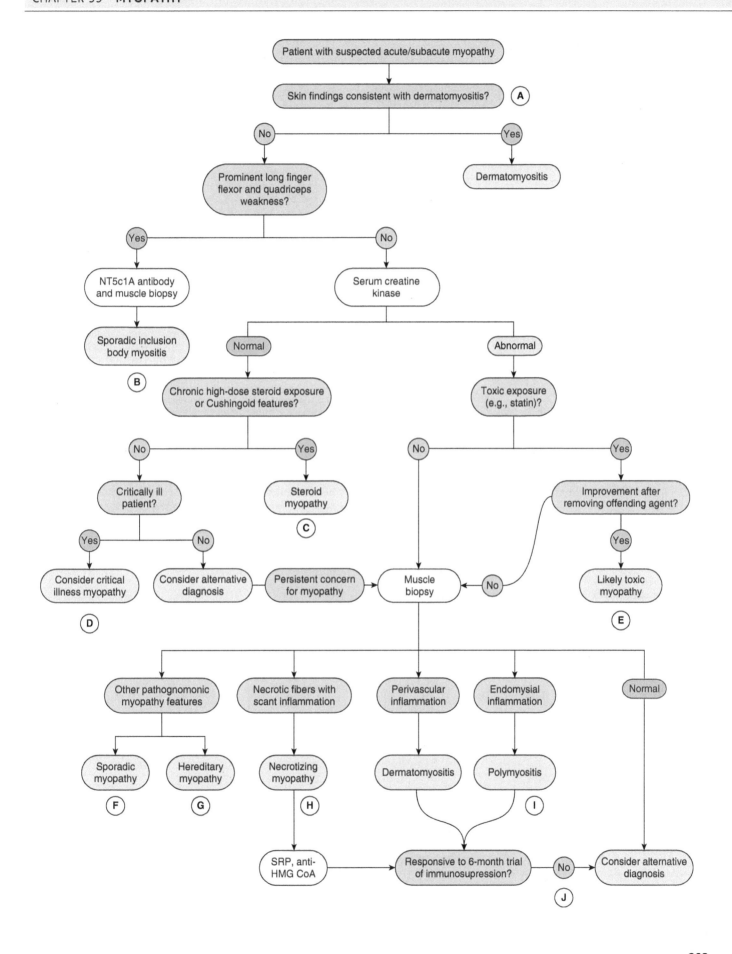

Chronic Myopathy

A. Sporadic inclusion body myositis is an acquired myopathy typically seen in older adults with a fairly distinct pattern of long finger flexor and/or quadriceps weakness. Patients may report difficulty climbing stairs or opening jars. Dysphagia is common. Characteristic changes on biopsy include rimmed vacuoles, inclusions, and the presence of inflammatory cells. NT5c1A antibodies are seen in 60%–70% of patients.

B. Fascioscapulohumeral muscular dystrophy (FSHD) is the second most common adult onset muscular dystrophy. Facial and scapular weakness are prominent, and elevation of the scapulae can cause the appearance of trapezius hypertrophy ("trap hump"). Triceps/biceps, abdominal, and ankle dorsiflexion weakness is also common. The deltoid is relatively spared. FSHD 1 is caused by a contraction of the D4Z4 region on the short arm of chromosome 4. About 5% of FSHD patients have FSHD 2 in which they have a normal number of D4Z4 repeats but instead have hypomethylation in this region.

C. Oculopharyngeal muscular dystrophy (OPMD) is an adult-onset muscular dystrophy that commonly affects extraocular movements, upper facial muscles (ptosis), and swallowing. Neck and proximal limb weakness is usually a later manifestation. OPMD is more commonly seen in French Canadians and New Mexicans of Latin American origin and is caused by a triple repeat expansion in the poly(A) binding protein (PABN2). As with other repeat disorders, it will not be detected by next-generation sequencing (NGS) and therefore must be tested separately.

D. Multiple genetic disorders affecting mitochondria may result in the progressive loss of eye movement and ptosis that define chronic progressive external ophthalmoplegia (CPEO). These defects may be seen in the context of other manifestations of mitochondrial disease (e.g., Kerns Sayre syndrome, which is characterized by CPEO, pigmentary retinopathy, and cardiomyopathy) or as an isolated finding. Testing may involve both nuclear and mitochondrial encoded genes affecting mitochondrial function.

E. Myotonic dystrophy type 1 (DM1) is the most common adult-onset muscular dystrophy. Patients typically present with distal limb and facial weakness, and may also describe action myotonia. DM1 is a multisystem disorder associated with cardiac conduction abnormalities, cataracts, endocrine abnormalities, sleep disturbance, and cognitive impairment. It is autosomal dominant and caused by excessive repeats in the *DMPK* gene.

F. Hereditary distal myopathies, caused by various genetic mutations, initially affect the muscles of the hand and forearm and/or ankle dorsal and plantar flexion. Ankle dorsiflexion is typically more impaired with the exception of "Miyoshi myopathies" (e.g., dysferlin, anoctamin), which have prominent atrophy of the medial gastrocnemius. There are many overlapping features, and NGS is typically the best testing approach when there is no family history of a specific mutation.

G. Myotonic dystrophy type 2 (DM2) is a myotonic myopathy that causes predominantly proximal weakness. It is sometimes referred to as proximal myotonic myopathy (PROMM). It is caused by an expansion of the CCTG repeat sequence in the *CNBP* gene. Weakness and action myotonia may be subtle; some patients present with isolated muscle pain. Other symptoms such as arrhythmias and cataracts overlap with DM1. Myotonic discharges are seen on EMG in 90% of patients.

H. Dystrophin mutations results in Duchenne and Becker muscular dystrophy. Dystrophinopathies are the most common causes of muscular dystrophy overall and should be considered in all patients with proximal weakness. Dystrophin is located on the X chromosome. While males are more commonly affected, females can present as manifesting carriers. Limb girdle muscular dystrophies (LGMDs) are defined by weakness of the shoulders and hips. There are many genetic causes of LGMD classified by inheritance pattern (LGMD1 = dominant, LGMD2 = recessive) and the order in which they were identified (indicated by a letter). NGS is the most efficient way to identify mutations causing muscular dystrophy. Large deletions, which are common in dystrophinopathies, can be missed on NGS; specific testing for these should be done as well.

I. If genetic testing is negative, an inherited myopathy may still be diagnosed based on biopsy characteristics. For example, myofibrillar myopathies are defined by disruption of the z disc and are associated with various gene mutations, not all of which have been identified. Mitochondrial myopathies may be suggested by light microcopy findings such as ragged red fibers or COX-/SDH+ fibers. If mitochondrial disease is suspected, testing of mitochondrial DNA can be performed directly on muscle tissue.

J. In patients with a suspected inflammatory myopathy that is unresponsive to treatment, reconsider the diagnosis. Alternatively, the cause of weakness (e.g., myopathic vs. neurogenic) may have been misidentified.

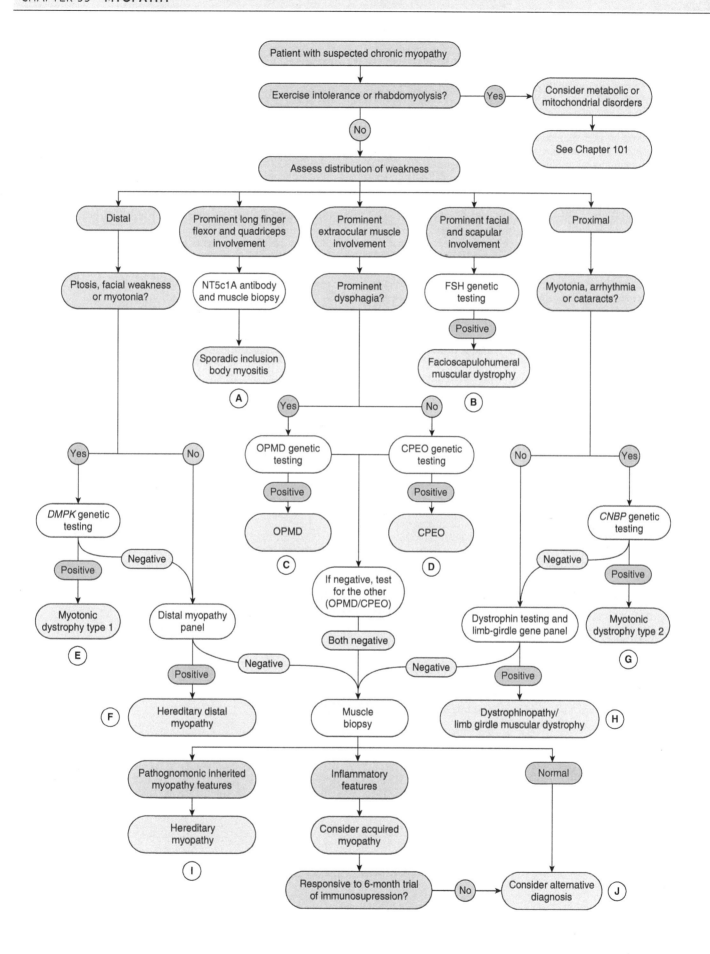

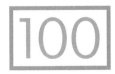

Myotonia

Colin Quinn and Raymond S. Price

Myotonia is a failure of muscle cell relaxation manifesting clinically as impaired relaxation after voluntary muscle contraction (e.g., grip myotonia, Video 100.1) or prolonged reflexive contraction during specific neurological examination testing (e.g., percussion myotonia, Video 100.2). The latter is most frequently evaluated by gently percussing the thenar eminence with a reflex hammer and assessing for sustained thumb abduction. Myotonia may be described as "stiffness" but is not typically associated with significant pain. This distinguishes it from muscle cramping, in which pain is prominent. Myotonic discharges can be seen during electromyography (EMG) and are characterized by spontaneous waxing and waning muscle cell discharges with variable amplitude and frequency (unlike cramping, which is due to spontaneous motor-unit firing). Clinical myotonia is most commonly associated with myotonic dystrophies and skeletal muscle channelopathies; myotonia seen on EMG is less specific and may be seen in other chronic disorders of muscle, particularly metabolic myopathies.

A. Periodic paralysis in the setting of myotonia is typically associated with mutations in the *SCN4A* gene, resulting in hyperkalemic periodic paralysis. Andersen-Tawil syndrome (ATS), a rare disorder associated with periodic paralysis, cardiac arrhythmias, and developmental abnormalities, should be considered in any patient manifesting at least two of these issues. Two-thirds of patients with ATS have mutations in the *KCNJ2* gene. Hypokalemic and thyrotoxic periodic paralysis are not addressed here, as these disorders are not associated with myotonia but should be considered in any patient presenting with episodes of periodic paralysis.

B. The pattern of weakness associated with clinical myotonia can be helpful in distinguishing myotonic dystrophy type 1, which typically causes facial and hand grip weakness, from other myotonic disorders, which are usually—though not invariably—associated with proximal weakness.

C. Myotonic muscular dystrophy, type 1 (DM1) is the most common myotonic disorder. It is an autosomal dominant condition caused by a trinucleotide (CTG) repeat expansion in the 3' untranslated region of the dystrophica myotonia type-1 protein kinase (*DMPK*) gene. DM1 may present from infancy (congenital DM1) to adulthood. Distal muscles are typically affected first, particularly in the upper extremities. The neck flexors and facial muscles are commonly involved. The classic facial appearance of DM1 patients is due to the combination of atrophy of the temporalis muscles, weakness of the muscles of jaw closure, and ptosis. Dysphagia is common. DM1 can be associated with other systemic issues including cardiac arrhythmias, cataracts, and intellectual impairment.

D. When prominent proximal weakness is present, myotonic dystrophy type 2 (DM2), also called proximal myotonic myopathy, is most likely. DM2 is an autosomal dominant disorder caused by a tetranucleotide (CCTG) repeat expansion in intron 1 of the *CNBP* gene. DM2 patients tend to have milder systemic features than are seen in DM1 and there is no congenital form. In the setting of proximal weakness and myotonia seen only on EMG, other chronic myopathic disorders, particularly metabolic myopathies like acid maltase deficiency and debranching enzyme deficiency, should be considered. McArdle disease, a disorder of glycogen metabolism, can be difficult to distinguish from a myotonic disorder clinically due to increasing muscle stiffness with exertion seen in this disorder, which may resemble a paramyotonic pattern.

E. Chloride channelopathies, also known as myotonia congenita, are the result of mutations in the *CLCN1* gene. They may be inherited in an autosomal dominant (Thomsen disease) or recessive (Becker disease) pattern. These patients have classic myotonia with initial impairment of muscle relaxation, which improves with repeated movements. Mutations do not appear to cause systemic effects or weakness, and patients have a normal life span. On occasion, DM2 can present without notable proximal muscle weakness, so this should be considered if testing for myotonia congenita is negative.

F. Most myotonia improves with exercise; patients who experience myotonia that worsens with exercise have "paradoxical myotonia" or paramyotonia. Symptoms are typically exacerbated by cold. Paramyotonia congenita is caused by mutations in the *SCN4A* gene. Paramyotonia congenita and hyperkalemic periodic paralysis are allelic disorders, and some families demonstrate clinical features of both.

G. Genetic testing panels are a useful tool in diagnosing myotonic disorders; however, it is important to recognize that DM1 and DM2 are nucleotide repeat disorders that are not effectively studied by large genetic muscular dystrophy next-generation sequencing panels.

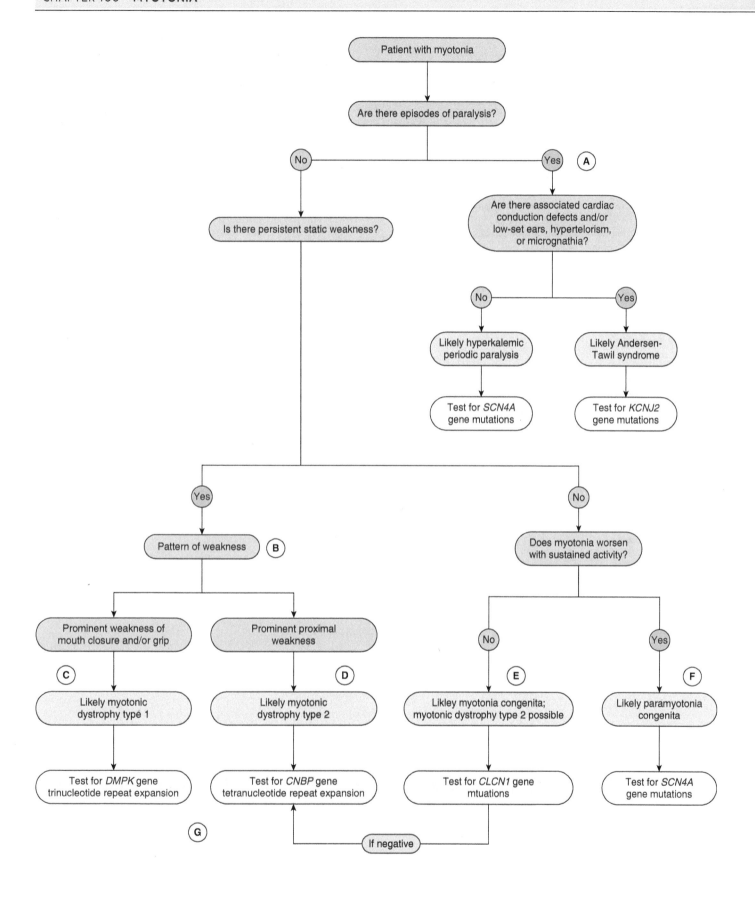

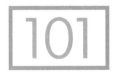

Rhabdomyolysis

Colin Quinn and Raymond S. Price

Acute rhabdomyolysis is a medical emergency that often requires hospitalization for infusion of intravenous fluids to protect from renal injury. In the acute period, the cause of rhabdomyolysis and the risk of recurrent episodes are often unknown. Many patients unnecessarily avoid exertion to prevent recurrence. An evaluation of baseline strength and creatine kinase (CK) once the patient has recovered from the acute episode will guide the diagnostic evaluation and prognosis.

A. Substantial trauma or prolonged immobilization causing diffuse muscle injury can lead to rhabdomyolysis. These events are often known at the time of presentation but should be screened for in the initial evaluation. Specific events of concern include falls resulting in prolonged immobilization, coma, compartment syndromes, and electrical injury from lightning or other high-voltage sources. In the presence of a substantial trauma or prolonged immobilization, further workup is not required and the patient may resume physical activity as tolerated.

B. Many toxic exposures have been associated with rhabdomyolysis, though much of the literature is limited to isolated case reports. Here we have included exposures with a clear and consistent association with rhabdomyolysis. In the presence of a clear toxic exposure, further workup is not required and the patient may resume physical activity as tolerated.

C. In the absence of trauma or toxic exposure, a thorough examination of motor strength is necessary to assess for baseline weakness. Additionally, a CK level should be drawn. Patients should refrain from strenuous exercise for one week to avoid artificially elevated CK levels. If the patient's strength is impaired or the CK is elevated at baseline, further testing is required to assess for acquired or inherited causes of myopathy.

D. In patients with subacute progressive weakness or skin changes concerning for dermatomyositis, a biopsy should be performed to exclude rhabdomyolysis in the setting of an acquired myopathy. In the setting of skin changes, a skin biopsy of an affected region can also be performed. If biopsy findings are not consistent with an inflammatory process, then inherited myopathies should be considered, although if there is clear subacute progression of weakness, concurrent empiric treatment may be warranted due to the risk of sampling error. It is important to note that biopsies performed within several months of an episode of rhabdomyolysis are likely to demonstrate fiber necrosis and regeneration related to the acute episode of muscle breakdown.

E. In patients with a single episode of rhabdomyolysis with preserved strength and a normal baseline CK level, further evaluation is not recommended, and these patients are encouraged to resume their prior level of activity. Education should be provided regarding signs of recurrent rhabdomyolysis, including muscle pain, constitutional symptoms, and dark urine, which would require immediate medical assessment.

F. Advances in genetic testing have revolutionized the assessment of various inherited myopathies. The use of next-generation sequencing (NGS) allows a large number of genes to be tested in a single disease panel. Some panels are focused on particular disease sets (e.g., "metabolic" vs. "muscular dystrophy") while others are broad and cover multiple disease categories ("comprehensive myopathy panels"). It is important to understand the strengths and weakness of individual panels. It is also important to know if large gene deletions and duplications are examined in the panel. Finally, NGS technology does not assess the two most common adult-onset muscular dystrophies, fascioscapulohumeral muscular dystrophy and myotonic dystrophy. It is important to consider these specific presentations, as they require separate specific genetic testing.

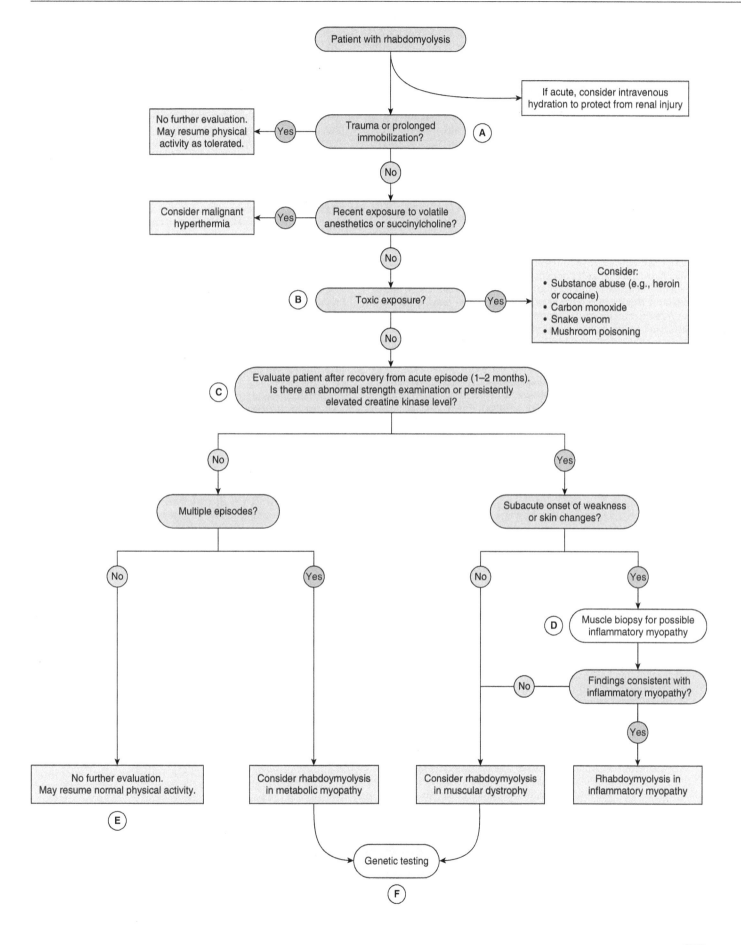

Patient with rhabdomyolysis

If acute, consider intravenous hydration to protect from renal injury

Trauma or prolonged immobilization? **A**

Yes → No further evaluation. May resume physical activity as tolerated.

No

Recent exposure to volatile anesthetics or succinylcholine?

Yes → Consider malignant hyperthermia

No

B Toxic exposure?

Yes → Consider:
- Substance abuse (e.g., heroin or cocaine)
- Carbon monoxide
- Snake venom
- Mushroom poisoning

No

C Evaluate patient after recovery from acute episode (1–2 months). Is there an abnormal strength examination or persistently elevated creatine kinase level?

No → Multiple episodes?

  No → No further evaluation. May resume normal physical activity. **E**

  Yes → Consider rhabdoymyolysis in metabolic myopathy

Yes → Subacute onset of weakness or skin changes?

  No → Consider rhabdoymyolysis in muscular dystrophy

  Yes → **D** Muscle biopsy for possible inflammatory myopathy

    Findings consistent with inflammatory myopathy?

    No → Consider rhabdoymyolysis in muscular dystrophy

    Yes → Rhabdoymyolysis in inflammatory myopathy

Genetic testing **F**

Glioma

Andrea Fuentes and Raymond S. Price

Diffusely infiltrating gliomas are a heterogenous group of central nervous system tumors arising from glial cells, such as astrocytes and oligodendrocytes. The diagnosis, classification, and treatment of gliomas have evolved significantly with increased understanding of the genetics of tumorigenesis. Seizures, focal neurologic deficits, and headache are common presenting signs and symptoms in patients with glial tumors. Initial diagnosis is typically based on contrast-enhanced brain magnetic resonance imaging (MRI).

A. High-grade gliomas include anaplastic gliomas (anaplastic astrocytomas and anaplastic oligodendrogliomas) and glioblastomas. These are typically hypointense on MRI T1-weighted sequences and hyperintense on T2-weighted sequences with heterogenous enhancement, surrounding vasogenic edema, and associated mass effect. A thick rim of enhancement with central clearing can be seen due to areas of central necrosis, cystic cavities, or blood products, particularly with glioblastomas. Antiepileptic therapy is indicated for clinical or subclinical seizures, but should not be given in patients with a newly diagnosed brain tumor who are seizure-free.

B. Low-grade gliomas include diffuse astrocytomas and oligodendrogliomas. They appear hyperintense on MRI T2-weighted sequences, typically without vasogenic edema or enhancement. Oligodendrogliomas may be partially calcified.

C. Surgical resection, rather than biopsy alone, allows for optimal tumor characterization and grading to guide further management. Advanced imaging, such as functional MRI and diffusion tensor imaging, can help identify eloquent cortex for surgical planning. Maximal surgical resection is favored in patients with a high-grade glioma or focal neurologic signs or symptoms. Although expectant management with serial imaging was previously used for patients with a low-grade glioma without symptoms or with medically controlled seizures, given inevitable tumor progression and evidence of improved median survival with more active, aggressive management, surgical resection is now also favored in patients with low-grade glioma. If an asymptomatic low-grade glioma is not amenable to resection, chemotherapy and/or radiation therapy may potentially be deferred until the time of clinical or radiographic progression.

D. Histopathologic and molecular data are used for glioma classification. The key molecular characteristics are deletions of the short arm of chromosome 1 (1p) and the long arm of chromosome 19 (19q) as well as isocitrate dehydrogenase (*IDH*) 1 or 2 missense mutations. Oligodendroglial tumors, which include oligodendrogliomas and anaplastic oligodendrogliomas, are defined by the presence of 1p and 19q codeletion and *IDH* mutation. They comprise 5%–20% of all gliomas and are typically particularly sensitive to chemotherapy.

E. Histopathology is used to differentiate oligodendrogliomas and anaplastic oligodendrogliomas. Anaplastic features, such as increased mitotic activity, necrosis, and endothelial proliferation, are required for a diagnosis of anaplastic oligodendroglioma.

F. Following anaplastic oligodendroglioma resection, focal radiation and adjuvant chemotherapy are recommended. Procarbazine, lomustine, and vincristine (PCV) chemotherapy are typically used; studies assessing the efficacy of temozolomide, which is often better tolerated, are ongoing.

G. Given the high risk of tumor progression with residual disease, focal radiation and adjuvant chemotherapy (with PCV or temozolomide) are recommended in patients with subtotally resected oligodendrogliomas. Surveillance imaging following treatment should be obtained every 3–6 months for 5 years, then at least once a year thereafter.

H. Astrocytomas, which are defined by the absence of 1p and 19q codeletion, are further divided into mutant and wild type *IDH* categories. *IDH* wild-type tumors are associated with a poorer prognosis.

I. Astrocytomas are further divided based on histopathologic features into low-grade and high-grade tumors, the latter including anaplastic astrocytoma and glioblastoma. Glioblastoma, a grade IV astrocytoma, is defined by the presence of necrosis. Glioblastomas that are *IDH* mutant are likely secondary to a transformed low-grade astrocytoma and have a better prognosis than de novo glioblastomas that are *IDH* wild-type. Anaplastic astrocytoma (grade III astrocytoma) will demonstrate endothelial proliferation and/or increased mitotic activity but will not demonstrate necrosis.

J. Focal radiation and temozolomide are recommended in most patients with low-grade astrocytomas. In patients under the age of 40 years with gross total resection, close clinical and radiographic follow-up without initial radiation or chemotherapy may be appropriate.

K. Temozolomide in combination with focal radiation therapy is indicated for anaplastic astrocytoma and glioblastoma, regardless of the extent of resection. Additionally, tumor-treating fields, low-intensity intermediate-frequency alternating electrical fields applied to the scalp with antimitotic properties prolong progression-free and overall survival when used with maintenance chemotherapy in patients with glioblastoma.

L. Radiographic surveillance following treatment completion is recommended at 4 weeks, then every 2–4 months for at least 2–3 years for high-grade astrocytomas and glioblastomas. At tumor recurrence, treatment options include repeat maximal safe surgical resection and repeat radiation and alternative chemotherapy, such as bevacizumab. Clinical trials should also be considered.

REFERENCES

1. Louis DN, Perry A, Reifenberger G, et al. The 2016 World Health Organization classification of tumors of the central nervous system: a summary. *Acta Neuropathol.* 2016;131(6):803–820.
2. Stupp R, Taillibert S, Kanner A, et al. Effect of tumor-treating fields plus maintenance temozolomide vs maintenance temozolomide alone on survival in patients with glioblastoma. *JAMA.* 2017;318(23):2306.
3. Weller M, van den Bent M, Tonn JC, et al. European Association for Neuro-Oncology (EANO) guideline on the diagnosis and treatment of adult astrocytic and oligodendroglial gliomas. *Lancet Oncol.* 2017;18(6):e315–e329.

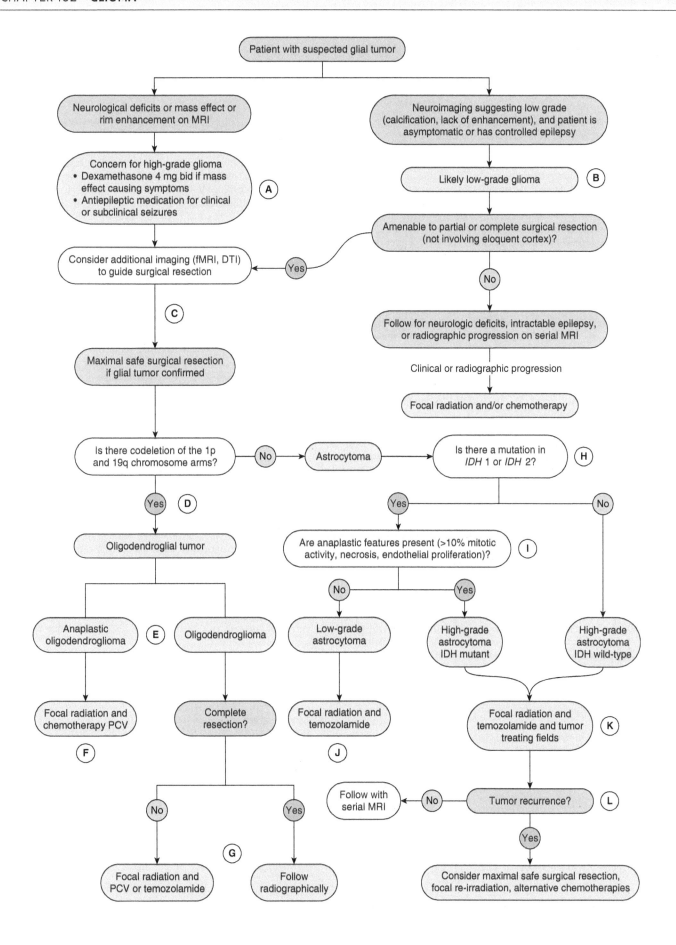

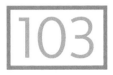

Meningioma

Andrea Fuentes and Raymond S. Price

Meningiomas are the most common primary central nervous system tumor. These extraaxial tumors can arise from the dura at any site along the neuroaxis, although are most frequently found at the skull base or in the parasagittal region. On magnetic resonance imaging (MRI), they typically appear iso- to slightly hypointense on T1-weighted sequences and hyperintense on T2-weighted sequences. Most characteristic is robust homogenous enhancement on postcontrast imaging; without contrast, small meningiomas may be easily missed. Calcifications may be present, and are best appreciated on computed tomography. A "dural tail," or an adjacent tapering dural thickening, can often be seen. Although these radiographic findings are quite specific for meningioma, very rarely lymphoma, sarcoidosis, and tuberculosis may produce similar-appearing radiographic lesions.

A. While most meningiomas are sporadic, identified risk factors for meningioma development include *NF2* gene deletion and ionizing radiation exposure. *NF2* is the tumor suppressor gene mutated in neurofibromatosis type 2, which can result in multiple meningiomas, schwannomas, and gliomas and has an autosomal dominant inheritance. Meningiomas are also associated with other tumor suppressor gene mutations, including *NF1*, *VHL*, and *PTEN* (which are present in neurofibromatosis type 1, Von Hippel-Lindau, and Cowden syndromes, respectively).

B. Meningiomas are often benign incidental findings on neuroimaging; however, progressive tumor growth can result in focal neurologic deficits from displacement or compression of adjacent cerebral and vascular structures. If causing significant mass effect with resulting neurologic symptoms, dexamethasone should be given. Meningiomas may also serve as a seizure focus, with seizure the presenting symptom in 20%–50% of patients. When seizures occur, antiepileptic medication is indicated. However, prophylactic antiepileptic use is not recommended.

C. In cases of persistent symptoms, refractory seizures and/or neuroimaging suggestive of high-grade features, surgical resection is the standard therapeutic option. However, radiation therapy alone can be considered if the mass is not amenable to surgery. If the patient is asymptomatic or has controlled epilepsy, serial MRI can be performed every 6–12 months for 2–3 years to assess for meningioma growth, followed by clinical monitoring if there is radiographic stability.

D. The World Health Organization (WHO) Classification of Central Nervous System Tumors, based on histopathologic features, is used for meningioma grading. About 90% of meningiomas are WHO grade I and histologically benign. If complete resection, including the dural attachment and potentially infiltrated bone, is achieved, the rate of recurrence is low (3%–10% at 5 years). However, this rate increases to 10%–50% with incomplete resection. Therefore, focal radiation should be considered for cases of subtotal resection. For incompletely resected grade I meningiomas, radiographic follow-up for tumor growth should be obtained approximately every 6–12 months. For completely resected grade I meningiomas, radiographic follow-up for tumor recurrence may be performed less frequently, such as annually for 5 years, then every 2 years.

E. WHO grade II meningiomas have atypical histologic features, characterized by mitotic activity or at least three of the following features: increased cellularity, small cells with a high nucleus to cytoplasm ratio, large and prominent nucleoli, abnormal growth pattern, and necrosis. Grade II meningiomas have a higher rate of recurrence (30%–40% at 5 years). While adjuvant radiation is standard in cases of subtotal resection, it may also be considered after complete resection; however, this remains controversial. Given the higher rate of tumor recurrence, radiographic surveillance following treatment should be performed more frequently than with grade I meningiomas, such as every 6 months for 5 years, then annually.

F. Only 1%–3% of meningiomas are WHO grade III. These are histologically anaplastic, featuring an increased number of mitotic figures (20 or more per 10 high-power field) or frank sarcomatous or carcinomatous features, and are clinically aggressive with recurrence rates of 50%–80% at 5 years. Adjuvant radiation therapy is recommended, regardless of the extent of resection. Radiographic surveillance following treatment should be obtained every 3–6 months.

G. In the case of tumor recurrence, repeat surgery and/or radiation therapy can be considered. There is otherwise limited evidence for systemic chemotherapy, immunotherapy, or hormonal therapy use in recurrent meningiomas. However, targeted therapy research is ongoing, and thus clinical trials should be considered.

REFERENCES

1. Apra C, Peyre M, Kalamarides M. Current treatment options for meningioma. *Expert Rev Neurother.* 2018;18(3):241–249.
2. Louis DN, Perry A, Reifenberger G, et al. The 2016 World Health Organization classification of tumors of the central nervous system: a summary. *Acta Neuropathol.* 2016;131(6):803–820.

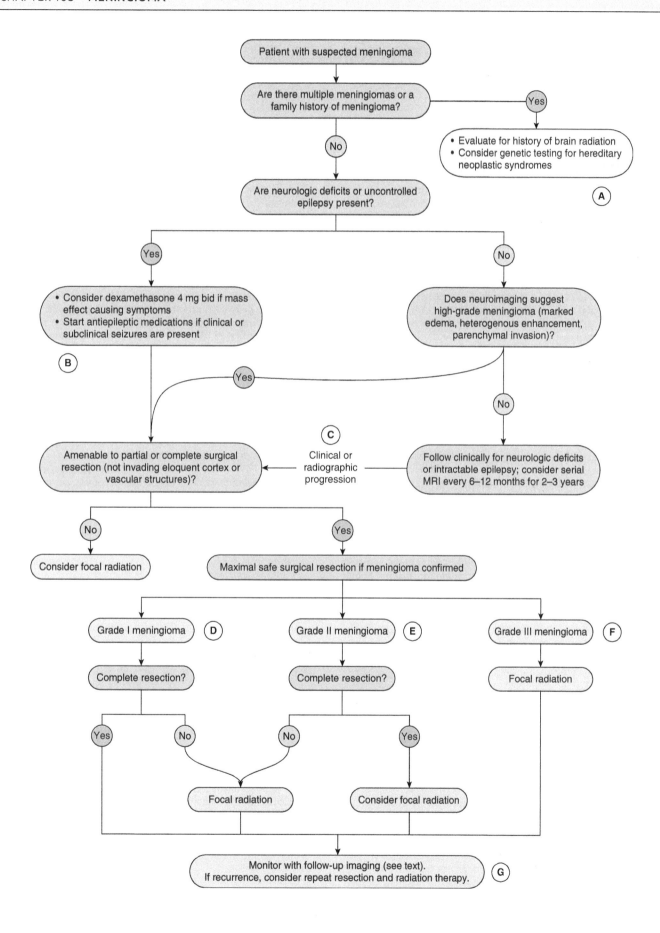

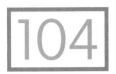

Paraneoplastic Syndromes

Alexander J. Gill and Raymond S. Price

Paraneoplastic neurologic syndromes are characterized by an immune response targeting the central or peripheral nervous system in the presence of an underlying malignancy. This autoimmune response is usually associated with an antibody targeting antigens shared by both the tumor and the nervous system. These antibodies are divided into two categories: (1) directly pathogenic antibodies that target neuronal cell surface or synaptic proteins, and (2) nonpathogenic antibodies that are directed against intracellular neuronal proteins and thus are a surrogate marker for a T-cell–mediated immune response against the nervous system. Diagnostic evaluation of the patient with a suspected paraneoplastic syndrome varies based on the presenting symptoms, but may include lumbar puncture, testing for serum or cerebrospinal fluid (CSF) paraneoplastic autoantibodies, magnetic resonance imaging (MRI) of brain and/or spine with contrast, and nerve conduction studies and electromyography (when peripheral nervous system involvement is suspected). Importantly, patients with cancer often have detectable nonpathogenic paraneoplastic antibodies without clinical manifestations of a paraneoplastic syndrome, and thus results of antibody testing must be interpreted with caution. However, as a paraneoplastic syndrome may precede the diagnosis of cancer, at times by several years, a thorough evaluation to identify occult malignancy is required in any patient with a positive paraneoplastic antibody regardless of clinical manifestations. Treatment of the underlying malignancy (when identified) to remove the antigen source should be undertaken, and immunosuppression (e.g., high-dose steroids, intravenous immunoglobulin, plasma exchange, and in some cases rituximab and cyclophosphamide) may be used. Paraneoplastic syndromes due to directly pathogenic antibodies are more likely to respond to these therapies, whereas those with antibodies targeting intracellular antigens often respond minimally.

A. Patients with anti-Hu sensory neuronopathy often present with painful paresthesias and subacute distal and proximal sensory loss across all modalities. They may exhibit pseudoathetosis in their hands secondary to severe loss of proprioception. Nerve conduction studies typically show reduced or absent sensory amplitudes with normal motor nerve conduction studies. Spine MRI may show dorsal root or posterior column T2 hyperintensity or contrast enhancement.

B. Lambert-Eaton myasthenic syndrome (LEMS) is associated with antibodies against the voltage-gated calcium channel. About 65% of patients with LEMS have a paraneoplastic syndrome associated with small cell lung cancer. These patients are more likely to be older and male (see Chapter 91).

C. Thymic tumors are present in up to 15% of patients with anti-AChR antibody-positive myasthenia gravis (MG), and occasionally in patients with seronegative MG. Patients with anti-MuSK antibody–positive MG are not at increased risk of thymoma (see Chapter 97).

D. A demyelinating polyneuropathy can occur in paraprotein-related diseases associated with an underlying hematologic malignancy, and should be considered in any patient not responding to treatment for chronic inflammatory demyelinating polyneuropathy (see Chapter 97).

E. Inflammatory myopathies are associated with various cancers, most commonly adenocarcinoma but also squamous cell carcinoma and hematologic malignancies. Patients with an inflammatory myopathy associated with cancer are older and progress more rapidly. About 50% of patients with a paraneoplastic inflammatory myopathy will have an antibody directed against transcriptional factor 1 gamma; these patients almost exclusively have dermatomyositis (see Chapter 99).

F. Paraneoplastic myelopathy should be considered in patients with symmetric and longitudinally extensive tract-specific T2 hyperintensity on MRI. In addition, anti-Hu antibodies have also been associated with gray-matter T2 hyperintensity. The majority of patients do not respond to treatment.

G. Both stiff-person syndrome (SPS) and progressive encephalomyelitis with rigidity and myoclonus (PERM) are characterized by progressive muscle rigidity, stimulus-induced muscle spasm (hyperekplexia), myoclonus, and autonomic dysfunction. PERM is distinguished from SPS by additional brainstem or other neurologic deficits and is usually more severe and progressive than SPS. SPS is classically an autoimmune disorder associated with antibodies against glutamic acid decarboxylase (GAD). The paraneoplastic variant of this disorder is extremely rare (<2% of cases), but should be considered in a patient suspected of having SPS who is negative for GAD antibodies. PERM is also classically an autoimmune disorder associated with antibodies against GAD or the glycine receptor. The paraneoplastic variant of PERM with glycine receptor antibodies is rare but has been associated with thymoma or lymphoma.

H. Isolated chorea can rarely represent a paraneoplastic syndrome. Bilateral symmetric choreoathetosis of neck and limbs similar to Huntington chorea, unilateral chorea, or orobuccal dystonia have been described. These patients do not typically have basal ganglia abnormalities on MRI at presentation.

I. Multiple well-characterized paraneoplastic antibodies (e.g., Hu, Ri, Ma2, Cv2) are associated with limbic encephalitis with brainstem or other nervous system involvement. The presence of retinitis and encephalitis is strongly suggestive of antibodies targeting Cv2 (CRMP5). Symptoms are often poorly responsive to immunosuppressive therapy. Patients with isolated limbic encephalitis and seizures are more likely to have an autoimmune etiology in which there is not an associated malignancy (see Chapter 115).

J. Paraneoplastic cerebellar degeneration (PCD) is associated with a wide range of antibodies and cancers, though only anti-Yo, anti-Tr, and anti-mGluR1 predominantly associate with isolated cerebellar dysfunction/ataxia without involvement of other areas of the nervous system. Patients with PCD initially present with dizziness, nausea, and vomiting and later develop gait instability, appendicular and truncal ataxia, and diplopia among other cerebellar signs. PCD is often refractory to immunosuppressive therapy, especially in cases associated with anti-Yo and anti-Hu antibodies.

K. Opsoclonus-myoclonus syndrome is characterized by rapid vertical and horizontal saccadic eye movements ("dancing eyes"), rapid involuntary movements, and sleep disturbance. In pediatric patients, it is frequently associated with neuroblastoma. In adult patients, it may be a paraneoplastic syndrome but can also be an immune-mediated process without an associated underlying malignancy.

REFERENCES

1. Graus F, Dalmau J. Paraneoplastic neurological syndromes. *Curr Opin Neurol.* 2012;25(6):795–801.
2. Dalmau J, Rosenfeld MR. Paraneoplastic syndromes of the CNS. *Lancet Neurol.* 2008;7(4):327–340.
3. Carvajal-González A, Leite MI, Waters P, et al. Glycine receptor antibodies in PERM and related syndromes: characteristics, clinical features, and outcomes. *Brain.* 2014;137(Pt 8):2178–2192.

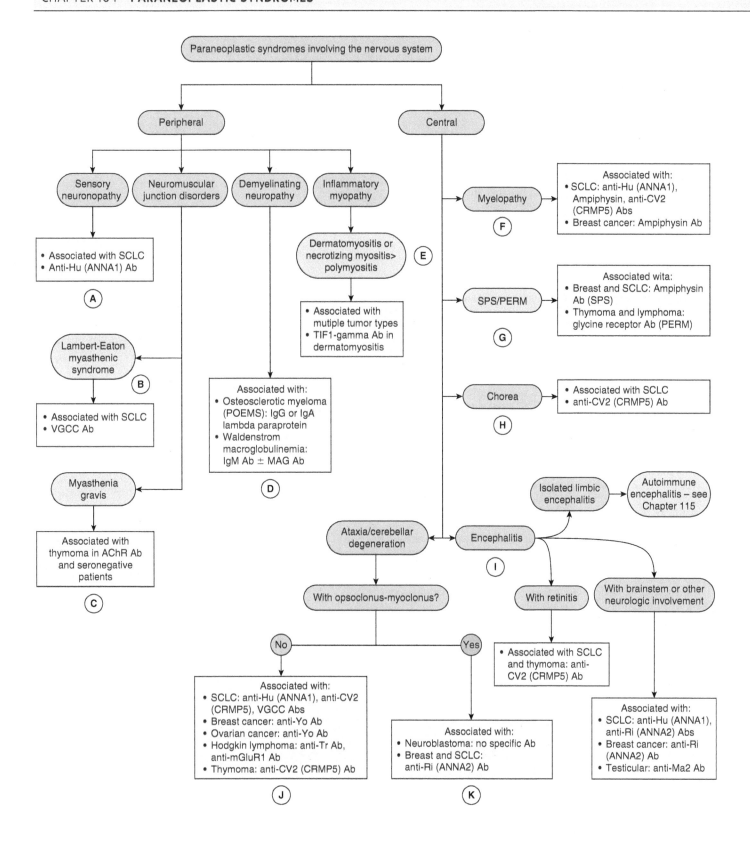

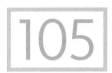

Encephalitis

Francisco Gomez and Ramani Balu

Encephalitis refers to a constellation of syndromes that present with brain inflammation and rapidly progressive neurologic symptoms. Although traditionally recognized as being caused by infection, a growing number of autoimmune encephalitis syndromes have been identified (see Chapter 115). Brain tumors, acute drug toxicities, metabolic encephalopathies, and vascular diseases can mimic encephalitis, making workup and management particularly challenging.

A. Suspect encephalitis in any patient with rapidly progressive (days to weeks) memory deficits, encephalopathy, behavioral symptoms, focal neurologic signs, or new unexplained seizures.

B. Obtain a detailed history including recent travel and possible exposures. Many causes of viral encephalitis have seasonal incidence patterns. Baseline laboratory testing helps identify systemic infections and toxic/metabolic encephalopathies that mimic encephalitis. Test human immunodeficiency virus (HIV) status, as acute HIV infection can cause encephalitis and immunocompromised patients are prone to opportunistic brain infections.

C. Start acyclovir empirically in patients with suspected encephalitis for coverage of herpes simplex virus (HSV) and varicella zoster virus (VZV) encephalitis. Patients with headaches, fevers, or stiff neck should also be started on empiric antibiotics for bacterial meningitis (see Chapter 106).

D. Head computed tomography (CT) is a useful initial screening test but is often normal in encephalitis, in which case lumbar puncture (LP) is necessary to evaluate for brain inflammation and assess for specific infectious causes. LP is contraindicated if CT shows evidence of increased intracranial pressure (i.e., mass effect, diffuse edema, or radiographic herniation); in this scenario, neurosurgical consultation for possible ventricular drainage and cerebrospinal fluid sampling should be obtained. If a unilateral focal brain lesion is seen on CT, this makes encephalitis less likely (although does not rule it out) and suggests an alternative etiology. Multifocal brain lesions seen on CT raise concern for a number of specific diagnoses which can present with symptoms similar to encephalitis. In both cases, magnetic resonance imaging (MRI) brain with contrast should be pursued to better characterize the visualized lesions. If this cannot be obtained promptly, or if there are signs of meningeal inflammation (stiff neck, fever), proceed directly to LP.

E. CSF pleocytosis (corrected white blood cell count > 5/mm^3) suggests encephalitis, although encephalitis can occur with normal WBC counts. Send cryptococcal antigen and HSV PCR for all patients with suspected encephalitis. Other testing depends on clinical presentation, risk factors, and geographical region (see Table 105.1).

F. If the diagnosis is not immediately obvious and MRI has not already been done, perform MRI as this can help with diagnosis. For instance, HSV encephalitis often shows asymmetric temporal lobe involvement with restricted diffusion and hemorrhage, and listeria meningoencephalitis shows brainstem edema and inflammatory changes.

TABLE 105.1	COMMON CAUSES OF ENCEPHALITIS
Herpes simplex virus	Temporal lobe hemorrhage or restricted diffusion on MRI. EEG may show periodic lateralized epileptiform discharges or temporal sharp waves. PCR has 98% sensitivity, 94%–100% specificity; may be falsely negative within first 48–72 hours. Treat with acyclovir 10–15 mg/kg IV q 8 hours for 14–21 days.
Varicella zoster virus	Reactivation of latent virus causes zoster (shingles), encephalitis, myelitis, and vasculopathy. Risk of encephalitis is higher in immunosuppressed and elderly patients. Detection of VZV DNA or anti-VZV IgG in CSF confirms diagnosis, but yield is higher for IgG.
Human herpes virus 6	Can cause encephalitis in immunosuppressed patients. HHV6 infection is associated with posttransplant acute limbic encephalitis.
Rabies	More common in Africa and Asia than North America. Transmitted by animal bite (dog and bat). Paresthesias occur at the inoculation site. "Encephalitic" rabies: agitation, bulbar signs, and hydrophobia. "Dumb/paralytic" rabies: flaccid paralysis. Both forms can progress to coma.
Japanese encephalitis virus	Most common cause of arboviral encephalitis worldwide, usually seen in periodic epidemics. Seizures and extrapyramidal signs common. Diagnosis with positive CSF IgM, treatment is supportive.
Zika virus	Emerging arboviral infection found in Asia, Africa, Polynesia, and the Americas. Associated with encephalitis, Guillain-Barré syndrome, and microcephaly (neonatal infection). Tests include CSF IgG/IgM and PCR.
West Nile virus	Can present as acute flaccid paralysis with superimposed encephalitis. MRI often shows involvement of basal ganglia and thalami. Diagnosis is confirmed by positive serum and CSF IgG/IgM.
Cryptococcus	Associated with immunosuppression; can occur in immunocompetent patients. Hydrocephalus is common. CSF cryptococcal antigen is 93%–100% sensitive, 93%–98% specific for diagnosis. Treat with liposomal amphotericin B (3–4 mg/kg IV daily) plus flucytosine (25 mg/kg orally q 6 hours).
Listeria	Most common infectious cause of rhombencephalitis. MRI may show brainstem involvement with contrast enhancement. Treat with ampicillin 2 g IV q 4 hours for 21 days.
Mycoplasma	Associated with encephalitis, transverse myelitis, cerebellitis. Symptoms may be from postinfectious inflammation. Diagnosis with CSF IgM/IgG. Treatment is largely supportive. Consider methylprednisolone 1 gram daily IV for 3–5 days.

CSF, Cerebrospinal fluid; *EEG,* electroencephalogram; *IV,* intravenous; *MRI,* magnetic resonance imaging; *PCR,* polymerase chain reaction; *VZV,* varicella zoster virus.

G. If infectious causes have been ruled out, consider primary autoimmune or paraneoplastic encephalitis (see Chapter 115).

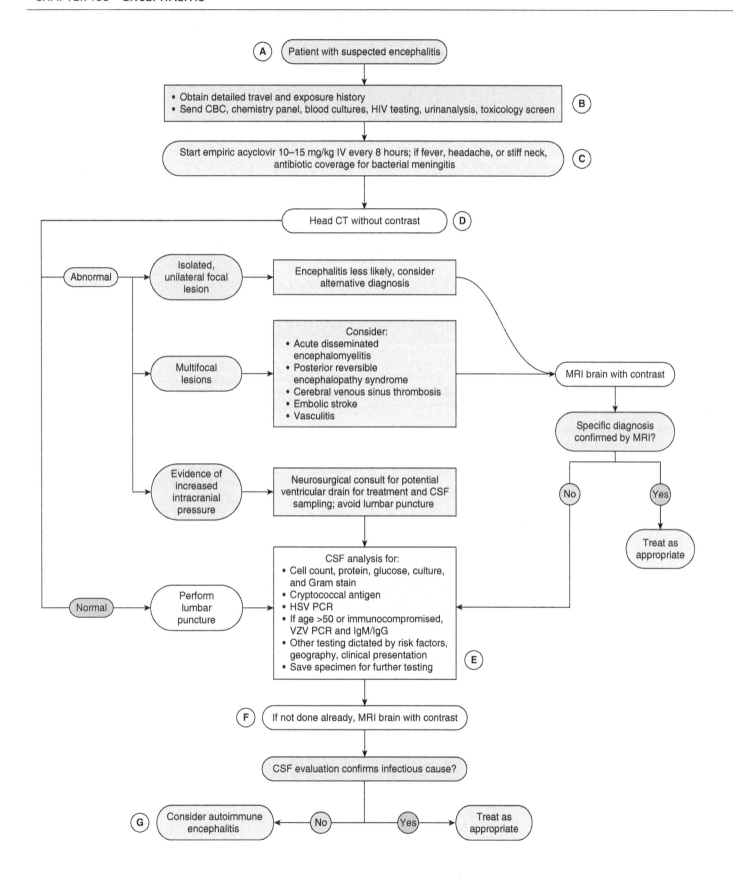

(A) Patient with suspected encephalitis

(B)
- Obtain detailed travel and exposure history
- Send CBC, chemistry panel, blood cultures, HIV testing, urinanalysis, toxicology screen

(C) Start empiric acyclovir 10–15 mg/kg IV every 8 hours; if fever, headache, or stiff neck, antibiotic coverage for bacterial meningitis

(D) Head CT without contrast

Abnormal

Isolated, unilateral focal lesion → Encephalitis less likely, consider alternative diagnosis

Multifocal lesions → Consider:
- Acute disseminated encephalomyelitis
- Posterior reversible encephalopathy syndrome
- Cerebral venous sinus thrombosis
- Embolic stroke
- Vasculitis

MRI brain with contrast

Specific diagnosis confirmed by MRI?

No   Yes

Treat as appropriate

Evidence of increased intracranial pressure → Neurosurgical consult for potential ventricular drain for treatment and CSF sampling; avoid lumbar puncture

Normal

Perform lumbar puncture

(E) CSF analysis for:
- Cell count, protein, glucose, culture, and Gram stain
- Cryptococcal antigen
- HSV PCR
- If age >50 or immunocompromised, VZV PCR and IgM/IgG
- Other testing dictated by risk factors, geography, clinical presentation
- Save specimen for further testing

(F) If not done already, MRI brain with contrast

CSF evaluation confirms infectious cause?

(G) Consider autoimmune encephalitis ← No   Yes → Treat as appropriate

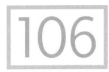

Acute Meningitis

Francisco Gomez and Ramani Balu

Acute meningitis is a neurological emergency. Clinical evaluation alone cannot accurately determine the cause of meningitis; lumbar puncture (LP) is essential and should be performed without delay. Empiric treatment should be started while waiting to confirm a pathogen, as earlier treatment reduces mortality and sequelae, particularly in bacterial meningitis.

A. Meningitis should be suspected in patients exhibiting any two of the following symptoms: decreased level of consciousness, headache, neck stiffness, fever, or unexplained seizures. Immunocompromised patients may present without neck rigidity or fever, so a high level of suspicion must be maintained. Emesis is an often-overlooked symptom that tends to accompany bacterial meningitis.

B. Obtain a detailed medical history including travel and exposures. Human immunodeficiency virus (HIV) or immunocompromised status must also be ascertained as they predispose to opportunistic infections such as cryptococcosis and tuberculosis. A comprehensive medication history is also indicated. Commonly used medications, including nonsteroidal antiinflammatory drugs, intravenous immunoglobulin, penicillins, and cephalosporins, can cause drug-induced aseptic meningitis. Recent antibiotic use should be assessed, as this may confound the results of cerebrospinal fluid cultures.

C. Prompt empiric treatment is imperative, as delay to antibiotic initiation worsens outcomes and increases mortality. Do not delay medications until after LP has been performed.

1. Empiric acyclovir until herpes simplex virus (HSV) encephalitis can be excluded. Dosage is 10–15 mg/kg every 8 hours.
2. Empiric therapy for acute bacterial meningitis
   a. Community acquired—vancomycin + third-generation cephalosporin.
   b. Recent neurosurgical instrumentation—requires coverage for *Pseudomonas*. Use vancomycin + fourth-generation cephalosporin or carbapenem.
   c. Immunocompromised, elderly, or young—requires coverage for *Listeria*. Add ampicillin.
   d. Concurrent otitis, mastoiditis or sinusitis—add metronidazole.
   e. Empiric steroids may improve mortality and outcome in adults with *Streptococcus pneumoniae* and *Neisseria meningitidis* infections, and reduce delayed hearing loss in children with *Haemophilus influenzae* infections. It is therefore reasonable to give steroids to patients with suspected bacterial meningitis due to these organisms (dexamethasone, 0.15 mg/kg up to 10 mg every 6 hours in developed countries, 0.4 mg/kg every 12 hours in developing countries, give first dose 15 minutes prior to starting antibiotics). The benefit of steroids is equivocal in developing countries where rates of HIV infection are high. Steroids should be stopped at 4 days, or immediately after disproving the mentioned organisms.

D. Obtain head computed tomography prior to LP in immunocompromised patients or those with signs of increased intracranial pressure, focal neurologic findings, or seizures. In the absence of these risk factors, LP may be performed without prior imaging.

E. LP should be performed without delay. Include opening and closing pressures, cell counts, protein and glucose measurement, Gram stain and culture, and cryptococcal antigen testing. It is useful to save cerebrospinal fluid for additional specific testing once the cell counts are available, as this may help focus diagnostic testing. Common tests to consider include polymerase chain reaction (PCR) for herpes simplex virus (HSV), varicella zoster virus (VZV), West Nile disease, Epstein-Barr virus, and enterovirus, as well as Lyme disease (if in an endemic region) and syphilis (Venereal Disease Research Lab, VDRL) testing. The latter are generally tested in both blood and cerebrospinal fluid (CSF). A variety of less common infectious organisms can be tested for in the proper clinical context. Low CSF glucose levels should raise suspicion for fungal or tuberculous meningitis. Neutrophilic-predominant pleocytosis suggests bacterial meningitis, while a lymphocytic predominance suggests viral meningitis (though the latter can be seen in early bacterial meningitis at times).

F. Further therapy should be guided by results of gram stain, culture, and other specific diagnostic testing. If cultures are negative but suspicion for bacterial meningitis remains, PCR and/or proteomics-based assays may aid in pathogen identification. If viral meningitis continues to be of concern, echovirus PCR from stool or throat samples can be of higher yield than that from CSF.

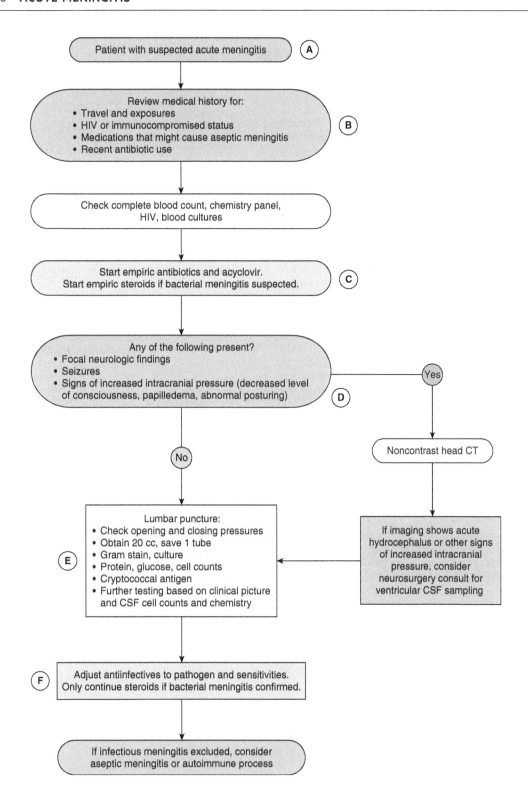

Patient with suspected acute meningitis Ⓐ

Review medical history for:
- Travel and exposures
- HIV or immunocompromised status
- Medications that might cause aseptic meningitis
- Recent antibiotic use

Ⓑ

Check complete blood count, chemistry panel, HIV, blood cultures

Start empiric antibiotics and acyclovir.
Start empiric steroids if bacterial meningitis suspected.

Ⓒ

Any of the following present?
- Focal neurologic findings
- Seizures
- Signs of increased intracranial pressure (decreased level of consciousness, papilledema, abnormal posturing)

Ⓓ

Yes

Noncontrast head CT

No

If imaging shows acute hydrocephalus or other signs of increased intracranial pressure, consider neurosurgery consult for ventricular CSF sampling

Lumbar puncture:
- Check opening and closing pressures
- Obtain 20 cc, save 1 tube
- Gram stain, culture
- Protein, glucose, cell counts
- Cryptococcal antigen
- Further testing based on clinical picture and CSF cell counts and chemistry

Ⓔ

Adjust antiinfectives to pathogen and sensitivities.
Only continue steroids if bacterial meningitis confirmed.

Ⓕ

If infectious meningitis excluded, consider aseptic meningitis or autoimmune process

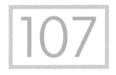

Subacute and Chronic Meningitis

Christopher Perrone and Brett L. Cucchiara

Patients with subacute or chronic meningitis typically have fluctuating but slowly progressive symptoms of fever, headache, neck pain or stiffness, vomiting, and/or cognitive changes over four or more weeks. Meningitis can also lead to focal neurologic deficits including cranial neuropathies such as facial palsy, radiculopathies, or seizures from focal cortical irritation. The persistence of symptoms is important, as there are forms of benign recurrent aseptic meningitis (such as Mollaret meningitis due to herpes simplex virus) in which symptoms resolve in between attacks even if they occur close together.

A. Lumbar puncture (LP) is necessary to establish that meningitis is present. Brain imaging to exclude a mass lesion should be considered prior to LP, particularly in patients age 60 years or older and those with focal neurologic deficits, seizures, known central nervous system disease, or who are immunocompromised. The majority of patients with a chronic meningitis will have normal brain imaging. Serum human immunodeficiency virus (HIV) testing should be performed on all patients. HIV seroconversion can present as a lymphocytic meningitis, and the range of infectious causes is significantly broader in immunocompromised patients. Cerebrospinal fluid (CSF) should be tested for cryptococcal antigen, venereal disease research laboratory (VDRL) test, cytology, and flow cytometry, as these will quickly identify more typical causes of a subacute meningitis.

B. An elevated CSF white blood cell count with neutrophilic predominance should raise concern for specific infections. In immunocompromised patients, a serum 1,3-beta-D-glucan assay and CSF fungal culture should be performed to assess for fungal infections such as aspergillus and candida. Some fungi, such as cryptoccocus and blastomycosis, have low levels of 1,3-beta-D-glucan in their cell walls, and thus will test negative. Nocardia should also be considered. Immunocompetent patients should be asked about exposure to unpasteurized milk for potential brucellosis (serology, blood culture), as well as recent oral trauma for actinomycosis (serology, culture).

C. Eosinophilia raises concern for parasitic meningitis. A thorough travel history should be obtained. Cysticercosis, strongyloidiasis, schistosomiasis, and trypanosomiasis can all be tested for by serologic tests. Coccidioides may also cause an eosinophilic meningitis.

D. The majority of patients with subacute or chronic meningitis will demonstrate a lymphocytic pleocytosis.

E. The CSF glucose is typically greater than two-thirds of the serum glucose, though this ratio may change in the setting of hypoglycemia. Low CSF glucose, defined as <50% of serum glucose, in the setting of subacute or chronic meningitis suggests fungal infection, tuberculosis, sarcoidosis, or neoplastic meningitis.

F. If the patient has a history of malignancy or systemic signs such as fever, night sweats, or weight loss that suggest malignancy, meningeal involvement should be suspected and assessed with CSF cytology and flow cytometry. To reduce the likelihood of a false-negative result, LP should be repeated if initial cytology is negative; compared to a single study, three serial LPs increases the diagnostic yield from ~70% to ~85%–90%. Primary central nervous system lymphoma can also be considered; lymphocytic pleocytosis may be absent in this scenario.

G. Iatrogenic causes of lymphocytic pleocytosis include recent spinal intervention (including epidural steroid injection), intravenous immunoglobulin, and nonsteroidal antiinflammatory drugs.

H. Travel to the northeast or midwest part of the United States (US), European countries (especially Austria, Estonia, Lithuania, the Netherlands, Slovenia), as well as Russia, China, and Japan, may indicate exposure to Lyme disease. *Histoplasma capsulatum* is found in the United States (Ohio River Valley), the Caribbean, southern Mexico, Central and South America, Africa, and Asia. Most cases of blastomycosis occur in people who have traveled to the southeastern or south central United States, Canada (bordering the Great Lakes), and Africa. Exposure to *Coccidiodes immitis* is restricted mostly to the southwestern United States and parts of Central and South America. Each of these infectious etiologies can be tested by serologies. If a patient has known exposure to tuberculosis or a positive screening test, CSF should be sent for acid-fast bacilli stains and mycobacterial culture, and consideration should be made for serial LPs.

I. Systemic signs may suggest an underlying autoimmune condition such as sarcoidosis, granulomatosis with polyangiitis, Behçet disease, or systemic lupus erythematosus.

J. Despite extensive focused serologic and CSF testing, a specific cause will not be identified in up to one-third of patients with a subacute/chronic meningitis. CSF from these patients can be assessed with unbiased next generation sequencing to identify nonhuman viral or parasitic genetic material. If a coexistent parenchymal lesion is identified, this lesion may be amenable to biopsy if an extensive evaluation is unrevealing and the patient is not responding to standard treatment.

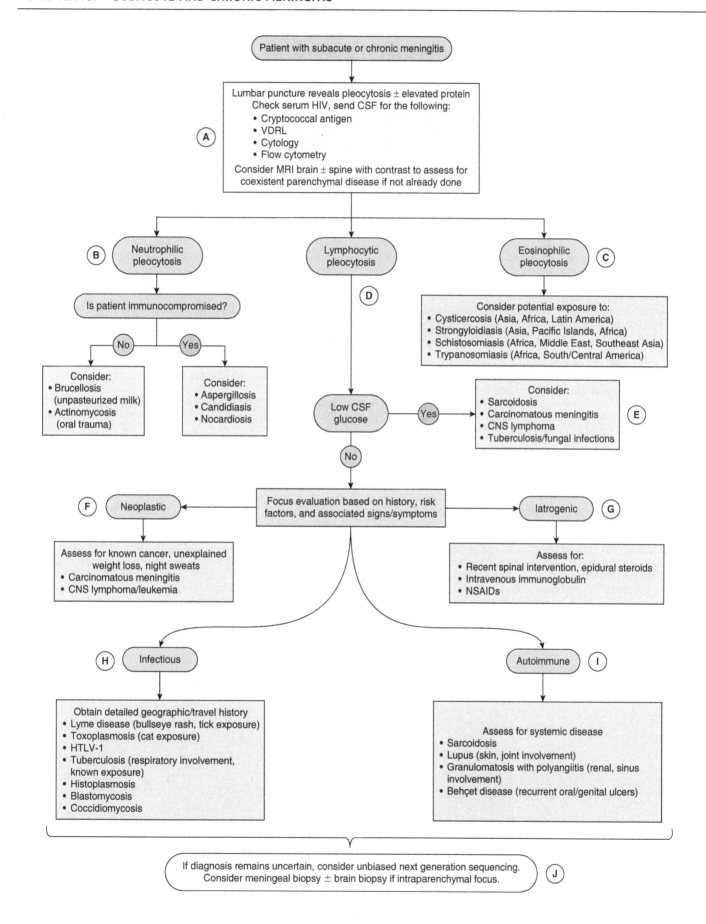

Patient with subacute or chronic meningitis

(A) Lumbar puncture reveals pleocytosis ± elevated protein
Check serum HIV, send CSF for the following:
- Cryptococcal antigen
- VDRL
- Cytology
- Flow cytometry

Consider MRI brain ± spine with contrast to assess for
coexistent parenchymal disease if not already done

(B) Neutrophilic pleocytosis

Lymphocytic pleocytosis

(C) Eosinophilic pleocytosis

(D)

Is patient immunocompromised?

No   Yes

Consider:
- Brucellosis (unpasteurized milk)
- Actinomycosis (oral trauma)

Consider:
- Aspergillosis
- Candidiasis
- Nocardiosis

Consider potential exposure to:
- Cysticercosis (Asia, Africa, Latin America)
- Strongyloidiasis (Asia, Pacific Islands, Africa)
- Schistosomiasis (Africa, Middle East, Southeast Asia)
- Trypanosomiasis (Africa, South/Central America)

Low CSF glucose   Yes

Consider:
- Sarcoidosis
- Carcinomatous meningitis
- CNS lymphoma
- Tuberculosis/fungal infections   (E)

No

(F) Neoplastic   ←   Focus evaluation based on history, risk factors, and associated signs/symptoms   →   Iatrogenic (G)

Assess for known cancer, unexplained weight loss, night sweats
- Carcinomatous meningitis
- CNS lymphoma/leukemia

Assess for:
- Recent spinal intervention, epidural steroids
- Intravenous immunoglobulin
- NSAIDs

(H) Infectious

Autoimmune (I)

Obtain detailed geographic/travel history
- Lyme disease (bullseye rash, tick exposure)
- Toxoplasmosis (cat exposure)
- HTLV-1
- Tuberculosis (respiratory involvement, known exposure)
- Histoplasmosis
- Blastomycosis
- Coccidiomycosis

Assess for systemic disease
- Sarcoidosis
- Lupus (skin, joint involvement)
- Granulomatosis with polyangiitis (renal, sinus involvement)
- Behçet disease (recurrent oral/genital ulcers)

If diagnosis remains uncertain, consider unbiased next generation sequencing.
Consider meningeal biopsy ± brain biopsy if intraparenchymal focus.   (J)

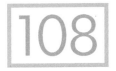

Tuberculosis Affecting the Nervous System

Christopher Perrone, Hamid Bassiri, and Brett L. Cucchiara

Neurologic manifestations of infection with tuberculosis (TB) are diverse and can be challenging to diagnose given the limitations of available diagnostic tests. Suspicion for TB should be heightened in patients with a history of travel to areas with high prevalence (such as India and Africa), known exposure to an individual infected with TB, or an immunocompromised state. All patients suspected of having TB should be tested for human immunodeficiency virus, as this may affect response to and type of treatment.

A. Tuberculous meningitis typically presents with a subacute course developing over weeks, and can cause cranial neuropathies, communicating hydrocephalus through impaired absorption of cerebrospinal fluid (CSF), and an infectious vasculitis leading to cerebral infarction, which is usually subcortical and often bilateral affecting the caudate, internal capsule, and anterior thalamus. Initial examination with brain magnetic resonance imaging (MRI) with contrast is indicated when any of these manifestations are suspected, particularly if a patient exhibits signs of progressive alteration of mental status. In that case, hydrocephalus is a major concern, and prompt neurosurgical intervention for placement of a ventricular drain may be necessary, at which time CSF can be obtained.

B. Tuberculoma, a conglomeration of tuberculous nodules following hematogenous spread of the organism, can lead to focal neurologic deficits or be a seizure focus.

C. Spinal cord involvement may be indirect with bony invasion of the vertebral bodies leading to fracture (Pott's disease) with resulting cord compression or direct due to spinal cord tuberculoma or arachnoiditis. The latter represents an inflammatory process along the arachnoid membrane, which leads to gradual encasement of the spinal cord with exudate. In the setting of acute paraparesis, computed tomography (CT) of the spine should be performed to assess for bony involvement; if acute fracture is present, urgent surgical consultation is indicated. Otherwise, and particularly with a more subacute course, MRI of the spine with contrast should be performed.

D. If hydrocephalus and mass effect are absent, CSF should be analyzed. A lymphocytic or mononuclear pleocytosis (white blood cells >100/mm³), highly elevated protein (>100 mg/dL), and low glucose (45 mg/dL) are commonly seen with neurologic involvement of TB, although absence of these findings does not rule out the disease.

E. Interferon-gamma release assays, which measure the release of interferon gamma by memory T-cells following stimulation with *Mycobacterium tuberculosis*–specific antigens, can provide evidence of exposure to this organism, even in individuals who have previously been inoculated with Bacille Calmette-Guérin (BCG) vaccine. Tuberculin skin tests, which involve intradermal injection of mycobacterial purified protein derivatives to stimulate a delayed hypersensitivity response, may also be used, although prior BCG receipt may provide cross-reactive false positivity. Neither test reliably distinguishes between active and latent infection, nor is either sufficiently sensitive to rule out TB infection. Chest radiographs or CT scanning can identify infiltrates, consolidations, or cavities (especially in the upper lungs), as well as hilar lymphadenopathy, to provide evidence of pulmonary involvement (most common). Sputum smears and culture for acid-fast bacilli can confirm a diagnosis of mycobacterial disease. If there is no pulmonary disease, look for lymphadenopathy, pleuritis, involvement of the liver/spleen on abdominal CT, choroidal tubercles on ophthalmologic examination, and/or osseous involvement on skeletal survey. Any of these may provide evidence of active extraneural TB, in which case treatment is indicated.

F. Empiric therapy with a combination of rifampin, isoniazid, pyrazinamide, and ethambutol (RIPE regimen) is standard initial therapy. Consider alternative regimens if disease may have been acquired from an area with high endemic levels of resistance to one or more of these drugs. All four medications are given for 2 months. Assuming a susceptible strain, isoniazid and rifampin are continued for an additional 7–10 months. Steroids have been shown to reduce mortality in TB meningitis and should also be administered; intravenous dexamethasone 0.3–0.4 mg/kg per day for 2 weeks followed by a taper over 6–8 weeks is a standard regimen.

G. If suspicion for TB remains high but the diagnosis remains unclear, serial lumbar punctures should be performed daily for 3 days. CSF acid-fast bacilli stains as well as culture should be sent. Yield is improved with large-volume CSF sampling. CSF nucleic acid amplification (NAA) can be confirmatory in the setting of negative cultures and should be sent, while CSF adenosine deaminase can support a diagnosis of CNS TB but cannot differentiate between TB and other types of bacterial meningitis.

H. Therapy should not be withheld in the setting of a strong clinical suspicion of CNS TB, as the sensitivity of CSF acid-fast bacilli staining with culture is only ~80%. CSF NAA has even poorer sensitivity (~60%) but very high specificity (nearly 100%), such that a positive result can be considered confirmatory of the diagnosis.

REFERENCE

1. Cherian A, Thomas SV. Central nervous system tuberculosis. *Afr Health Sci.* 2011;11(1):116–127.

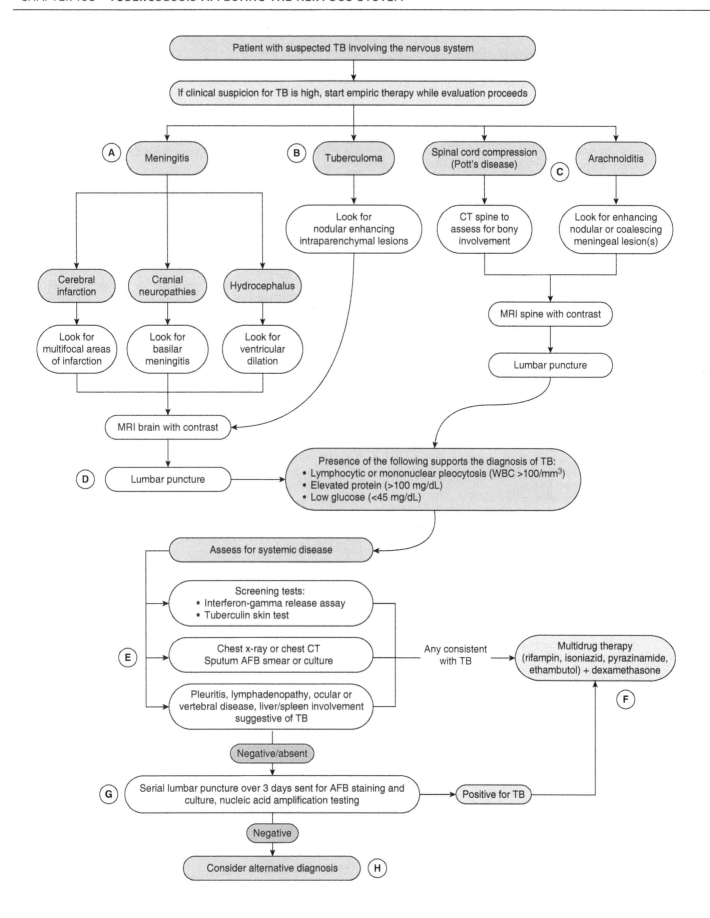

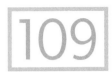

Neurosyphilis

Cody Nathan and Brett L. Cucchiara

Syphilis, caused by the bacterium *Treponema pallidum*, is able to invade the central nervous system early in the course of infection. As many as 40% of patients will have neuroinvasion of syphilis but most will not exhibit symptoms of neurosyphilis. Early neurosyphilis typically occurs within the first years of infection and can manifest as meningitis (symptomatic or asymptomatic), otosyphilis, ocular syphilis, and meningovascular syphilis. Later phase syphilis (usually one to two decades after initial infection) can result in the syndromes of tabes dorsalis and general paresis.

A. Symptomatic meningitis can present with headache, neck stiffness, photophobia, and confusion. Multiple cranial neuropathies may occur. Otosyphilis and ocular syphilis may occur independently or in conjunction with meningitis. Symptoms of otosyphilis include hearing loss, tinnitus, and vertigo. Vision loss secondary to uveitis, chorioretinitis, or optic nerve involvement may occur with ocular syphilis.

B. Meningovascular syphilis represents an infectious arteritis typically affecting the medium to large arteries and leading to cerebral or spinal cord infarction. It may occur early after primary infection or years later. Involvement may be limited to the intracranial vessels, with the middle cerebral artery often preferentially involved, or may affect extracranial vessels as well, including the aorta and its branches. Diagnosis is with computed tomography or magnetic resonance angiography.

C. In tabes dorsalis, syphilitic infection damages the dorsal columns of the spinal cord and dorsal roots of the spinal nerves. Findings include impaired vibration and proprioception in lower extremities causing an ataxic gait and positive Romberg sign, shooting pain in the legs and abdomen, bladder dysfunction, areflexia in lower extremities, and Argyll Robertson pupils (constrict to accommodation but not to light).

D. General paresis manifests as progressive dementia, personality change, and other psychiatric symptoms including depression, delusions, and hallucinations. Other neurologic deficits may include dysarthria, tremor, hyperreflexia, and Argyll Robertson pupils.

E. Diagnosis of syphilis is made using two types of tests: (1) nontreponemal serum screening tests, such as the rapid plasma reagin (RPR) and Venereal Disease Research Laboratory (VDRL) test; and (2) treponemal-specific tests such as the fluorescent treponemal antibody absorption test (FTA-ABS), *T. pallidum* particle agglutination assay (TP-PA), and microhemagglutination test for antibodies to *T. pallidum* (MHA-TP). Non-treponemal tests have lower sensitivity for late forms of syphilis, and are more likely to produce false-positive results, but have the advantage of providing a semiquantitative titer that correlates with infectious activity. Treponemal-specific tests are more sensitive for later forms of syphilis, and will remain positive for life once infection has occurred. Thus patients previously treated for syphilis with a positive treponemal test may or may not have active infection; evaluation of the non-treponemal test titer can help with this determination. The classic testing pathway is to perform the non-treponemal test first with positive results confirmed using a treponemal assay. More recently with advances in laboratory instrumentation, a reversed testing protocol has been introduced in some institutions starting with the treponemal-specific assay and, in positive subjects, subsequently testing the non-treponemal assay.

F. Patients with positive syphilis testing and suspected neurosyphilis should undergo lumbar puncture to assess for central nervous system infectious activity. Human immunodeficiency virus (HIV) testing should also be performed as up to 40% of people with syphilis are coinfected with HIV. In the absence of HIV infection, an elevated cerebrospinal fluid (CSF) protein (>45 mg/dL) OR pleocytosis (white blood cells, WBC >5 cells/mm^3) OR a positive CSF VDRL indicates possible neurosyphilis and is an indication for treatment.

G. Interpretation of CSF studies in patients with HIV infection is challenging as HIV infection itself may cause elevated protein and mononuclear pleocytosis. If CSF WBC are ≤5 cells/mm^3 and the CSF VDRL is negative, neurosyphilis can be reliably excluded. If the CSF VDRL is positive OR WBC >20 cells/mm^3 are present, the patient should be treated for neurosyphilis. In cases with intermediate pleocytosis, consultation with an infectious disease expert is reasonable to decide on treatment.

H. Treatment of neurosyphilis is more intensive than that for patients with syphilis not affecting the nervous system. Patients with penicillin allergy should undergo penicillin desensitization followed by treatment with penicillin. Efficacy of non-penicillin treatment for treatment of neurosyphilis is limited.

I. Monitoring includes repeat lumbar puncture at 6, 12, and 24 months posttreatment. Re-treatment should be considered if the CSF WBC count has not normalized by 6 months, the CSF VDRL has not become negative or decreased fourfold by 12 months, or CSF abnormalities persist at 24 months.

REFERENCES

1. Marra CM. Neurosyphilis. *Continuum (Minneap Minn).* 2015;21:1714–1728.
2. Hook E. Syphilis. *Lancet.* 2017;389(10078):1550–1557.

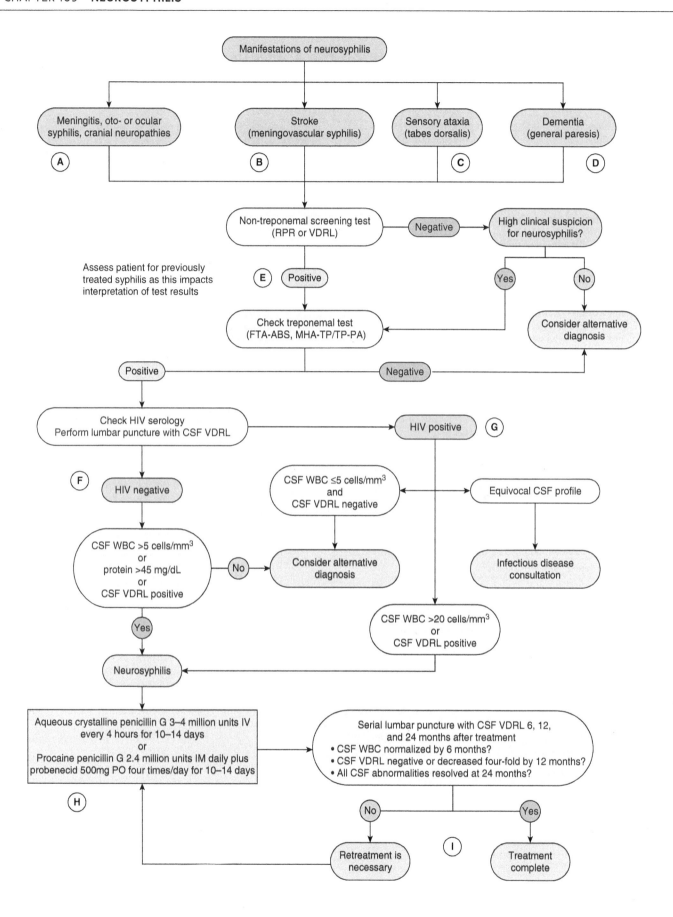

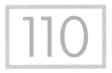

Lyme Disease Involving the Nervous System (Neuroborreliosis)

John Best and Brett L. Cucchiara

Lyme disease is caused by an infection with the spirochete *Borrelia burgdorferi* transmitted via tick bites (*Ixodes ricinus* in Europe and *Ixodes scapularis* in the United States). Primary infection is normally associated with an erythematous ring-shaped "bullseye" rash (erythema migrans); fever, headaches, and fatigue may also occur. Neurologic involvement (neuroborreliosis) occurs in 10%–15% of patients, and is more common in the absence of early treatment for primary infection. Onset of neurologic symptoms beyond the first few months after initial infection is rare.

A. Meningitis, cranial neuropathies, and painful radiculitis are common neurologic manifestations of Lyme disease. Approximately two-thirds of patients with neurologic involvement will develop meningitis with slowly progressive headache and neck stiffness and a lymphocytic pleocytosis in the cerebrospinal fluid (CSF). Cranial nerve involvement occurs with similar frequency. While almost any cranial nerve can be affected, facial nerve involvement is by far the most frequent, and may occasionally be bilateral. A painful radiculitis occurs in ~50% of patients with neuroborreliosis. It is an acute-onset radicular pain, often involving more than one dermatome.

B. Intracranial hypertension and encephalomyelitis are very rare neurologic manifestations of Lyme disease. Intracranial hypertension, seen more commonly in children than adults, presents with headaches and occasionally vision loss, with papilledema present on examination. Unlike typical benign intracranial hypertension (pseudotumor cerebri), the CSF demonstrates pleocytosis consistent with meningitis, which is felt to be the operative mechanism. Encephalomyelitis may be associated with focal signal abnormalities on magnetic resonance imaging; there is often associated radiculitis. It appears to be more common in Europe than in the United States. Mild cognitive impairment, often associated with fatigue and generalized nonspecific malaise, is common with active disseminated Lyme disease (as it is with many infectious/inflammatory diseases) but does not indicate active brain infection and should not be considered Lyme encephalitis.

C. The *Ixodes* tick, carrier of the tick-borne spirochetes that cause Lyme disease, are endemic across temperate regions of northern and central Europe and Asia and the northeast and north-central United States. Among the three spirochete species, *Borrelia garinii*, *Borrelia afzelii*, and *Borrelia burgdorferi sensu stricto*, only *B. burgdorferi sensu stricto* is found in the United States. Lyme disease should be considered only in those with plausible exposure to an *Ixodes* tick, recognizing that both tick bite and erythema migrans may go unnoticed by patients.

D. Serologic testing for Lyme disease starts with a screening enzyme-linked immunosorbent assay (ELISA). If this is negative, no further testing is indicated. If positive, confirmatory western blot testing for immunoglobulin (Ig)G and IgM antibodies is performed. IgM antibodies generally are present by about 2 weeks after infection, with IgG antibodies taking up to 6 weeks to appear. In patients with symptom duration of 6 weeks or greater, positive IgM but negative IgG testing is likely to represent a false-positive test.

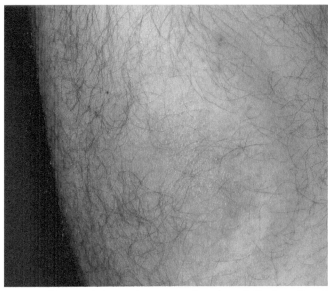

FIG. 110.1 Characteristic erythematous ring-shaped "bullseye" rash (erythema migrans) from Lyme disease.

E. Individuals with a history of a recent tick bite and characteristic erythema migrans ("bullseye" rash, Fig. 110.1) who have neurologic symptoms suspected due to Lyme disease may be tested with a serum Lyme titer but should be treated regardless of the results. While the vast majority of cases will be seropositive by the time neurologic symptoms of Lyme develop, occasionally a detectable antibody response is delayed for up to 6 weeks. Note that negative serologic testing is common early in the disease course when only rash is present, particularly if treated with antibiotics.

F. For most patients with neuroborreliosis, first-line treatment is oral doxycycline for 14–28 days. Previously, intravenous ceftriaxone was commonly used when neurologic manifestation of Lyme disease were present; however, subsequent data have demonstrated that oral doxycycline is as effective as intravenous antibiotics. If there a contraindication to doxycycline or in the setting of rare but more severe neurologic manifestations such as encephalomyelitis, intravenous ceftriaxone for 14–21 days may be used. There is no evidence of benefit for more prolonged courses of antimicrobial therapy in Lyme disease.

REFERENCE

1. Halperin JJ. Neuroborreliosis and neurosyphilis. *Continuum (Minneap Minn).* 2018;24:1439–1458.

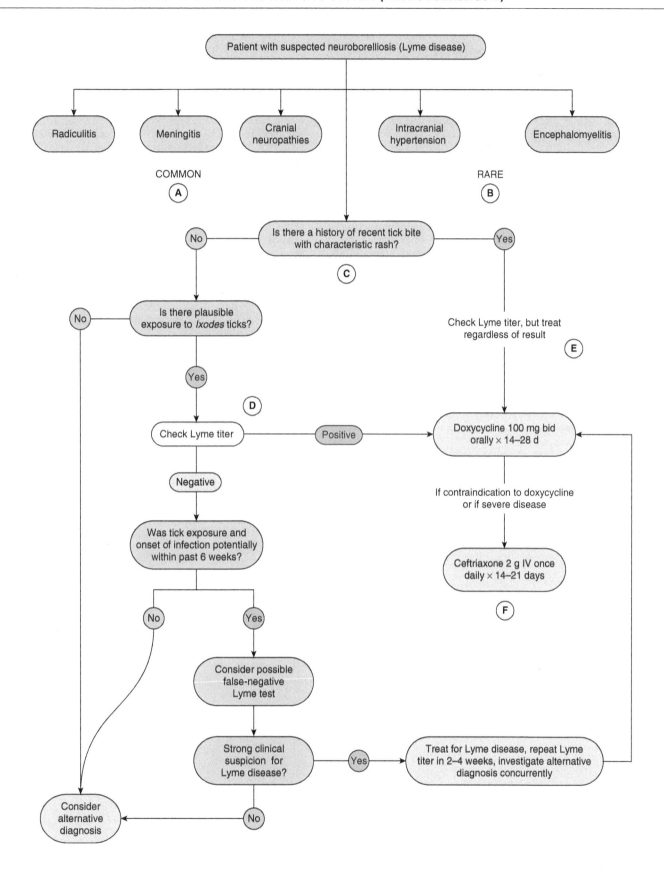

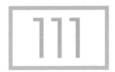

Optic Neuritis

Ali G. Hamedani

Optic neuritis is an inflammatory optic neuropathy that may be idiopathic or associated with underlying demyelinating disease. The typical presentation is one of subacute vision loss and dyschromatopsia (impairment of color vision) over hours to days. Pain with eye movement accompanies these symptoms in the overwhelming majority of patients. The fundoscopic examination is normal in two-thirds of patients, indicating retrobulbar optic nerve inflammation; in the remaining one-third, there is mild disc margin blurring without hemorrhages or exudates. As dyschromatopsia is an important feature, careful testing with color plates must be done to identify impairment in color vision. Treatment with intravenous corticosteroids hastens visual recovery in optic neuritis but does not affect the final visual outcome. In the Optic Neuritis Treatment Trial, at 2 years' follow-up, intravenous corticosteroids also delayed the development of clinically definite multiple sclerosis (MS), but this benefit did not persist at 5 years.

A. A lack of pain with eye movement and severe optic disc swelling should prompt consideration of alternative diagnoses, namely nonarteritic ischemic optic neuropathy (NAION). This is also more common in older individuals with vascular risk factors. Leber's hereditary optic neuropathy is a mitochondrial disease that causes subacute, painless vision loss in one eye followed weeks to months later by involvement of the other eye, primarily in young men. Acute fundus findings—mild disc margin blurring (pseudoedema) and peripapillary telangiectasias—are subtle and can mimic optic neuritis, so a lack of pain with eye movement and/or suggestive family history are important features to consider. Acute idiopathic blind spot enlargement is a group of autoimmune retinopathies characterized by enlargement of the physiologic blind spot. They may be accompanied by mild optic disc edema and as such may mimic optic neuritis; however, they are distinguished by prominent symptoms of photopsias out of proportion to vision loss and typically lack dyschromatopsia.

B. While MS is associated with an increased risk of uveitis, especially intermediate uveitis, concurrent uveitis and optic neuritis should raise suspicion for atypical inflammatory causes such as sarcoidosis. Neuroretinitis is an inflammatory disorder affecting both the optic nerve and retina and is often postinfectious (especially *Bartonella henselae* or "cat-scratch disease") in etiology. It presents with unilateral optic disc edema followed by the development of a macular star, which reflects lipid leakage from capillaries. Macular stars can also occur in other optic neuropathies when optic disc swelling is severe (e.g., NAION), but this would not be expected in optic neuritis.

C. Neuromyelitis optica (NMO) is a demyelinating disease that causes severe, often recurrent attacks of optic neuritis and longitudinally extensive transverse myelitis. Testing of aquaporin-4 autoantibodies should be considered in any patient optic neuritis, especially when vision loss is severe (no light perception), bilateral or chiasmal, or does not begin to improve after 1–2 weeks. The distinction between NMO and MS is important not only prognostically but also for choosing long-term immunomodulatory treatment, as most disease-modifying treatments for MS are ineffective in NMO, and some (IFN-β, fingolimod, natalizumab) may actually worsen it.

D. Magnetic resonance imaging (MRI) of the orbits is very sensitive in demonstrating optic nerve thickening, T2 signal abnormality, and gadolinium enhancement, and therefore the absence of these findings should also lead one to question the diagnosis of optic neuritis.

E. Patients with optic neuritis have an approximately 30% probability of developing MS within 5 years. By far the strongest predictor of MS is the presence of demyelinating-appearing lesions on MRI; in the Optic Neuritis Treatment Trial, the 15-year risk of MS was 72% for patients with abnormal brain MRI compared with 22% with normal brain MRI.

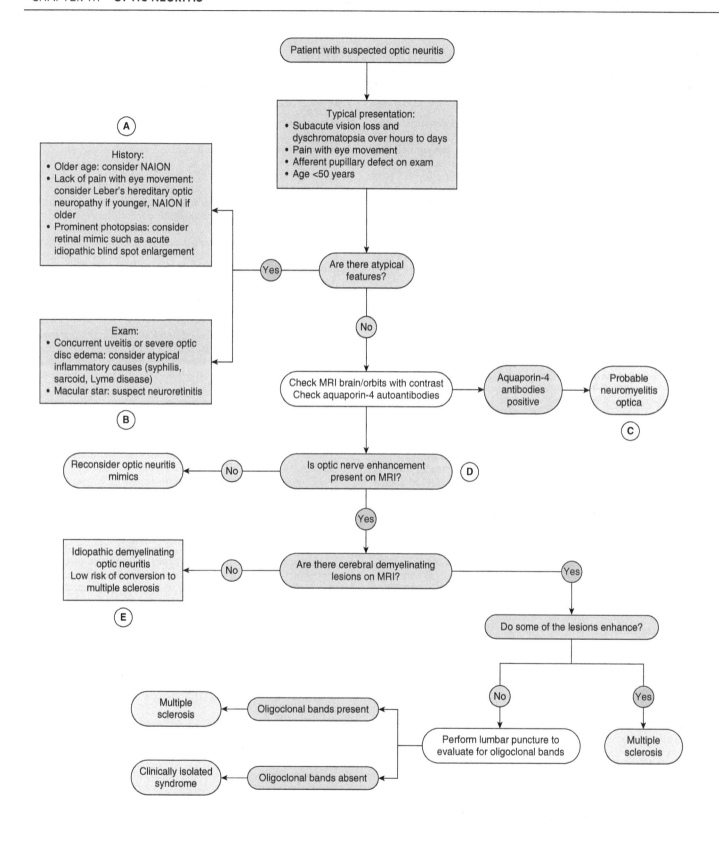

Patient with suspected optic neuritis

Typical presentation:
- Subacute vision loss and dyschromatopsia over hours to days
- Pain with eye movement
- Afferent pupillary defect on exam
- Age <50 years

Ⓐ

History:
- Older age: consider NAION
- Lack of pain with eye movement: consider Leber's hereditary optic neuropathy if younger, NAION if older
- Prominent photopsias: consider retinal mimic such as acute idiopathic blind spot enlargement

Exam:
- Concurrent uveitis or severe optic disc edema: consider atypical inflammatory causes (syphilis, sarcoid, Lyme disease)
- Macular star: suspect neuroretinitis

Ⓑ

Are there atypical features? — Yes

No

Check MRI brain/orbits with contrast
Check aquaporin-4 autoantibodies → Aquaporin-4 antibodies positive → Probable neuromyelitis optica Ⓒ

Is optic nerve enhancement present on MRI? Ⓓ — No → Reconsider optic neuritis mimics

Yes

Are there cerebral demyelinating lesions on MRI? — No → Idiopathic demyelinating optic neuritis. Low risk of conversion to multiple sclerosis Ⓔ

Yes

Do some of the lesions enhance?

No → Perform lumbar puncture to evaluate for oligoclonal bands

Yes → Multiple sclerosis

Oligoclonal bands present → Multiple sclerosis

Oligoclonal bands absent → Clinically isolated syndrome

112 Treatment of Multiple Sclerosis

Eric Williamson

Treatment of multiple sclerosis (MS) is aimed at slowing disease progression and preventing development or worsening of disability. New neurologic symptoms ("relapses") or progression of disability indicate ongoing disease activity. Further, the presence of new lesions on brain magnetic resonance imaging (MRI) serves as a surrogate of disease activity even in the absence of new symptoms, and thus has implications for modifying treatment. Medications (Table 112.1) used to treat MS primarily target the adaptive immune response system. When considering which treatment to use, it is important to assess (1) the degree of disease activity, (2) the side effect and risk profile of specific therapies, (3) patient preferences in terms of route of administration or risk/benefit profile, and (4) insurance coverage and financial resources, as MS therapies can be very expensive.

A. All agents approved to treat MS have shown benefit in the relapsing-remitting form of the disease and are also felt to be useful in secondary progressive MS with evidence of disease activity. In primary progressive MS, however, disability slowly accrues despite the absence of discrete relapses, At present, only ocrelizumab and, in rare cases, mitoxantrone are approved for primary progressive MS. Mitoxantrone use is limited by dose-related cardiac toxicity and requires monitoring with echocardiography.

B. Steroids (methylprednisolone, 1 g/day × 3–5 days, given intravenously) may hasten recovery in the case of clinical relapse, and can be given with or without an oral steroid taper. Typical side effects of steroids may occur and should be considered when weighing the decision to treat. Alternatives (if patient has side effects from steroids or they are deemed ineffective) include adrenocorticotropic hormone (dosed intravenously) or plasma exchange; both of these are more expensive and are used sparingly.

C. Disease activity can be broadly divided into (1) mild disease, in which the clinician interprets radiographic and/or clinical burden along with concern for future disease to be lower; (2) moderate disease, in which there is greater concern about future disease course or accumulation of disease activity; and (3) markedly active disease, in which there is neurologic or radiographic worsening or demonstration of significant burden of disease in the recent past. With more severe disease, more aggressive immunomodulating therapies are warranted despite an increased risk of serious side effects with these agents.

D. β-Interferons and glatiramer acetate are given via subcutaneous injection. They have excellent safety profiles and, among approved MS therapies, have been in use the longest. They have often been termed *platform therapies* for these reasons. Liver function tests (LFTs) should be checked every 3–6 months in patients on interferons; no monitoring is required with glatiramer acetate. Teriflunomide and dimethyl fumarate are both oral medications and are preferred by some patients for this reason. These have similar or slightly better efficacy than the interferons or glatiramer acetate, but do carry some risks (specifically pregnancy concerns with teriflunomide, gastrointestinal upset, flushing, and rare infections with dimethyl fumarate). Teriflunomide requires frequent monitoring of LFTs, a screen for tuberculosis prior to starting therapy, and contraceptive counseling, as pregnancy must be avoided due to potential teratogenicity. Blood count monitoring for lymphopenia must be done every 3–6 months with dimethyl fumarate.

E. In moderate disease, the oral agent fingolimod is effective, but cardiac monitoring must be performed with the initial dose due to the occurrence of bradycardia in some patients. Varicella immunization and screening every 3–6 months for lymphopenia and macular edema must also be performed. Ocrelizumab is a potent antiinflammatory given intravenously at 6-month intervals. Premedication with acetaminophen, methylprednisolone, and antihistamines is required to decrease the not infrequent occurrence of infusion reactions, and pretreatment screening for hepatitis should be performed. Natalizumab, dosed intravenously at monthly intervals, is one of the most potent agents for MS but carries a small risk of progressive multifocal leukoencephalopathy (PML), which is caused by the JC virus. Testing for JC virus antibody may help stratify risk, as antibody-negative patients appear to be at lower risk of PML than those with positive antibodies. When used long term, antibody status should be assessed two to three times per year along with surveillance MRI to evaluate for PML.

F. In cases of marked disease activity (typically despite use of less potent agents), natalizumab may be considered and a greater risk for PML may be tolerated, or alemtuzumab may be used. Alemtuzumab, which is given once yearly, appears to have efficacy even when used in a discontinuous fashion, i.e., some treated patients may not need to continue it beyond the first or second yearly dose. Unfortunately, it not infrequently leads to other medical issues (thyroid disease develops in one-third of patients subsequent to treatment), and close monitoring for rare but potentially serious complications (e.g., thrombocytopenia and renal disease) is required. Monthly blood count, urinalysis, LFTs, and 3-monthly thyroid function testing are recommended.

G. Potent immune suppressants and/or chemotherapeutics such as cyclophosphamide and methotrexate have been used off-label in some patients with MS who have not responded to conventional agents.

H. In the absence of new symptoms, imaging with MRI of the brain (and in select cases spinal cord) should typically be done yearly to assess for disease activity. When present, therapy may need to be modified, and repeat short-term interval imaging is indicated. It may also be helpful to have imaging at start or change of therapy for comparison in the future. Deescalation of therapy (such as moving from a more to less potent agent) can be considered when the concern for disease activity is reduced, such as in a patient with stable imaging for a number of years, older patients, or in those more likely to encounter or more vulnerable to serious side effects.

Drug	Route of administration	Dose	Schedule
Interferon-β1b	SC	250 mcg	Every other day
Interferon-β1a	SC	30 mcg, 22 and 44 mcg, 125 mcg pegylated	Weekly (lower efficacy), 3 × weekly, every other week
Glatiramer acetate	SC	20 mg or 40 mg	Daily or 3 × weekly
Fingolimod	Oral	0.5 mg	Daily
Teriflunomide	Oral	14 mg (or 7 mg, but of lower efficacy)	Daily
Dimethyl fumarate	Oral	240 mg	Twice daily
Natalizumab	IV	300 mg	Every 4 weeks
Mitoxantrone	IV	5–12 mg/m²	Every 3 months, maximum 2 years
Alemtuzumab	IV	12 mg daily × 5 d (× 3 d after year one)	Yearly, possibly discontinuous
Ocrelizumab	IV	600 mg (initially 300 mg q2 wk × 2)	Every 6 months after initial dose

TABLE 112.1 MEDICATIONS USED FOR TREATING MULTIPLE SCLEROSIS

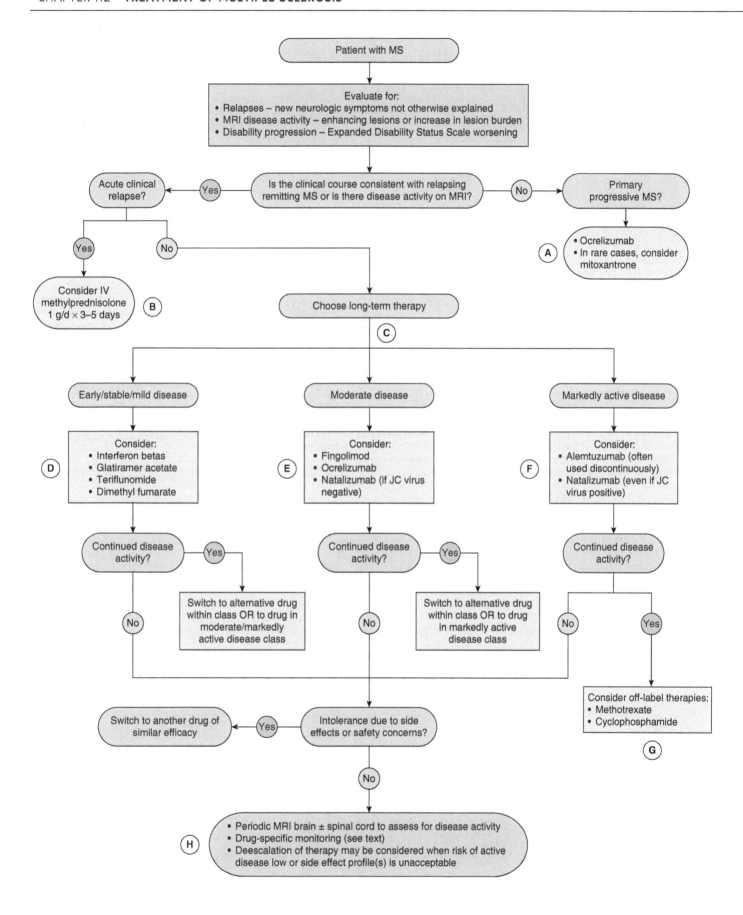

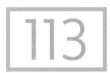

Transverse Myelitis

Dennis L. Kolson and Raymond S. Price

Transverse myelitis (TM) refers to a segmental inflammatory process involving the spinal cord, and may be idiopathic or secondary to a variety of specific disease processes. It typically presents with acute or subacute flaccid paraparesis, sensory abnormalities, and bowel/bladder dysfunction. When complete, both the anterior and posterior regions of the cord are involved; partial TM cord syndromes (those not involving the transverse span of the cord or those with mild symptoms of myelitis) are more commonly associated with multiple sclerosis than are complete TM syndromes. On examination, patients with acute TM may have bilateral lower motor neuron weakness, hyporeflexia, a spinal sensory level, and impaired joint position discrimination. Hyperacute onset and sparing of joint position discrimination should raise suspicion for anterior spinal artery cord infarction. Subacute and chronic TM typically evolves to demonstrate hyperreflexia and other upper motor neuron signs weeks after initial presentation.

A. Compressive spinal cord lesions may present with the same symptoms as TM and must be identified, as emergent decompressive surgery is indicated in such cases. Spine magnetic resonance imaging (MRI) is the preferred diagnostic test; in patients unable to undergo MRI, computed tomography (CT) or CT myelography may be used. Spinal cord infarction (see Chapter 47) and, rarely, spinal cord edema/ischemia from a spinal cord dural arteriovenous fistula can clinically mimic TM. Central T2 hyperintensity, particularly involving the anterior horns, is the classic MRI finding in cord infarction. Flow voids on the cord surface on T2 sequences are commonly but not uniformly seen in dural fistulas. Additional imaging such as cord MRI diffusion weighted imaging or catheter angiography may be necessary to clarify the diagnosis. If MRI is normal, consider Guillain-Barré syndrome.

B. If a lesion consistent with TM is found, start high-dose intravenous steroids immediately to reduce cord inflammation. Progression from onset to nadir in TM occurs between 4 hours and 21 days. Steroids may prevent progression and improve recovery. It is acceptable to start and continue steroids while determining the underlying cause of TM. Even if an infectious cause is present, steroids are generally safe.

C. Cerebrospinal fluid (CSF) examination is required for specific testing and to evaluate for inflammation. In addition to routine studies, check oligoclonal bands, IgG index, and cytology. Additional testing should be tailored to individual patient features (see below).

D. An intrinsic cord lesion spanning three or more segments suggests certain specific causes are more likely, but it does not absolutely rule in or out any type of inflammatory myelitis.

E. Neuromyelitis optica spectrum disorders (NMOSDs) are severe inflammatory diseases with a predilection for the spinal cord and optic nerves. Most cases are associated with aquaporin-4 antibodies (known as NMO antibody). Up to 40% of NMOSD patients with a negative NMO antibody have anti-myelin oligodendrocyte glycoprotein (MOG) antibodies.

F. TM related to multiple sclerosis is rarely associated with significant CSF pleocytosis. If suspected, brain MRI should be performed to look for cerebral demyelinating lesions. When >20 white blood cells (WBC)/mm^3 are present in the CSF, consider infectious agents, noting that noninfectious conditions such as NMOSD and neurosarcoidosis can also have significant pleocytosis.

G. Serologic testing is indicated to identify common and uncommon cause of TM, many of which are often overlooked. For most TM patients, this should include testing for human immunodeficiency virus (HIV), syphilis, Lyme disease (if in an endemic area), and antinuclear, antiphospholipid, Sjogren's Syndrome A/Ro (SS-A), Sjogren's Syndrome B/La (SS-B), NMO, and MOG antibody testing. B12 and copper deficiency typically cause a more chronic myelopathy, but they should be checked if there is uncertainty about the temporal course. In rare cases, TM may be associated with paraneoplastic disorders, particularly in association with lung and breast cancer. Specific autoantibodies associated with myelitis are collapsing response mediator protein-5-IgG (CRMP5 or anti-CV2), amphiphysin-IgG, anti-Hu (ANNA-1), anti-Ri (ANNA-2), and ANNA-3. Infectious causes should be evaluated in patients with significant CSF pleocytosis (>20 WBC/mm^3) or with clinical features suggesting infection. Herpes simplex, varicella zoster, and Epstein-Barr virus polymerase chain reaction (PCR), and in immunocompromised patients, cytomegalovirus PCR, can be checked in CSF. In motor-predominant TM (acute flaccid paralysis), West Nile (if in an endemic area), and enterovirus PCR should be considered.

H. Other tests that are useful in certain patients to determine the underlying cause are chest CT (sarcoidosis, malignancy), salivary gland or lip biopsy (Sjögren syndrome), and meningeal biopsy (undiagnosed, persistent meningeal enhancement).

I. Patients with no or poor response to steroids within ~15 days should be offered plasmapheresis, typically given as five treatments over 10–14 days. Anti-MOG NMSOD patients may respond to prolonged courses of steroids. Some degree of recovery is eventually seen in most patients with idiopathic TM, though residual disability is not uncommon. Recovery from myelitis associated with specific infections is highly variable.

REFERENCES

1. Cree BA. Acute inflammatory myelopathies. *Handb Clin Neurol.* 2014;122:613–667.
2. Weinshenker BG, Wingerchuk DM. Neuromyelitis spectrum disorders. *Mayo Clin Proc.* 2017;92(4):663–679.

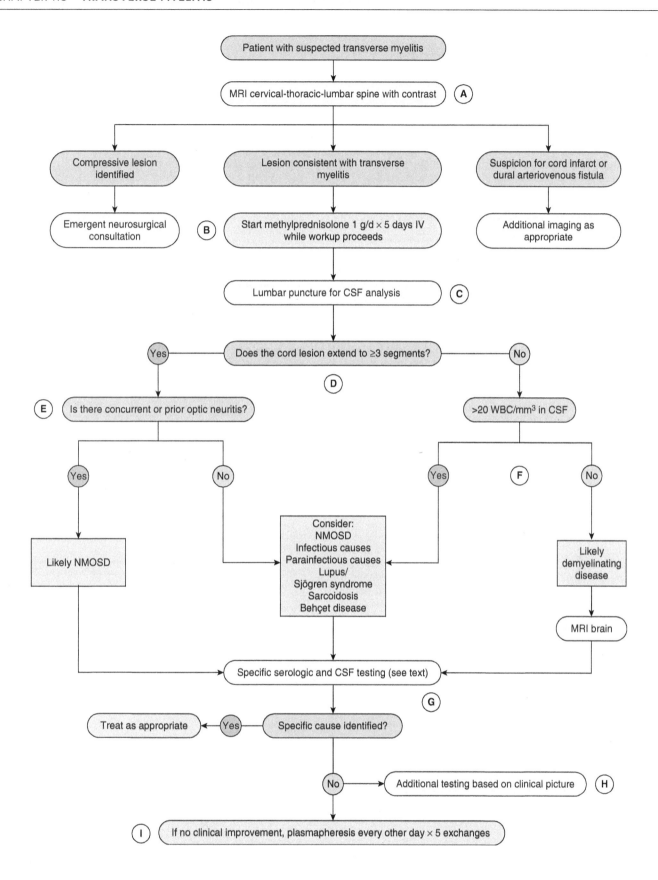

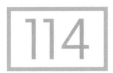

Neurosarcoidosis

Christopher Perrone and Brett L. Cucchiara

Sarcoidosis is an autoimmune disease of unknown cause characterized by the formation of noncaseating granulomas. It can affect multiple organ systems, although pulmonary involvement is most common. Ocular and neurologic involvement can be the presenting symptom of sarcoidosis, or can occur in patients with known systemic sarcoidosis. For obvious reasons, evaluation of the patient with known sarcoidosis and neurologic symptoms will differ from that outlined here, which applies to patients presenting with neurologic or ocular symptoms but without a prior sarcoidosis diagnosis.

A. Patients may present with decreased vision and floaters, resulting from granulomatous inflammation of the posterior chamber, iris, sclera, or conjunctiva. An orbital inflammatory syndrome with edema, erythema, and proptosis can also occur. Facial weakness is the most common cranial neuropathy seen; optic neuritis, eye movement abnormalities, hearing loss, and anosmia may also occur from cranial nerve involvement. Leptomeningeal involvement can also cause radiculitis or communicating hydrocephalus. Hypothalamic involvement may lead to increased thirst and polyuria (from diabetes insipidus) or sexual dysfunction. When brain parenchyma is affected, seizures, encephalopathy, or focal neurologic deficits may occur. Perivascular inflammation may lead to a vasculopathy; rarely, infarction or hemorrhage may ensue. Spinal cord involvement may present as myelitis, including a longitudinally extensive transverse myelitis with a predilection for the surface of the cord. Enhancement of the spinal cord may be multifocal or exhibit a "trident sign"—a crescent-shaped posterior enhancement accompanied by central canal enhancement leading to a three-pronged appearance. Very rarely, sarcoidosis may be associated with a neuropathy or myopathy.

B. The majority of patients will have abnormal cerebrospinal fluid (CSF), with elevated protein and a mononuclear pleocytosis the most common findings. Elevated opening pressure (~10%) and low CSF glucose (10%–20%) may occur, but are uncommon. Elevated CSF angiotensin converting enzyme is not sensitive, but is specific if found (>90%). When abnormal CSF is present, thorough testing to exclude alternative infectious or inflammatory diagnoses should be pursued.

C. Biopsy of affected nervous system tissue provides definitive diagnosis of neurosarcoidosis. However, biopsy of ocular, brain, or spinal cord lesions is often high risk. A diagnosis of probable neurosarcoidosis can be made in a patient with the above neurological manifestations and a positive biopsy of non–nervous system tissue, which is more easily sampled. Since pulmonary involvement is common, a chest computed tomography (CT) scan should be performed looking for hilar adenopathy. When present, pulmonary biopsy can usually be performed safely with good diagnostic yield.

D. If chest CT is unrevealing, consider fluorodeoxyglucose-positron emission tomography (FDG-PET) to look for other sites of systemic involvement that might be amenable to biopsy. If none are found, then biopsy of brain (or other affected neural tissue, such as meninges) should be considered.

E. Treatment of the patient with neurosarcoidosis should begin with corticosteroids. A short course of intravenous high-dose steroids should be used for patients with severe neurologic symptoms, otherwise oral prednisone may be used. The duration of oral steroid treatment varies based on the extent and severity of neurologic involvement, but most cases should receive at least 1 month of high-dose prednisone before considering dose reduction. Steroid taper should be slow and adjusted based on the patient's clinical response. Alternative immunosuppressants can be considered in patients intolerant of or unable to taper off steroids.

REFERENCES

1. Stern BJ, Royal W, Gelfand JM, et al. Definition and consensus diagnostic criteria for neurosarcoidosis. *JAMA Neurol.* 2018;75(12):1546–1553. https://doi.org/10.1001/jamaneurol.2018.2295.
2. Fritz D, van de Beek D, Brouwer MC. Clinical features, treatment, and outcome in neurosarcoidosis: systematic review and meta-analysis. *BMC Neurol.* 2016;16:220.
3. Rao DA, Dellaripa PF. Extrapulmonary manifestations of neurosarcoidosis. *Rheum Dis Clin North Am.* 2013;39(2):277–297.
4. Gelfand JM, Bradshaw MJ, Stern BJ, et al. Infliximab for the treatment of CNS sarcoidosis: a multi-institutional series. *Neurology.* 2017;89(20):2092–2100.

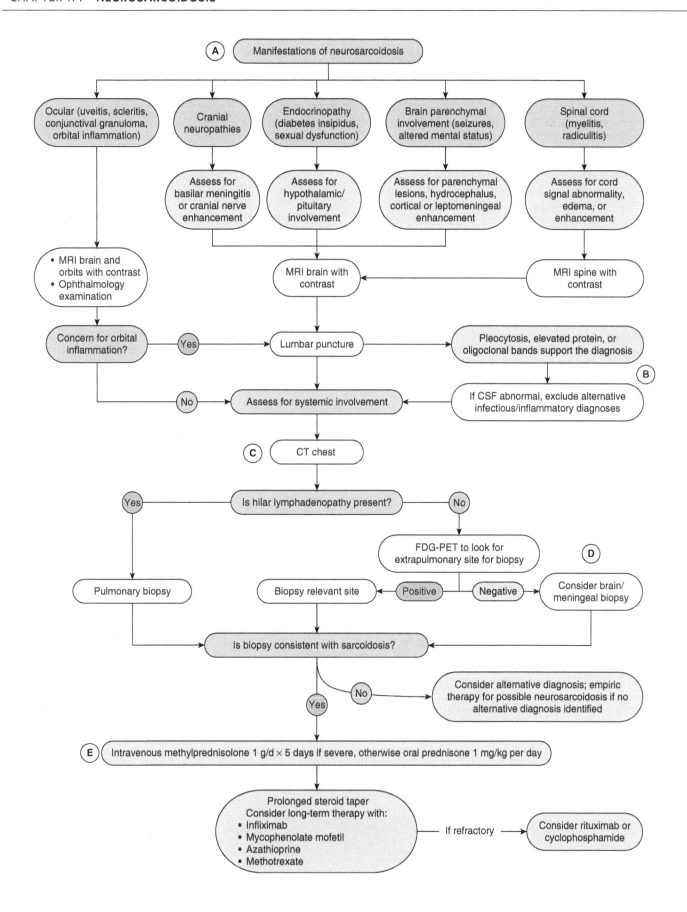

A — Manifestations of neurosarcoidosis

Ocular (uveitis, scleritis, conjunctival granuloma, orbital inflammation)

Cranial neuropathies

Endocrinopathy (diabetes insipidus, sexual dysfunction)

Brain parenchymal involvement (seizures, altered mental status)

Spinal cord (myelitis, radiculitis)

Assess for basilar meningitis or cranial nerve enhancement

Assess for hypothalamic/ pituitary involvement

Assess for parenchymal lesions, hydrocephalus, cortical or leptomeningeal enhancement

Assess for cord signal abnormality, edema, or enhancement

- MRI brain and orbits with contrast
- Ophthalmology examination

MRI brain with contrast

MRI spine with contrast

Concern for orbital inflammation?

Yes → Lumbar puncture → Pleocytosis, elevated protein, or oligoclonal bands support the diagnosis

B

No → Assess for systemic involvement ← If CSF abnormal, exclude alternative infectious/inflammatory diagnoses

C — CT chest

Yes ← Is hilar lymphadenopathy present? → No

FDG-PET to look for extrapulmonary site for biopsy

D

Pulmonary biopsy

Biopsy relevant site ← Positive ← Negative → Consider brain/ meningeal biopsy

Is biopsy consistent with sarcoidosis?

No → Consider alternative diagnosis; empiric therapy for possible neurosarcoidosis if no alternative diagnosis identified

Yes

E — Intravenous methylprednisolone 1 g/d × 5 days if severe, otherwise oral prednisone 1 mg/kg per day

Prolonged steroid taper
Consider long-term therapy with:
- Infliximab
- Mycophenolate mofetil
- Azathioprine
- Methotrexate

If refractory → Consider rituximab or cyclophosphamide

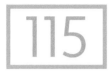

Autoimmune Encephalitis

Eric Lancaster

A. Autoimmune encephalitis (AE) is a rare form of reversible brain inflammation that may present with psychosis, seizures, altered consciousness, dystonia, and a diverse spectrum of other neurologic symptoms. Tests for specific antibodies to brain proteins may assist in diagnosis of some of the most common forms of the disease, many of which are associated with specific malignancies (i.e., paraneoplastic disease). Most cases improve substantially with immune therapy.

B. Certain clinical features may suggest disorders associated with the presence of particular antibodies, although there is considerable overlap in clinical presentation between different forms of AE. NMDAR antibodies strongly predominate in patients under 30 years, and often associate with psychosis, dystonia, catatonia, seizures, respiratory failure, and autonomic instability. AMPAR antibodies may cause similar symptoms but are rarer and affect older adults, often with lung, breast, or thymic tumors. LGI1 antibodies affect mostly older adults and may cause fasciobrachial dystonic seizures, hyponatremia, and insidious memory impairment. GABA-B receptor antibodies are the most common cause of AE in patients with small cell lung cancer and cause particularly severe seizures. GABA-A receptor antibodies associate with characteristic brain lesions and status epilepticus or epilepsy partialis continua. Caspr2 antibodies associate with Morvan syndrome (encephalitis with neuromyotonia). DPPX antibodies associate with central nervous system (CNS) and gastrointestinal hyperexcitability. Ophelia syndrome is a rare form of encephalitis associated with Hodgkin lymphoma and mGluR5 antibodies. Bickerstaff encephalitis is closely related to Miller Fisher syndrome and Gq1b antibodies. Hashimoto encephalitis is a steroid-responsive encephalopathy associated with high-titer thyroid antibodies; however, it should be noted that thyroid antibodies may be found in other forms of AE and also the general population.

C. The presence of autoantibodies to specific brain antigens together with clinical symptoms can be diagnostic and help guide therapy. Some of the higher-yield tests include autoantibodies to NMDAR, LGI1, AMPAR, Caspr2, GABA-B, and GAD65. GABA-A, glycine, mGluR5, and DPPX antibodies also have value in some cases but may not be commercially available. GQ1b antibodies should sent if Bickerstaff encephalitis is considered. Thyroid antibodies (antithyroid peroxidase [TPO], and anti-thyroglobulin, [TG]) may support the diagnosis of Hashimoto encephalopathy but are not specific. In cases with a strong suspicion for AE, consider testing in a research laboratory. Antibody testing should be refined if a tumor is identified, as certain antibodies associate with certain malignancies and this can enhance diagnostic confidence.

D. Clinical criteria for possible autoimmune encephalitis and definite autoimmune encephalitis are available,[1] and empiric treatment for patients who meet criteria for possible or definite AE can be started while awaiting results of antibody testing. "Possible AE" requires: (1) <3 months of altered mental status, memory loss, or psychiatric symptoms and (2) new focal CNS findings, CSF pleocytosis or magnetic resonance imaging (MRI) showing features of AE and (3) exclusion of other causes. "Definite AE" requires (1) <3 months altered mental status, memory loss, or psychiatric symptoms and (2) increased T2 signal in the temporal lobes, electroencephalogram (EEG) with focal temporal abnormalities or CSF pleocytosis and (3) exclusion of alternative causes. Specific criteria for probable and definite anti-NMDAR AE have similarly been proposed[1] and should be considered in children, where anti-NMDAR encephalitis is much more common than the other diseases in this group.

E. Initial immune therapy typically consists of intravenous steroids plus either intravenous immunoglobulin (IVIG) or plasmapheresis (PLEX). The former may be preferred in patients with agitation in whom maintaining a pheresis access may be difficult. Seizures are common and should be treated with antiepileptic drugs. Autonomic instability, especially in patients with NMDAR antibodies, requires careful management of blood pressure and heart rate during autonomic storms. Respiratory failure may necessitate mechanical ventilation. Psychosis and agitation may be managed with neuroleptics that do not have strong dopamine antagonism, since this can worsen movement disorders. Muscle relaxants and benzodiazepines may be considered for muscle spasms. Focal botulinum toxin may be useful for severe, refractory dystonia, particularly of the jaw. The level of care and possible transfer to a specialized center should be regularly considered.

F. Close clinical follow-up is necessary to adjust immune therapy based on symptoms. Antibody titers should in general not be used to guide treatment. Additional immunosuppression with rituximab or cyclophosphamide may be necessary in refractory cases. The side effects of immune suppression need to be addressed (e.g., prophylaxis against opportunistic infection, mitigating effects of steroids on bone density, etc.). Relapse is always a risk. Steadily wean symptomatic medications that are no longer needed.

G. Consider repeat cancer screening at 3, 6, 12, 24, and 36 months, with the specific tests influenced by the precise antibody diagnosis if there is one.

REFERENCE

1. Graus F, Titulaer MJ, Balu R, et al. A clinical approach to diagnosis of autoimmune encephalitis. *Lancet Neurol.* 2016;15(4):391–404.

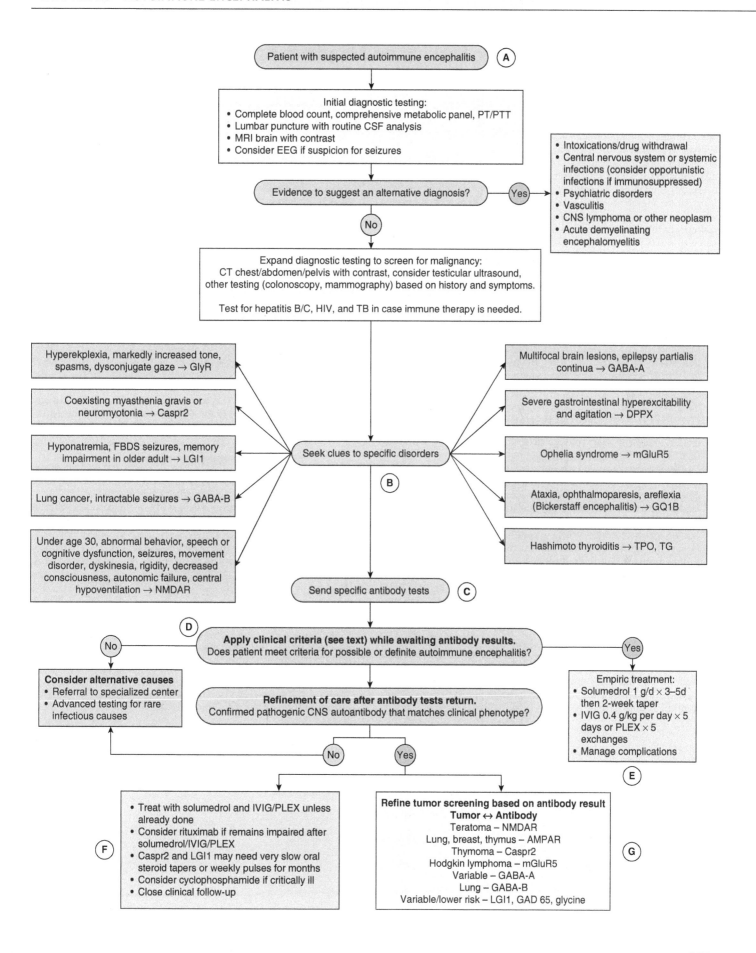

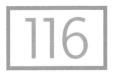

White Matter Lesions on Magnetic Resonance Imaging

Koto Ishida and Brett L. Cucchiara

White matter lesions (WMLs), also called white matter hyperintensities, are a common finding on T2 and fluid-attenuated inversion recovery (FLAIR) sequences on brain magnetic resonance imaging (MRI). WMLs are most often due to small vessel ischemia, though may also occur with demyelinating or other inflammatory diseases and a variety of more obscure pathologies. In population-based studies enrolling midlife subjects, the prevalence of at least one WML on MRI is approximately 40%. Prevalence increases with older age, hypertension, smoking, and diabetes. In those older than 70 years, prevalence of WML of presumed vascular etiology exceeds 90%. Although at times symptomatic, more often WMLs are incidentally discovered and not directly related to current active focal neurologic symptoms. An example is the patient with migraine or nonspecific neurologic symptoms who undergoes MRI. Radiographic pattern and location, along with clinical features of the patient, help to identify the most likely underlying etiology of WML.

A. When WMLs are accompanied by restricted diffusion on diffusion weighted imaging, acute infarction is by far the most likely explanation. Rarely, acute demyelinating lesions may mimic infarction in this setting, but the clinical presentation is usually one of gradually evolving (as opposed to abrupt onset) symptoms, allowing differentiation.

B. The vast majority of clinically silent lesions in the subcortical white matter represent the consequences of small vessel ischemia (Fig. 116.1). Hypertension is the most important risk factor. Migraine, particularly with aura, is associated with an increased prevalence of WML and is an important consideration in younger patients without vascular risk factors found to have WML. Lesions tend to be juxtacortical or periventricular and usually spare the callosal and subcallosal regions. Infectious and inflammatory disease can be associated with WML; suggestive systemic symptoms or focal neurologic symptoms are almost always present in these cases. In the immunocompromised patient, rare causes of WML include progressive multifocal leukoencephalopathy (caused by the JC virus), primary human immunodeficiency virus (HIV) encephalopathy, and central nervous system (CNS) lymphoma, among others. The characteristic radiographic appearance of these conditions may be variable in the immunocompromised. For instance, CNS lymphoma typically enhances homogenously but can demonstrate a rim of enhancement in immunocompromised patients. Progressive multifocal leukoencephalopathy usually does not enhance in markedly immunocompromised patients but can enhance in patients with milder immunosuppression or during immune reconstitution.

C. Demyelinating disease (i.e., multiple sclerosis) causes WMLs that tend to be periventricular and extend perpendicular to the corpus callosum ("Dawson's fingers") as shown in Fig. 116.2. Lesions are often associated with the "central vein sign" on T2* weighted imaging.

D. Perivascular spaces (also called Virchow-Robin spaces) are normal, benign findings in the subcortical white matter that can on occasion be quite dramatic in appearance (Fig. 116.3). They are of cerebrospinal fluid intensity and typically have a cystic appearance.

E. Susac syndrome (Fig. 116.4) is a rare autoimmune endotheliopathy causing encephalopathy, hearing loss, and branch retinal artery occlusions. WMLs are seen on MRI and have a predilection for the corpus callosum with a characteristic "snowball" appearance.

F. Cerebral autosomal dominant arteriopathy with subcortical infarcts (CADASIL) and retinal vasculopathy with cerebral leukodystrophy (RVCL) are two distinct clinical syndromes associated with multiple WML. CADASIL is far more common, and is associated with clinical stroke, migraine with aura, and early dementia. As the disease advances, extremely characteristic anterior temporal lobe and external capsule white matter hyperintensities appear which strongly suggest the disease (Fig. 116.5). RVCL is distinguished by the presence of retinal and systemic involvement. Diagnosis of both diseases is by genetic testing.

G. Symmetric and confluent WMLs may represent severe small vessel ischemic disease, particularly in an older patient with long-standing hypertension, but can also be due to a variety of other causes. These should be suspected based on younger age or the particular clinical context. In most such cases there are clinical symptoms associated with the WML. For instance, posterior reversible encephalopathy syndrome typically presents with headache, visual disturbances, and altered mental status, often in the setting of immunosuppressive therapy (Fig. 116.6).

REFERENCES

1. Sati P, Oh J, Constable RT, et al. The central vein sign and its clinical evaluation for the diagnosis of multiple sclerosis: a consensus statement from the North American Imaging in Multiple Sclerosis Cooperative. *Nat Rev Neurol.* 2016;12:714–722.
2. Palm-Meinders IH, Koppen H, Terwindt GM, et al. Structural brain changes in migraine. *JAMA.* 2012;308(18):1889–1896.
3. Wardlaw JM, Hernandez MCV, Munoz-Maneiga S. What are white matter hyperintensities made of? *J Am Heart Assoc.* 2015;4(6):e001140.

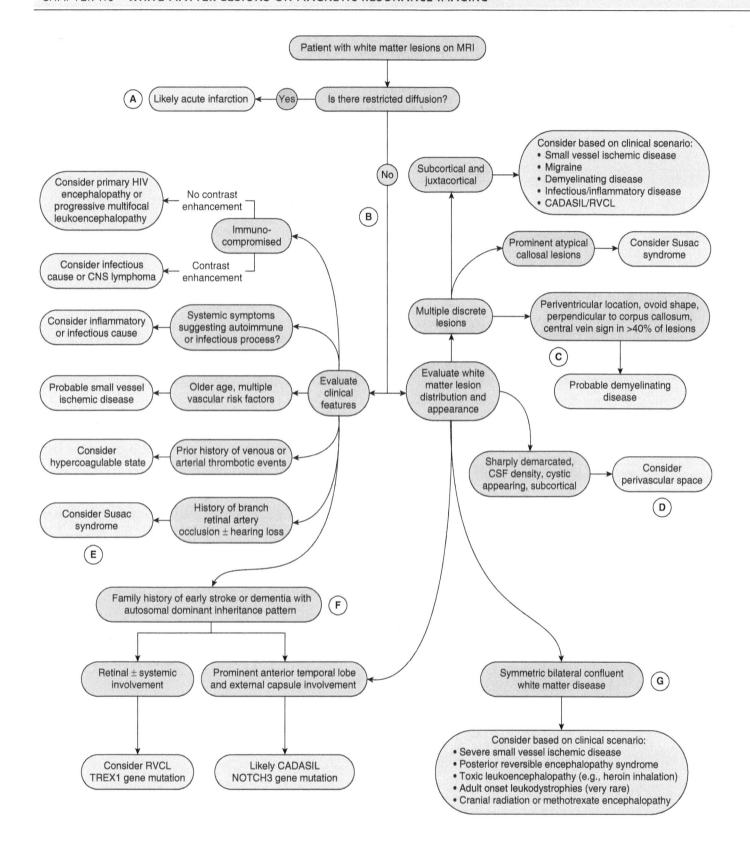

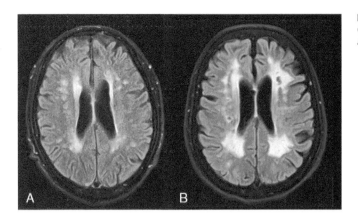

FIG. 116.1 Magnetic resonance axial fluid-attenuated inversion recovery (FLAIR) images showing moderate small vessel ischemic disease *(left)* and severe small vessel ischemic disease *(right)*.

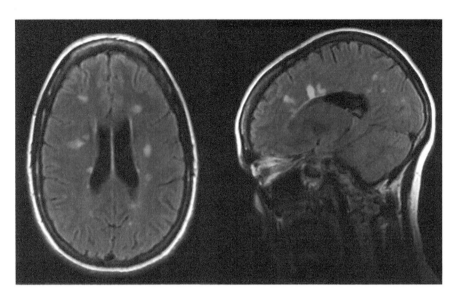

FIG. 116.2 Magnetic resonance axial *(left)* and sagittal *(right)* FLAIR sequences showing typical white matter lesions in multiple sclerosis.

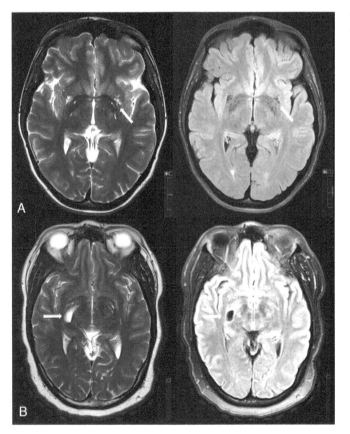

FIG. 116.3 Magnetic resonance axial T2 *(left)* and FLAIR *(right)* sequences showing an example of (A) multiple small perivascular spaces bilaterally (arrows), and (B) a large perivascular space (arrows).

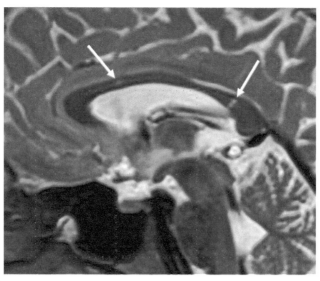

FIG. 116.4 Magnetic resonance sagittal T2 image showing characteristic callosal lesions *(arrows)* in Susac syndrome.

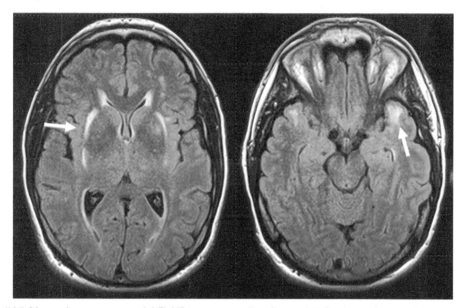

FIG. 116.5 Magnetic resonance axial FLAIR sequences showing typical findings of external capsule *(left panel, arrow)* and anterior temporal *(right panel, arrow)* white matter abnormalities seen in cerebral autosomal dominant arteriopathy with subcortical infarcts and leukoencephalopathy (CADASIL).

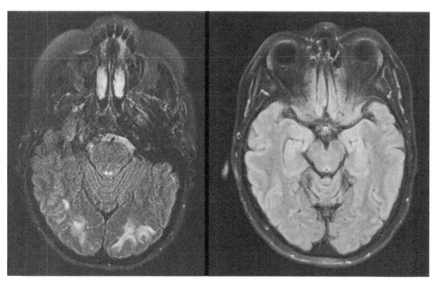

FIG. 116.6 Magnetic resonance axial FLAIR image showing posterior reversible encephalopathy syndrome. Initial imaging is shown *(left)*, with follow-up imaging 3 months later demonstrating resolution of the abnormal white matter signal *(right)*.

Ring-Enhancing Lesions on Magnetic Resonance Imaging

Raymond S. Price and Joshua P. Klein

Gadolinium-based intravenous contrast agents used in magnetic resonance imaging (MRI) appear hyperintense on T1 sequences. These agents do not cross the blood–brain barrier in normal patients, and thus T1 hyperintensity from contrast should primarily be present in the brain vasculature and regions of brain without a blood–brain barrier, such as the choroid plexus. When an enhancing lesion is present, this indicates either breakdown of the existing blood–brain barrier or angiogenesis of blood vessels without a blood–brain barrier (as may be seen with a tumor or after cerebral infarction). If a lesion has enhancement of its peripheral rim but not its central core, it is frequently referred to as a ring-enhancing (or more accurately "rim-enhancing") lesion.

A. Active demyelinating lesions in multiple sclerosis can have different enhancement patterns, including complete enhancement, heterogenous enhancement, or an incomplete rim of enhancement (Fig. 117.1). The latter refers to a pattern where the enhancing rim around the lesion is not completely circumferential; the segment of the rim that is not enhancing typically faces the ventricle. An incomplete rim of enhancement is unusual in a neoplasm or abscess, and thus its presence suggests demyelinating disease. Active demyelinating lesions in multiple sclerosis typically enhance for about 3 weeks. Thus, if clinical uncertainty persists as to whether a lesion with an incomplete rim of enhancement is secondary to demyelination, follow-up imaging in about one month can be helpful. If enhancement has resolved at that point, this is most consistent with demyelination.

B. Restricted diffusion on diffusion weighted imaging indicates decreased mobility of water molecules, which can be caused by increased intracellular water as seen in cytotoxic edema or by increased cell density as can be seen in high-grade malignancies. In glioblastoma, where the central core is typically necrotic, the enhancing rim may show restricted diffusion indicating high density of tumor cells at the growing periphery. This may also be seen in lymphoma, particularly in immunocompromised patients.

C. The classic appearance of an abscess is a complete rim of enhancement due to the angiogenesis required by the fibroblasts to create the wall of the abscess, and restricted diffusion in its core due to high cellularity of pus (Fig. 117.2). An abscess also typically has associated vasogenic edema out of proportion to the size of the abscess.

D. Neurocysticercosis, a central nervous system infection by *Taenia solium* tapeworm larvae, is one of the most common causes of seizures in the world. Cysts containing the live larvae do not enhance. As the cysts degenerate, they are surrounded by edema and will demonstrate nodular enhancement or a marked rim of enhancement delineating the cyst from normal brain parenchyma. With further degeneration, the cysts may calcify and become gliotic nodules without enhancement. In contrast, a glioblastoma, which is a diffusely infiltrating tumor, will frequently demonstrate an irregular rim of enhancement around its necrotic core, as there is not a sharp demarcation between normal brain and tumor (Fig. 117.3).

E. Perfusion imaging is not typically included in routine MRI. In the setting of an enhancing mass lesion, however, perfusion imaging may be diagnostically useful. High-grade neoplasms (including glioblastoma and metastases), abscesses, and other active infections will typically demonstrate increased perfusion to meet increased metabolic demand. Low-grade neoplasms, inflammatory lesions, and demyelination can cause variable perfusion changes, and thus perfusion imaging is less helpful in the evaluation of these entities.

F. When there is uncertainty about the cause of a ring-enhancing lesion, follow-up imaging in 4–6 weeks is indicated. Subacute cerebral infarction, demyelinating disease, and inflammatory lesions will show resolution of enhancement over time, unlike tumors. Radiation necrosis may also show improvement in enhancement over time. Subacute cerebral infarction bears specific consideration, as it is an occasional source of diagnostic error. Parenchymal enhancement can appear ~5–7 days after infarction occurs; this may persist for 2–3 months. A ring-enhancing pattern may be seen, particularly with deep subcortical infarct locations. Abnormal signal on diffusion weighted imaging, a critical diagnostic feature supporting infarction, resolves after 10–14 days. Therefore, when subacute/chronic cerebral infarction is imaged between 2 and 12 weeks postevent, particularly in patients without a clear clinical presentation of ischemic stroke, the lesion may be misinterpreted as tumor (Fig. 117.4). Resolution of enhancement on follow-up imaging in 4–6 weeks will clarify the diagnosis. Another common diagnostic challenge is distinguishing radiation necrosis, a complication of brain radiation therapy, from tumor recurrence. Delayed radiation necrosis can demonstrate a rim of enhancement due to radiation-induced endothelial injury. Again, resolution of enhancement on follow-up imaging supports the diagnosis, though lack of resolution does not exclude the possibility of radiation necrosis. Perfusion imaging may also be helpful, as decreased cerebral blood volume may be seen in radiation necrosis and the opposite with active tumor.

REFERENCES

1. Baig MA, Klein JP, Mechtler LL. Imaging of brain tumors. *Continuum (Minneap Minn).* 2016;22(5):1529–1552.
2. Balashov K. Imaging of central nervous system demyelinating disorders. *Continuum (Minneap Minn).* 2016;22(5):1613–1635.
3. Garcia HH, Nash TE, Del Brutto OH. Clinical symptoms, diagnosis, and treatment of neurocysticercosis. *Lancet Neurol.* 2014;13(12):1202–1215.

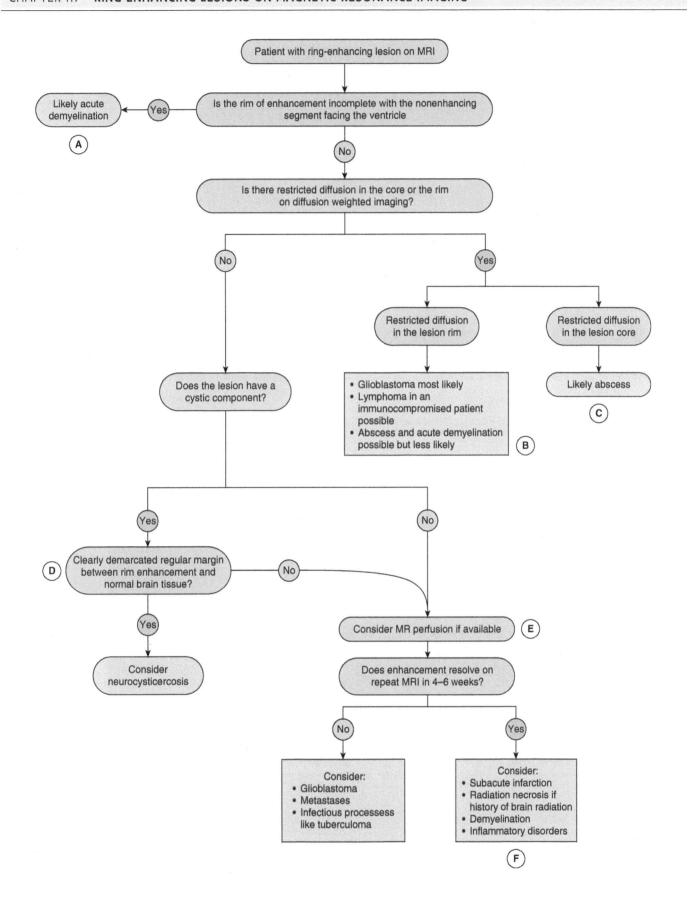

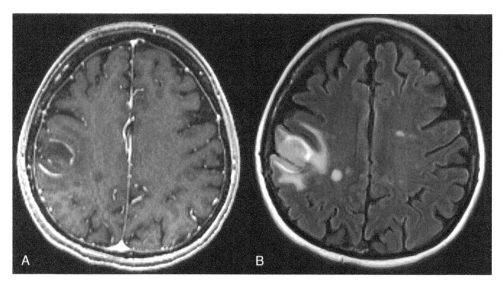

FIG. 117.1 Magnetic resonance imaging axial T1 with contrast sequence showing a lesion with an incomplete rim of enhancement in the right parietal lobe (A), which is more typical of tumefactive demyelination. There is also a T1 hypointense lesion without enhancement in the right corona radiata. Fluid-attenuated inversion recovery (FLAIR) imaging (B) shows T2 hyperintensity within this right parietal lesion, as well as multiple bilateral white matter T2 hyperintensities more typical of relapsing-remitting multiple sclerosis.

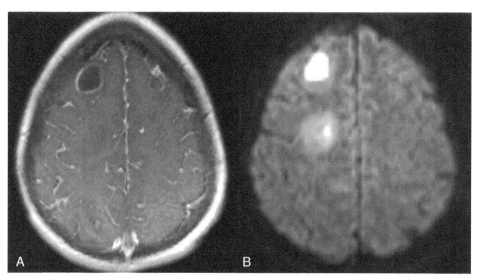

FIG. 117.2 Magnetic resonance imaging axial T1 with contrast sequence showing a lesion with a complete rim of enhancement in the right frontal lobe (A). Diffusion weighted imaging (B) shows restricted diffusion in its core. These are the classic neuroimaging findings of an abscess. There is a second abscess in the right corona radiata, which is not completely seen on these slices.

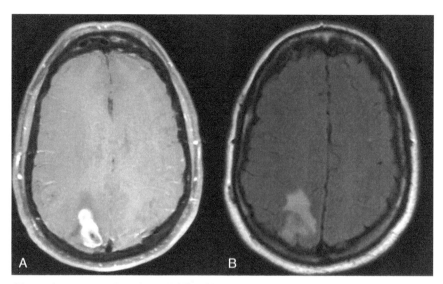

FIG. 117.3 Magnetic resonance imaging axial T1 with contrast sequence showing a typical appearance of a glioblastoma with a complete but irregular rim of enhancement and a partially hypointense core consistent with necrosis (A). There is also a rim of T1 hypointensity in the white matter surrounding the lesion, with corresponding T2 hyperintensity seen on T2 FLAIR image (B), consistent with vasogenic edema.

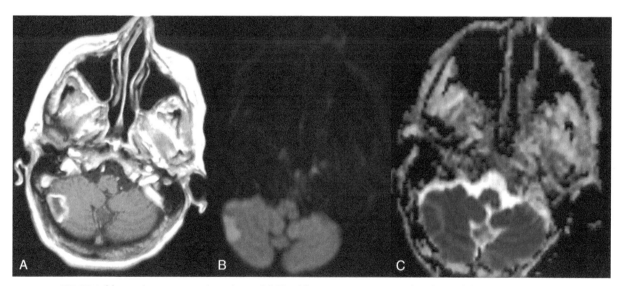

FIG. 117.4 Magnetic resonance imaging axial T1 with contrast sequence showing a right cerebellar hemisphere lesion with a complete rim of enhancement (A). Diffusion weighted imaging (B) shows hyperintensity. Apparent diffusion coefficient imaging (C) is relatively isointense in the region that was bright on diffusion weighted imaging. This combination of findings are typically seen in a subacute infarction (around 2 weeks after the infarction) and can be confused for mass lesions.

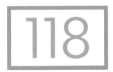

Sellar Lesions on Magnetic Resonance Imaging

Raymond S. Price and Joshua P. Klein

The pituitary gland resides in the sella turcica, a depression in the sphenoid bone, and is subdivided into an anterior portion, composed of hormone-secreting cells, and a posterior portion, composed of axons from hypothalamic neurons that secrete oxytocin and vasopressin. The hypothalamic axons form the pituitary stalk (infundibulum) that enters the sella through a perforation in the overlying dura (diaphragma sellae). On unenhanced magnetic resonance imaging (MRI) T1-weighted sequences, the anterior pituitary is isointense to gray matter whereas the posterior pituitary is hyperintense (pituitary bright spot). The anterior pituitary enhances with contrast. The potential space between the anterior and posterior portions of the pituitary is known as the Rathke cleft. Patients with mass lesions confined to the sella (intrasellar lesions) are frequently asymptomatic. However, with a hormone-secreting pituitary microadenoma, symptoms may occur from the excess secreted hormone. The area directly above the sella turcica (the suprasellar region) contains the optic nerves and optic chiasm anteriorly, the hypothalamus with its infundibulum superiorly, and the third ventricle posteriorly. Mass lesions can be purely suprasellar or begin in either the sellar or suprasellar region and grow into the other region. Those that cross between sellar and suprasellar regions frequently show pinching in the middle due to constriction by the diaphragma sellae giving an hourglass appearance. Suprasellar lesions may cause headache secondary to elevated intracranial pressure from involvement of the third ventricle or central or bitemporal vision loss due to involvement of the optic nerve or chiasm, respectively. Lateral growth of sellar or suprasellar lesions can involve the cavernous sinus and may cause pupillary abnormalities, ocular motility deficits, facial numbness in the ophthalmic/maxillary divisions of the trigeminal nerve, or cerebral ischemia from compression of the cavernous carotid artery.

A. Acute infarction or hemorrhage in the pituitary is referred to as pituitary apoplexy; abrupt headache and visual symptoms suggest the diagnosis. An underlying adenoma is present in most cases. Emergent neurosurgical consultation is indicated.

B. A Rathke cleft cyst (Fig. 118.1) is a congenital lesion that is nearly always an incidental asymptomatic finding. The cystic fluid is proteinaceous and usually hyperintense on T1-weighted imaging, but can also be T1 hypointense. There is either no enhancement or a small rim of enhancement. Larger Rathke cleft cysts can extend into the suprasellar region. If there is diagnostic uncertainty, follow-up imaging can be performed to ensure stability.

C. Pituitary hyperplasia is an enlargement of the pituitary gland to 10–15 mm due to either increased physiologic requirements for hormone secretion (e.g., pregnancy) or decreased responsiveness of end-organ glands such as the adrenal glands. Imaging characteristics are the same as normal pituitary tissue. The pituitary gland can also appear enlarged in intracranial hypotension due to increased blood volume.

D. Pituitary microadenomas are <10 mm in size, typically isointense or hypointense on T1 sequences, and often have decreased enhancement compared to normal pituitary tissue. A microadenoma causes asymmetric enlargement of the pituitary gland displacing it from the midline, and the infundibulum is often deflected contralaterally, best seen on coronal images.

E. Meningiomas are frequently found in the parasagittal region, arising from the diaphragma sella, the walls of the cavernous sinus, or the sphenoid or petroclival dura. On MRI, they typically appear iso- to slightly hypointense on T1 sequences and have robust homogenous enhancement. Internal calcifications may be present. An adjacent tapering dural thickening (a "dural tail") can often be seen. If there is extension laterally to the cavernous sinus, there can be encasement of the cavernous carotid artery limiting surgical resection.

F. Pituitary macroadenomas (Fig. 118.2), the most common mass in the suprasellar region, are >10 mm in size with sellar and suprasellar components, and thus frequently exhibit the hourglass sign. They cause asymmetric enlargement of the pituitary gland displacing it and the pituitary stalk from the midline. They are typically isointense or hypointense on T1 sequences and will enhance. If there is extension laterally to the cavernous sinus, there can be encasement of the cavernous carotid artery.

G. Large aneurysms arising from the circle of Willis can be mistaken for a suprasellar mass lesion on MRI without accompanying vascular imaging. An aneurysm is suggested by marked internal T1 and T2 hypointensity (flow voids) and enhancement with contrast.

H. Inflammatory processes may mimic a mass lesion. Autoimmune hypophysitis is a rare inflammatory condition of the pituitary stalk that presents with headache and bitemporal visual field loss, predominantly in women or patients treated with ipilimumab. Neurosarcoidosis and neuromyelitis optica spectrum disorder (NMOSD) frequently involves the hypothalamic-pituitary axis. One of the core characteristics of NMOSD is a diencephalic syndrome with T2 hyperintensities involving the hypothalamus, periependymal surface of the third ventricle, or thalamus. Primary germ cell tumors are rare slow growing tumors that have a predilection for the suprasellar region, more specifically the floor of the third ventricle and the pituitary stalk. They are isointense on T1 sequences and enhance homogenously.

I. A hypothalamic hamartoma (Fig. 118.3) is a congenital benign suprasellar mass lesion arising from the floor of the third ventricle. Patients may present with gelastic (laughing) seizures or hormonal abnormalities. Hypothalamic hamartomas are isointense on T1 sequences and do not enhance. Low-grade astrocytomas arising from the optic nerve or hypothalamus may present as a suprasellar infiltrating mass lesion that is hyperintense on T2 sequences.

J. A craniopharyngioma (Fig. 118.4) is a suprasellar tumor seen in children and patients over age 50 years. Craniopharyngiomas, especially the adamantinomatous subtype, have both cystic and solid components. The cystic fluid is usually hyperintense on T1 and T2 sequences. The rim of the cyst and the solid component will enhance. The rim of the cyst is also usually calcified.

K. A dermoid cyst is a congenital usually midline lesion in which the cystic cavity has high fat content causing T1 hyperintensity.

L. Arachnoid and epidermoid cysts are congenital usually nonmidline lesions. An arachnoid cyst contains cerebrospinal fluid and thus will be hypointense on T1 and FLAIR sequences and hyperintense on T2 sequences. An arachnoid cyst will not restrict on diffusion weighted imaging. An epidermoid cyst contains keratin and is hypointense on T1 imaging with restricted diffusion on diffusion weighted imaging.

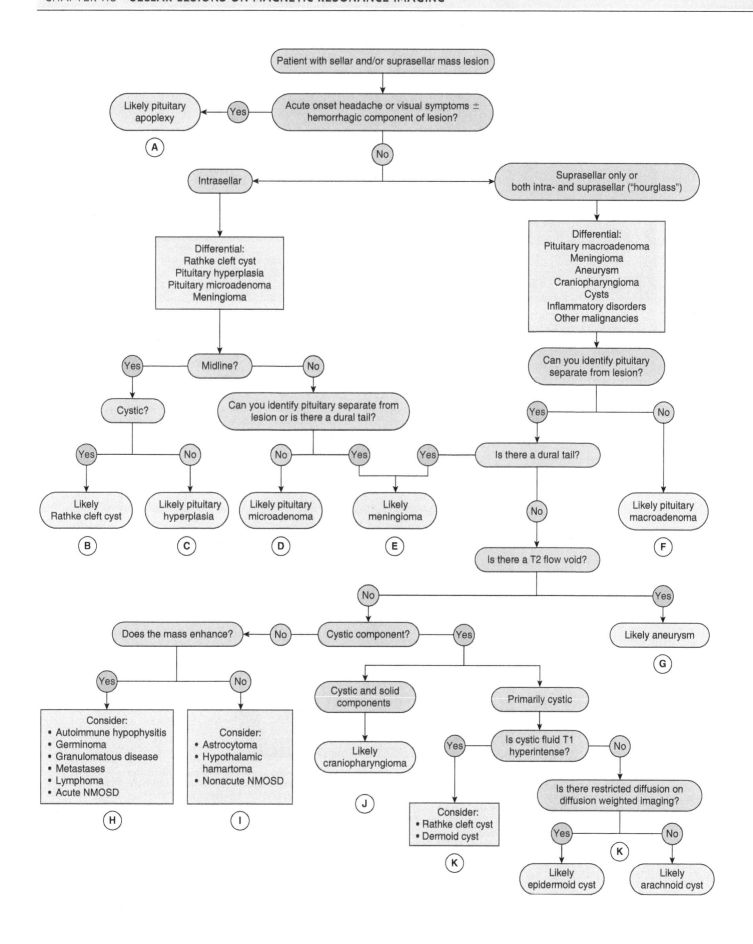

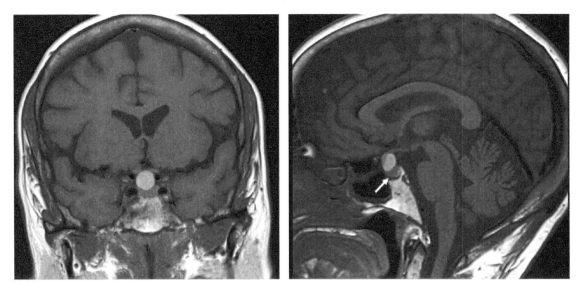

FIG. 118.1 Magnetic resonance imaging coronal *(left panel)* and sagittal *(right panel)* T1 without contrast sequence showing a large midline sellar lesion extending into the suprasellar region that is hyperintense to brain, which is typical for a Rathke cleft cyst containing proteinaceous fluid. The anterior and posterior pituitary gland can be seen inferior to the cyst on the sagittal image *(arrow)*.

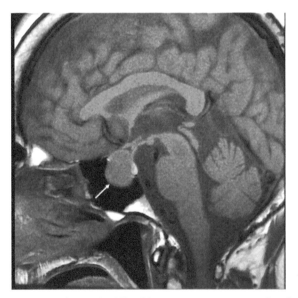

FIG. 118.2 Magnetic resonance imaging sagittal T1 without contrast sequence showing a large sellar lesion extending into the suprasellar region that is isointense to brain (arrow), which is typical for a pituitary macroadenoma. The bright spot of T1 signal between the posterior aspect of the mass and the clivus is the normal appearance of the posterior pituitary gland.

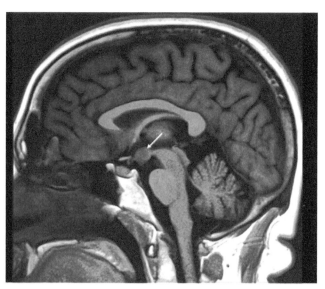

FIG. 118.3 Magnetic resonance imaging sagittal T1 without contrast sequence showing a suprasellar lesion that is isointense to brain arising from the anterior floor of the third ventricle (arrow), which is typical for a hypothalamic hamartoma. This lesion would not enhance with contrast.

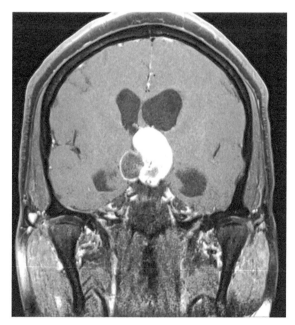

FIG. 118.4 Magnetic resonance imaging coronal T1 with contrast sequence showing a suprasellar lesion with both cystic and solid components. The solid component avidly enhances and the rim of the cyst enhances. There are the typical findings of an adamantinomatous craniopharyngioma. This image also demonstrated enlarged lateral ventricles, especially on the left, as can be seen obstruction of outflow from the third ventricle by suprasellar lesions.

Cerebellopontine Angle Mass Lesions on Magnetic Resonance Imaging

Raymond S. Price and Joshua P. Klein

The cerebellopontine angle (CPA) is formed by the lateral pons and the cerebellum around the level of the middle cerebellar peduncle. At the CPA, there is a triangular extraaxial subarachnoid space known as the cerebellopontine angle cistern. The normal contents of the cerebellopontine angle cistern include the facial and vestibulocochlear cranial nerves, the anterior inferior cerebellar artery, and the flocculus of the cerebellum. CPA masses are relatively common with most related to congenital lesions or tumors arising from the normal contents of the CPA cistern.

A. Normal anatomic structures can occasionally be confused with a CPA mass. The flocculus of the cerebellum is one of the normal components of the CPA cistern. The foramen of Luschka connects the fourth ventricle with the CPA cistern. Choroid plexus from the fourth ventricle can extend into the CPA cistern and occasional calcify, mimicking a mass lesion. The jugular bulb is the initial segment of the jugular vein, which receives blood from the inferior petrosal and sigmoid venous sinuses. The right jugular bulb is larger than the left jugular bulb in around two-thirds of patients and this asymmetry can cause it to be mistaken for an asymmetric mass lesion. The jugular bulb is typically inferior to the CPA cistern but rarely can be more superior in the CPA cistern.

B. Vertebrobasilar artery ectasia indicates enlargement of the normal vertebral or basilar arterial diameter, often with a tortuous, atypical course. It can be asymptomatic, associated with brainstem and cerebellar ischemia, or can cause direct compression on the cranial nerves. An aneurysm or arteriovenous malformation is suggested by marked internal T1 and T2 hypointensities (flow voids) (Fig. 119.1) and enhancement with contrast. When uncertainty is present, magnetic resonance angiography should be performed to confirm the visualized structure is vascular. A dural arteriovenous fistula can be suggested by dilated subarachnoid pial vessels on magnetic resonance imaging (MRI); catheter angiography is required to confirm the diagnosis.

C. Meningiomas (Fig. 119.2) are the second most common extraaxial CPA mass. On MRI, they typically appear iso- to slightly hypointense on T1 sequences and hyperintense on T2 sequences, and there is robust homogenous enhancement. Internal calcifications may be present and this can be particularly helpful in differentiating a meningioma from a schwannoma, which does not typically calcify. A broad "dural tail," or an adjacent tapering dural thickening, can often be seen.

D. More than 80% of extraaxial CPA masses are schwannomas, with the vast majority originating from the vestibular portion of the vestibulocochlear nerve (vestibular schwannomas) (Fig. 119.3). Trigeminal or facial schwannomas are much rarer. A vestibular schwannoma usually presents initially with sensorineural hearing loss. When confined to the internal auditory canal (IAC), it will have a round or oval appearance. When extending out of the IAC into the CPA, its growth is no longer restricted by bone and thus the component in the CPA has a spherical appearance. The overall appearance of a vestibular schwannoma extending out of the IAC is frequently described as having an "ice cream cone" appearance, with the cone representing the IAC component. Meningiomas, by comparison, can occasionally grow from the CPA into the IAC but do not typically have this ice cream cone appearance. A vestibular schwannoma is isointense on T1 sequences; on T2 sequences it will be hypointense in comparison to cerebrospinal fluid, but hyperintense compared to the pons. Small vestibular schwannomas typically enhance homogenously whereas larger ones may have heterogeneous enhancement.

E. Ependymomas are tumors arising from the ependymal cells lining the ventricular system, and are most commonly located in the fourth ventricle. They may extend from the fourth ventricle through the foramen of Luschka into the CPA cistern. Ependymomas frequently have cystic components, enhance heterogeneously, and calcify. Paraganglia are collections of autonomic neurons in the peripheral nervous system. Paragangliomas are tumors arising from these neurons and can extend into the CPA, typically demonstrating heterogenous enhancement. Extradural tumors arising from the skull base can occur at the CPA. A chordoma is a malignant midline tumor arising from the clivus and will be markedly hyperintense on T2 imaging and enhance heterogeneously. Less common than chordomas, a chondrosarcoma is a malignant cartilaginous tumor arising at the joint between the occipital bone and the petrous temporal bone, which is off midline. The MRI characteristics are otherwise similar to a chordoma.

F. A dermoid cyst is a congenital lesion in which the cystic cavity has high fat content, causing T1 hyperintensity. A lipoma is a congenital asymptomatic lesion composed entirely of fat and will also have appear hyperintense on T1 sequences. The facial or vestibulocochlear nerve may run through the lipoma. Neither dermoid cysts nor lipomas enhance with contrast.

G. Arachnoid and epidermoid cysts are congenital lesions. An arachnoid cyst contains cerebrospinal fluid and thus will be hypointense on T1 and T2 FLAIR sequences and hyperintense on T2. An arachnoid cyst will not restrict on diffusion weighted imaging. An epidermoid cyst contains keratin and is hypointense on T1 imaging and shows restricted diffusion on diffusion weighted imaging (Fig. 119.4).

REFERENCES

1. Sriskandan N, Connor SE. The role of radiology in the diagnosis and management of vestibular schwannoma. *Clin Radiol.* 2011;66:357–365.
2. Chen HJ. Cerebellopontine angle cisterns. In: Small JE, Schaefer PW, eds. *Neuroradiology: Key Differential Diagnoses and Clinical Questions.* Philadelphia, PA: Saunders; 2013:73–79.

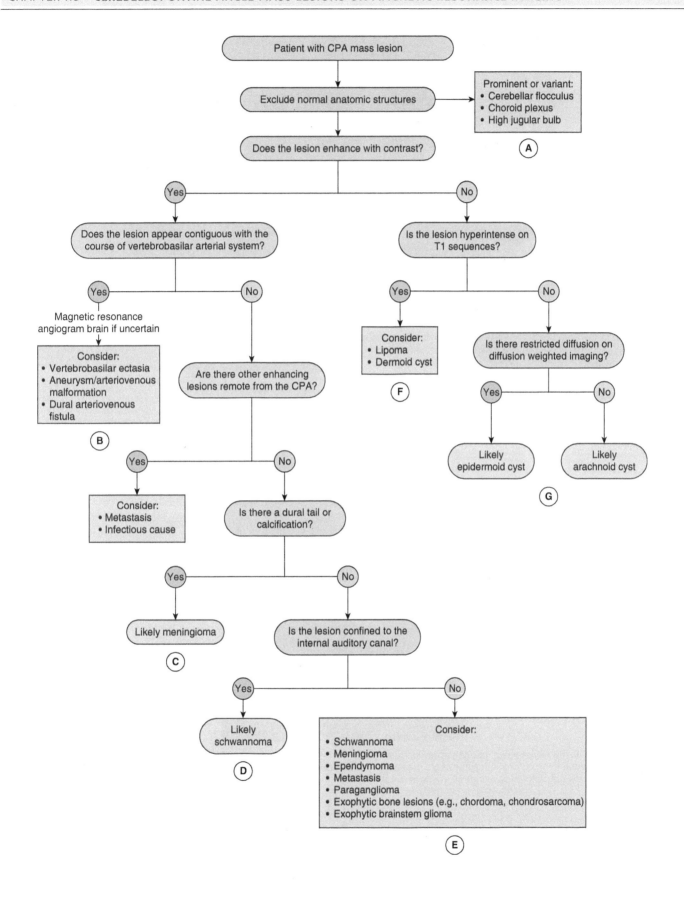

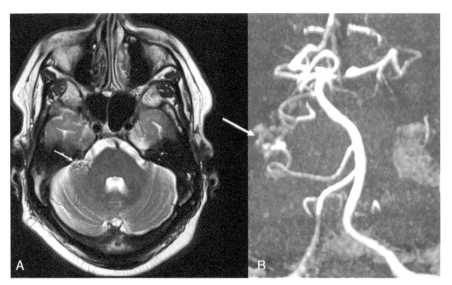

FIG. 119.1 Magnetic resonance (MR) imaging axial T2 sequence showing multiple rounded T2 hypointensities in the right cerebellopontine angle suggesting vascular flow voids *(left panel)*. MR angiogram *(right panel)* confirms an arteriovenous malformation with feeding arteries arising from the right anterior inferior cerebellar artery and right superior cerebellar artery.

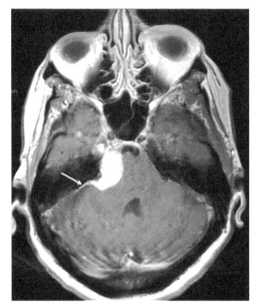

FIG. 119.2 Magnetic resonance imaging axial T1 with contrast sequence showing a homogenously enhancing cerebellopontine angle mass with dural thickening *(arrow)* consistent with "dural tail." These imaging findings are characteristic of a meningioma.

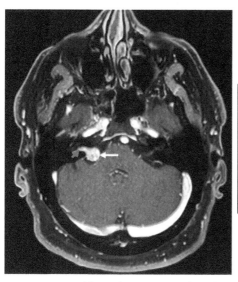
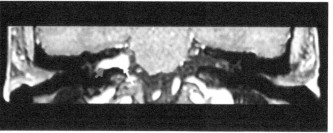

FIG. 119.3 Magnetic resonance imaging axial *(left panel)* and coronal *(right panel)* T1 with contrast sequence showing an enhancing right cerebellopontine angle mass with a cylindrical appearance in the internal auditory canal *(red arrow head)* and spherical appearance in the cerebellopontine angle *(arrow)*. These findings are characteristic of a vestibular schwannoma.

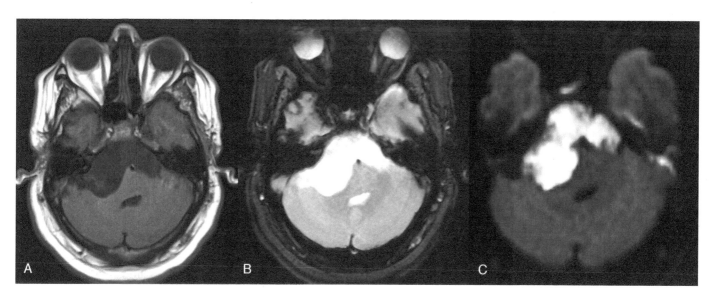

FIG. 119.4 Magnetic resonance imaging axial T1 without contrast *(left panel)* and axial T2 *(center panel)* showing a large extraaxial mass in the right greater than left cerebellopontine angle with mass effect on the brainstem. Note the hypointense flow void of the basilar artery between the pons and the mass on both of these sequences. Diffusion weighted imaging *(right panel)* shows restricted diffusion. These findings in this location are characteristic of an epidermoid cyst.

APPENDIX 1
Additional Tables

TABLE 10.1 MEDICATIONS COMMONLY USED FOR DELIRIUM[a]

Medication	Dosing <65 years	Dosing >65 years	QT prolongation	Dopamine receptor antagonism	Sedation	Route
Antipsychotics*						
Haloperidol	Initial 1–5 mg q30 min IM/IV or q2 hrs PO prn. Maintenance 1–10 mg q8–12 hrs w/prn Maximum 30 mg q24 hrs	Initial 0.5–2 mg q30 min IM/IV or q2 hrs PO prn. Maintenance 0.5–10 mg q8–12 hrs w/prn Maximum 30 mg q24 hrs	+++	+++	–	PO, IM, IV
Olanzapine	Initial 5–10 mg q30 min IM or q2 hrs PO prn. Maintenance 5–10 mg q12–24 hrs w/prn Maximum 30 mg q24 hrs	Initial 2.5–5 mg q30min IM or q2 hrs PO prn. Maintenance 2.5–10mg q12–24 hrs w/prn Maximum 20 mg q24 hrs	+	+	++	PO, IM
Quetiapine	Initial 25–50 mg q12 hrs Maintenance Increase by 25–50 mg q12 hrs PRN Maximum 600 mg q24 hrs	Initial 12.5–25 mg q12 hrs Increase 25 mg q24 hrs prn. Maintenance Increase by 25 mg q12 hrs PRN Maximum 600 mg q24 hrs	+	+	+++	PO
Antiepileptics						
Valproic acid (note: check baseline LFTs, CBC, lipase, pregnancy test; check level 72 hrs from first dose)	Initial 250 mg AM/250 mg afternoon/500 mg PM Maintenance Increase 500–1000 mg daily divided q8 hrs prn Maximum 2500 mg/24 hrs	Initial 125 mg AM/250 mg PM Maintenance Increase 250–500 mg daily divided bid PRN Maximum 1500 mg/24 hrs	–	–	+	PO, IV
Delirium Secondary to Stimulant Intoxication or Alcohol Withdrawal						
Benzodiazepines	Stimulant Intoxication	Alcohol withdrawal				
Lorazepam	2–4 mg prn.	CIWA >8: 2–4 mg IV q30 min or PO q4 hrs	–	–	+++	IV,PO, IM
Diazepam	5–10 mg prn.	CIWA >8: 5–10 mg IV q30 min or PO q4 hrs	–	–	+++	IV,PO, IM
Delirium Secondary to Opiate Intoxication						
Naloxone	**Initial:** 0.05–0.4 mg, 0.4–2 mg if apneic **Maintenance:** Repeat dose q2–5 min prn., consider starting infusion (0.2–6 mg/hr) and ICU transfer					IV,IM, SC

QTc <460: check EKG for 2 days then stop if stable.
QTc 460–500: check EKG for 3 days then stop if stable.
QTc >500: consider dose reduction, telemetry, daily EKG/electrolytes, stop other QT prolonging agents.
CBC, Complete blood count; *EKG*, electrocardiogram; *IM*, intramuscular; *IV*, intravenous; *LFT*, liver function tests; *PO*, per os; *SC*, subcutaneous injection.
*For antipsychotics, once maintenance dose reached:
[a]There is no universal dosing regimen for above medications. Use table as a guideline not a fixed protocol.

TABLE 41.1 CRITERIA FOR SELECTING PATIENTS WITH ACUTE ISCHEMIC STROKE FOR THROMBOLYSIS

Intravenous thrombolysis contraindications

1. Time of symptom onset/last known normal >4.5 hours
2. Platelets <100,000/mm^3
3. INR >1.7 if patient is on warfarin
4. Heparin use within 48 hours and elevated aPTT
5. BP >185/110 mmHg
6. Neuroimaging (CT) evidence of intracranial hemorrhage
7. Extensive region of clear hypodensity on CT which reflects well-developed infarct
8. History of ischemic stroke within 3 months
9. Severe head trauma within 3 months
10. Intracranial or spinal surgery within 3 months
11. Arterial puncture at noncompressible site in previous 7 days
12. Any history of intracranial hemorrhage
13. Signs or symptoms clinically most consistent with subarachnoid hemorrhage
14. Signs or symptoms concerning for infective endocarditis
15. Signs/symptoms or vascular imaging concerning for aortic dissection
16. Known history or imaging evidence of intracranial neoplasm
17. Gastrointestinal bleeding within 3 weeks
18. Therapeutic dose LMWH within 24 hours
19. Therapeutic dose direct thrombin inhibitor or factors Xa inhibitor within 48 hours, unless appropriate assay or coagulation testing is normal.

Additional consideration and relative contraindications

1. Seizure at onset should raise concern for postictal (Todd) paralysis, but if there is high suspicion for stroke, it is reasonable to treat with intravenous thrombolysis.
2. Early clinical improvement does not preclude treatment with thrombolysis if clinically debilitating deficit remains at the time of evaluation.
3. If initial blood glucose is <50 or >400 mg/dL but imaging confirms acute stroke, it is reasonable to consider treatment with thrombolysis.
4. In the case of systemic (nonneurologic) trauma within 14 days, risk of hemorrhage may be increased, so risks and benefits must be weighed in each individual case.
5. With surgery (non-neurologic) within 14 days, risk of hemorrhage may be increased, so risks and benefits must be weighed in each individual case.
6. In pregnancy, thrombolysis may increase the risk of uterine bleeding so individualized risk benefit analysis is appropriate.
7. If there is a history of MI in the past 3 months, thrombolysis can be considered in the case of right-sided or inferior wall infarct or in the case of a non-STEMI. Thrombolysis after left-sided STEMI may increase risk of cardiac rupture or fatal cardiac tamponade.
8. In patients presents with concomitant MI and stroke, thrombolysis is appropriate if eligible from a stroke perspective, followed by PCI and cardiac stenting if indicated.
9. If there is a known history of >10 cortical microbleeds, there may be an increased risk of intracranial hemorrhage with thrombolysis.
10. If there is a known unruptured aneurysm <10 mm, thrombolysis is likely reasonable, but in the case of a large unruptured aneurysms (>10 mm), the risk/benefit of thrombolysis is unclear.

aPTT, Activated partial thromboplastin time; *BP,* blood pressure; *INR,* international normalized ratio; *LMWH,* low-molecular-weight heparin; *MI,* myocardial infarction; *PCI,* percutaneous coronary intervention; *STEMI,* ST elevation myocardial infarction.

TABLE 65.1 MEDICATIONS FOR TREATING MIGRAINE HEADACHE

Medication	Dosing	Special considerations
General analgesics		
Acetaminophen	500–1000 mg q4–6 h	Maximum 4000 mg/24 h
Ibuprofen	400–800 mg q6–8 h	General NSAID precautions
Naproxen sodium	500 mg q12 h	General NSAID precautions
Diclofenac potassium	50 mg PO as a single dose	General NSAID precautions
Combination analgesics		
Aspirin 250 mg + acetaminophen 250 mg + caffeine 65 mg	Two tablets q24 h	Use with caution to prevent medication overuse headache
Butalbital 50 mg + acetaminophen 300 mg or aspirin 325 mg + caffeine 40 mg	One to two capsules q4 h; max six capsules/day	Significant potential to cause medication overuse headache
Triptans		
Sumatriptan	50–100 mg PO 4–6 mg SC 20 mg IN	Max two doses/24 h SC formulation preferred if nausea and vomiting present
Almotriptan	6.25–12.5 mg PO	Max 25 mg/24 h
Rizatriptan	5–10 mg PO	Max 30 mg/24 h
Frovatriptan	2.5 mg PO	Max 7.5 mg/24 h
Zolmitriptan	2.5–5 mg PO 2.5–5 mg IN	Max 10 mg/24 h
Dihydroergotamine	1 mg IM, SC q h IN 0.5 mg (one spray) q 15 min 1 mg IV	Max 3 mg/d Potential serious side effects with daily use
Antiemetics		
Metoclopramide	5–10 mg PO q6–8 h prn 10 mg IV	Max 40 mg/d Risk of tardive dyskinesia with chronic use
Prochlorperazine	5–10 mg PO q6–8 h prn	Max 40 mg/d Risk of tardive dyskinesia with chronic use
Chlorpromazine	10–25 mg PO q4–6 h prn 25–50 mg IM, IV q4–6 h prn	Risk of tardive dyskinesia with chronic use
Additional ED therapies		
Ketorolac	60 mg IM 30 mg IV	General NSAID precautions
Droperidol	2.5 mg IV q30 min × 3 or 2.75 mg IM × 1	Monitor for QT prolongation
Valproic acid	1000 mg IV	Teratogenic risk
Magnesium	1000 mg IV over 1 h	
Dexamethasone	1–25 mg IV	To prevent headache recurrence

ED, emergency department; *IM*, intramuscular; *IN*, intranasal; *IV*, intravenous; *NSAID*, nonsteroidal antiinflammatory drug; *PO*, per os; *SC*, subcutaneous.

APPENDIX 2

Clinical Institute Withdrawal Assessment for Alcohol Scale (CIWA-Ar Protocol)

Nausea and Vomiting

Ask: "Do you feel sick to your stomach? Have you vomited?"

Observation
0: No nausea and no vomiting
1: Mild nausea with no vomiting
2:
3:
4: Intermittent nausea with dry heaves
5:
6:
7: Constant nausea, frequent dry heaves and vomiting

Tactile Disturbances

Ask: "Have you any itching, pins and needles sensations, any burning, any numbness or do you feel bugs crawling on or under your skin?"

Observation
0: None
1: Very mild itching, pins and needles, or burning/numbness
2: Mild itching, pins and needles, or burning/numbness
3: Moderate itching, pins and needles, or burning/numbness
4: Moderately severe hallucinations
5: Severe hallucinations
6: Extremely severe hallucinations
7: Continuous hallucinations

Tremor

Arms extended and fingers spread apart.

Observation
0: No tremor
1: Not visible but can be felt fingertip to fingertip
2:
3:
4: Moderate with arms extended
5:
6:
7: Severe, present with arms not extended

Auditory Disturbances

Ask: "Are you more aware of sounds around you? Are they harsh? Do they frighten you? Are you hearing anything that is disturbing to you? Are you hearing things you know are not there?"

Observation
0: Not present
1: Very mild harshness or ability to frighten
2: Mild harshness or ability to frighten
3: Moderate harshness or ability to frighten
4: Moderately severe hallucinations
5: Severe hallucinations
6: Extremely severe hallucinations
7: Continuous hallucinations

Paroxysmal Sweats

Observation
0: No sweat visible
1: Barely perceptible sweating, moist palms
2:
3:
4: Beads of sweat obvious on forehead
5:
6:
7: Drenching sweats

Visual Disturbances

Ask: "Does the light appear to be too bright? Is its color different? Does it hurt your eyes? Are you seeing anything that is disturbing to you? Are you seeing things you know are not there?"

Observation
0: Not present
1: Very mild photosensitivity
2: Mild photosensitivity
3: Moderate photosensitivity
4: Moderately severe hallucinations
5: Severe hallucinations
6: Extremely severe hallucinations
7 Continuous hallucinations

Anxiety

Ask: "Do you feel nervous?"

Observation
0: No anxiety, at ease
1: Mildly anxious
2:
3:
4: Moderately anxious, or guarded, so anxiety is inferred
5:
6:
7: Acute panic state consistent with delirium or psychosis

Headache

Ask: "Does your head feel different? Does it feel like there is a band around your head?" Do not rate for dizziness or lightheadedness. Otherwise, rate severity.
0: Not present
1: Very mild
2: Mild
3: Moderate
4: Moderate–severe
5: Severe
6: Very severe
7: Extremely severe

Agitation

Observation
0: Normal activity
1: Somewhat more than normal activity
2:
3:
4: Moderately fidgety and restless
5:
6:
7: Pacing back and forth or constantly thrashes about

Orientation and Clouding of Sensorium

Ask: "What day is this? Where are you? Who am I?"
0: Oriented and can do serial additions
1: Cannot do serial additions or is uncertain about date
2: Disoriented for date by no more than 2 calendar days
3: Disoriented for date by more than 2 calendar days
4: Disoriented to place and/or person

Total CIWA Score (Maximum 67)_____

Reassess every 30 to 60 minutes.

< 10: Very mild withdrawal
10–15: Mild Withdrawal
16–20: Moderate Withdrawal
> 20: Severe withdrawal

The Clinical Institute Withdrawal Assessment of Alcohol Scale, Revised (CIWA-Ar) is not copyrighted and may be reproduced freely.
Modified from Sullivan JT, Sykora K, Schneiderman J, et al. Assessment of alcohol withdrawal: the revised Clinical Institute Withdrawal Assessment for Alcohol scale (CIWA-Ar). *Br. J. Addict.* 1989; 84:1353–1357.

NIH Stroke Scale

Administer stroke scale items in the order listed. Record performance in each category after each subscale examination. Do not go back and change scores. Follow directions provided for each examination technique. Scores should reflect what the patient does, not what the clinician thinks the patient can do. The clinician should record answers while administering the examination and work quickly. Except where indicated, the patient should not be coached (i.e., repeated requests to patient to make a special effort).

Instructions	Scale Definition	Score
1a. Level of Consciousness (LOC): The investigator must choose a response if a full evaluation is prevented by such obstacles as an endotracheal tube, language barrier, orotracheal trauma/bandages. A 3 is scored only if the patient makes no movement (other than reflexive posturing) in response to noxious stimulation.	0 = **Alert**; keenly responsive. 1 = **Not alert**; but arousable by minor stimulation to obey, answer, or respond. 2 = **Not alert**; requires repeated stimulation to attend, or is obtunded and requires strong or painful stimulation to make movements (not stereotyped). 3 = Responds only with reflex motor or autonomic effects or totally unresponsive, flaccid, and areflexic.	_____
1b. LOC Questions: The patient is asked the month and his/her age. The answer must be correct—there is no partial credit for being close. Aphasic and stuporous patients who do not comprehend the questions will score 2. Patients unable to speak because of endotracheal intubation, orotracheal trauma, severe dysarthria from any cause, language barrier, or any other problem not secondary to aphasia are given a 1. It is important that only the initial answer be graded and that the examiner not "help" the patient with verbal or nonverbal cues.	0 = **Answers** both questions correctly. 1 = **Answers** one question correctly. 2 = **Answers** neither question correctly.	_____
1c. LOC Commands: The patient is asked to open and close the eyes and then to grip and release the nonparetic hand. Substitute another one step command if the hands cannot be used. Credit is given if an unequivocal attempt is made but not completed due to weakness. If the patient does not respond to command, the task should be demonstrated to him or her (pantomime), and the result scored (i.e., follows none, one or two commands). Patients with trauma, amputation, or other physical impediments should be given suitable one-step commands. Only the first attempt is scored.	0 = **Performs** both tasks correctly. 1 = **Performs** one task correctly. 2 = **Performs** neither task correctly.	_____
2. Best Gaze: Only horizontal eye movements will be tested. Voluntary or reflexive (oculocephalic) eye movements will be scored, but caloric testing is not done. If the patient has a conjugate deviation of the eyes that can be overcome by voluntary or reflexive activity, the score will be 1. If a patient has an isolated peripheral nerve paresis (CN III, IV, or VI), score a 1. Gaze is testable in all aphasic patients. Patients with ocular trauma, bandages, preexisting blindness, or other disorder of visual acuity or fields should be tested with reflexive movements, and a choice made by the investigator. Establishing eye contact and then moving about the patient from side to side will occasionally clarify the presence of a partial gaze palsy.	0 = **Normal**. 1 = **Partial gaze palsy**; gaze is abnormal in one or both eyes, but forced deviation or total gaze paresis is not present. 2 = **Forced deviation**, or total gaze paresis not overcome by the oculocephalic maneuver.	_____
3. Visual: Visual fields (upper and lower quadrants) are tested by confrontation, using finger counting or visual threat, as appropriate. Patients may be encouraged, but if they look at the side of the moving fingers appropriately, this can be scored as normal. If there is unilateral blindness or enucleation, visual fields in the remaining eye are scored. Score 1 only if a clear-cut asymmetry, including quadrantanopia, is found. If patient is blind from any cause, score 3. Double simultaneous stimulation is performed at this point. If there is extinction, patient receives a 1, and the results are used to respond to item 11.	0 = **No visual loss**. 1 = **Partial hemianopia**. 2 = **Complete hemianopia**. 3 = **Bilateral hemianopia** (blind including cortical blindness).	_____
4. Facial Palsy: Ask – or use pantomime to encourage – the patient to show teeth or raise eyebrows and close eyes. Score symmetry of grimace in response to noxious	0 = **Normal** symmetrical movements. 1 = **Minor paralysis** (flattened nasolabial fold, asymmetry on smiling).	

Instructions	Scale Definition	Score
stimuli in the poorly responsive or noncomprehending patient. If facial trauma/bandages, orotracheal tube, tape or other physical barriers obscure the face, these should be removed to the extent possible.	2 = **Partial paralysis** (total or near-total paralysis of lower face). 3 = **Complete paralysis** of one or both sides (absence of facial movement in the upper and lower face).	____
5. **Motor Arm:** The limb is placed in the appropriate position: extend the arms (palms down) 90 degrees (if sitting) or 45 degrees (if supine). Drift is scored if the arm falls before 10 seconds. The aphasic patient is encouraged using urgency in the voice and pantomime, but not noxious stimulation. Each limb is tested in turn, beginning with the nonparetic arm. Only in the case of amputation or joint fusion at the shoulder, the examiner should record the score as untestable (UN), and clearly write the explanation for this choice.	0 = **No drift**; limb holds 90 (or 45) degrees for full 10 seconds. 1 = **Drift**; limb holds 90 (or 45) degrees, but drifts down before full 10 seconds; does not hit bed or other support. 2 = **Some effort against gravity**; limb cannot get to or maintain (if cued) 90 (or 45) degrees, drifts down to bed, but has some effort against gravity. 3 = **No effort against gravity**; limb falls. 4 = **No movement**. UN = **Amputation** or joint fusion, explain: _____ 5a. Left Arm 5b. Right Arm	____ ____ ____
6. **Motor Leg:** The limb is placed in the appropriate position: hold the leg at 30 degrees (always tested supine). Drift is scored if the leg falls before 5 seconds. The aphasic patient is encouraged using urgency in the voice and pantomime, but not noxious stimulation. Each limb is tested in turn, beginning with the nonparetic leg. Only in the case of amputation or joint fusion at the hip, the examiner should record the score as untestable (UN), and clearly write the explanation for this choice.	0 = **No drift**; leg holds 30-degree position for full 5 seconds. 1 = **Drift**; leg falls by the end of the 5-second period but does not hit bed. 2 = **Some effort against gravity**; leg falls to bed by 5 seconds, but has some effort against gravity. 3 = **No effort against gravity**; leg falls to bed immediately. 4 = **No movement**. UN = **Amputation** or joint fusion, explain: _____ 6a. Left Leg 6b. Right Leg	 ____ ____
7. **Limb Ataxia:** This item is aimed at finding evidence of a unilateral cerebellar lesion. Test with eyes open. In case of visual defect, ensure testing is done in intact visual field. The finger-nose-finger and heel-shin tests are performed on both sides, and ataxia is scored only if present out of proportion to weakness. Ataxia is absent in the patient who cannot understand or is paralyzed. Only in the case of amputation or joint fusion, the examiner should record the score as untestable (UN), and clearly write the explanation for this choice. In case of blindness, test by having the patient touch nose from extended arm position.	0 = **Absent**. 1 = **Present in one limb**. 2 = **Present in two limbs**. UN = **Amputation** or joint fusion, explain: _____	 ____
8. **Sensory:** Sensation or grimace to pinprick when tested, or withdrawal from noxious stimulus in the obtunded or aphasic patient. Only sensory loss attributed to stroke is scored as abnormal, and the examiner should test as many body areas (arms [not hands], legs, trunk, face) as needed to accurately check for hemisensory loss. A score of 2, "severe or total sensory loss," should only be given when a severe or total loss of sensation can be clearly demonstrated. Stuporous and aphasic patients will, therefore, probably score 1 or 0. The patient with brainstem stroke who has bilateral loss of sensation is scored 2. If the patient does not respond and is quadriplegic, score 2. Patients in a coma (item 1a=3) are automatically given a 2 on this item.	0 = **Normal**; no sensory loss. 1 = **Mild-to-moderate sensory loss**; patient feels pinprick is less sharp or is dull on the affected side; or there is a loss of superficial pain with pinprick, but patient is aware of being touched. 2 = **Severe to total sensory loss**; patient is not aware of being touched in the face, arm, and leg.	 ____
9. **Best Language:** A great deal of information about comprehension will be obtained during the preceding sections of the examination. For this scale item, the patient is asked to describe what is happening in the attached picture, to name the items on the attached naming sheet, and to read from the attached list of sentences. Comprehension is judged from responses here, as well as to all of the commands in the preceding general neurological examination. If visual loss interferes	0 = **No aphasia**; normal. 1 = **Mild-to-moderate aphasia**; some obvious loss of fluency or facility of comprehension, without significant limitation on ideas expressed or form of expression. Reduction of speech and/or comprehension, however, makes conversation about provided materials difficult or impossible. For example, in conversation about provided materials, examiner can identify picture or naming card content from patient's response.	 ____

Instructions	Scale Definition	Score
with the tests, ask the patient to identify objects placed in the hand, repeat, and produce speech. The intubated patient should be asked to write. The patient in a coma (item 1a=3) will automatically score 3 on this item. The examiner must choose a score for the patient with stupor or limited cooperation, but a score of 3 should be used only if the patient is mute and follows no one-step commands.	2 = **Severe aphasia**; all communication is through fragmentary expression; great need for inference, questioning, and guessing by the listener. Range of information that can be exchanged is limited; listener carries burden of communication. Examiner cannot identify materials provided from patient response. 3 = **Mute, global aphasia**; no usable speech or auditory comprehension.	
10. **Dysarthria**: If patient is thought to be normal, an adequate sample of speech must be obtained by asking patient to read or repeat words from the attached list. If the patient has severe aphasia, the clarity of articulation of spontaneous speech can berated. Only if the patient is intubated or has other physical barriers to producing speech, the examiner should record the score as untestable (UN), and clearly write an explanation for this choice. Do not tell the patient why he or she is being tested.	0 = **Normal.** 1 = **Mild-to-moderate dysarthria**; patient slurs at least some words and, at worst, can be understood with some difficulty. 2 = **Severe dysarthria**; patient's speech is so slurred as to be unintelligible in the absence of or out of proportion to any dysphasia, or is mute/anarthric. UN = **Intubated** or other physical barrier, explain: _____	_____
11. **Extinction and Inattention (formerly Neglect)**: Sufficient information to identify neglect may be obtained during the prior testing. If the patient has a severe visual loss preventing visual double simultaneous stimulation, and the cutaneous stimuli are normal, the score is normal. If the patient has aphasia but does appear to attend to both sides, the score is normal. The presence of visual spatial neglect or anosognosia may also be taken as evidence of abnormality. Since the abnormality is scored only if present, the item is never untestable.	0 = **No abnormality.** 1 = **Visual, tactile, auditory, spatial, or personal inattention** or extinction to bilateral simultaneous stimulation in one of the sensory modalities. 2 = **Profound hemi-inattention or extinction to more than one modality**; does not recognize own hand or orients to only one side of space.	_____

From National Institute of Neurological Disorders and Stroke, National Institutes of Health, Bethesda, Maryland.

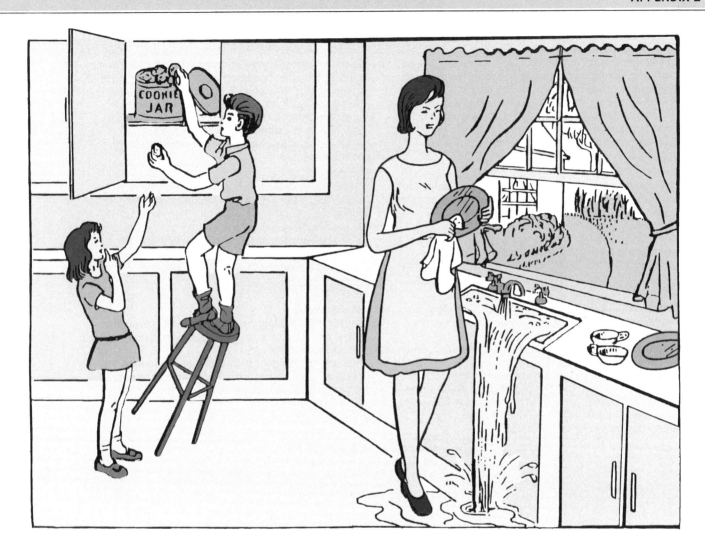

You know how.
Down to earth.
I got home from work.
Near the table in the dining room.
They heard him speak on the radio last night.

MAMA
TIP-TOP
FIFTY-FIFTY
THANKS
HUCKLEBERRY
BASEBALL PLAYER

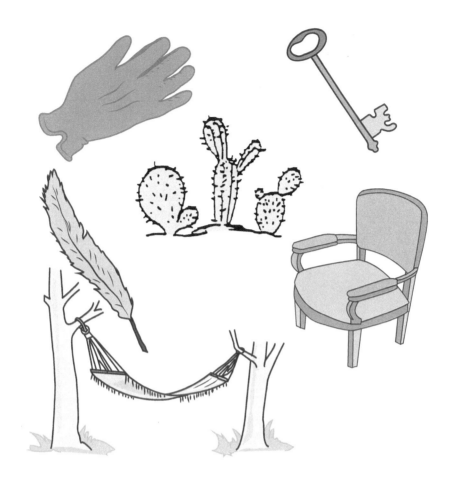

Index

Note: Page numbers followed by *f* indicate figures and *t* indicate tables.